Localized Micro/Nanocarriers for Programmed and On-Demand Controlled Drug Release

Authored by

Seyed Morteza Naghib

Samin Hoseinpour

&

Shadi Zarshad

Nanotechnology Department
School of Advanced Technologies
Iran University of Science and Technology (IUST)
P.O. Box 16846-13114
Tehran, Iran

Localized Micro/Nanocarriers for Programmed and On-Demand Controlled Drug Release

Authors: Seyed Morteza Naghib, Samin Hoseinpour & Shadi Zarshad

ISBN (Online): 978-981-5051-63-6

ISBN (Print): 978-981-5051-64-3

ISBN (Paperback): 978-981-5051-65-0

need for a court order if at any point you breach any terms of this License Agreement. In no event will any delay or failure by Bentham Science Publishers in enforcing your compliance with this License Agreement constitute a waiver of any of its rights.

3. You acknowledge that you have read this License Agreement, and agree to be bound by its terms and conditions. To the extent that any other terms and conditions presented on any website of Bentham Science Publishers conflict with, or are inconsistent with, the terms and conditions set out in this License Agreement, you acknowledge that the terms and conditions set out in this License Agreement shall prevail.

Bentham Science Publishers Pte. Ltd.
80 Robinson Road #02-00
Singapore 068898
Singapore
Email: subscriptions@benthamscience.net

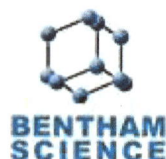

BENTHAM SCIENCE

CONTENTS

PREFACE

In the healthcare field, providing optimal treatment to individual patients is of primary concern. Drug delivery systems can regulate drug release rate to get the desired profile, ensure high therapeutic effectiveness, and reduce side effects that are very interesting in pharmaceutical and biomedical applications. The localized drug delivery presents various factors designed to enable the delivery of therapeutic agents, such as drugs, genes, proteins, etc., directly to the site of disease in a controlled manner, sparing off-target cell/tissue toxicities. In this context, one of the considerable challenges in systemic drug delivery systems is to get the desired drug concentration at the specific organ, reduce side effects, and prevent drug inefficiency. The present book entitled "smart stimuli-responsive micro/nanocarriers for programmed and on-demand localized controlled drug release" is one of the first books on the market that focuses on localized drug delivery with enhanced drug release at the target site, reduced local toxicity, and better patient compliance in order to inspire readers to design and create novel drug delivery systems for the treatment of a wide range of diseases.

In this book, the present chapters provide a detailed introduction to polymers, nanostructures, and stimuli-responsive materials and their great potential for opening new avenues to address several challenges in conventional dosage forms in localized drug delivery systems. This book is ideally designed for researchers working in pharmaceuticals, bionanotechnologies, biomedical engineering, materials science, and related industries.

CONSENT FOR PUBLICATION

Not applicable.

CONFLICT OF INTEREST

The author declares no conflict of interest, financial or otherwise.

ACKNOWLEDGEMENT

Declared none.

Seyed Morteza Naghib
Nanotechnology Department, School of Advanced Technologies
Iran University of Science and Technology (IUST)
P.O. Box 16846-13114, Tehran
Iran

CHAPTER 1

Introduction to Localized Controlled Drug Delivery Systems (LCDDSs)

Abstract: Localized controlled drug delivery systems (LCDDS) that can control drug release profiles to ensure high therapeutic efficacy and reduced side effects are highly desired in the pharmaceutical and biomedical fields. Biodegradable drug delivery depots have been investigated over the last several decades as the means to improve tumor targeting and severe systemic morbidities associated with intravenous chemotherapy treatments. These localized therapies exist in a variety of factors designed to facilitate the controlled drug delivery, directly to the disease site, sparing off-target tissue toxicities. Many of these depots are biodegradable and designed to maintain therapeutic concentrations of drugs at the tumor site for a prolonged period of time. The depots are placed inside the body through a single implantation procedure, sometimes simultaneously with the tumor excision surgery, following the complete release of the loaded active agent. Even though localized depot delivery systems have been widely investigated, only a small subset have demonstrated curative preclinical results for cancer applications, from which just a few have reached commercialization.

Keywords: Biomedical field, Drug delivery system, Localized controlled drug delivery, Pharmaceutical application.

1.1. HISTORY AND STATISTICAL TRENDS IN LCDDS

Typical drug delivery systems may have some challenges which must be considered to obtain the best results. One of these challenges is to obtain the desired drug concentration in certain organs (Gooneh-Farahani *et al.*, 2020, Gooneh-Farahani *et al.*, 2019, Kalkhoran *et al.*, 2018, Zeinali Kalkhoran *et al.*, 2018). Another issue may be the degradation of the drug before reaching the intended organ or tissue. These challenges might cause failure even in adequate drug doses. However, with the development of local delivery, unstable drugs, which had to be delivered through frequent daily dosing, can be delivered once a week or even once a year (Singh *et al.*, 2019, Aj *et al.*, 2012, Singh *et al.*, 2009). In this regard, Densby and Parkes developed the idea of implantable drug delivery systems by describing the effect of subcutaneous implantation of compressed pellets of crystalline estrone upon castrated male chickens in 1938. Furthermore,

Folkman and Long investigated biocompatible implantable drug release formulations with the use of silicone rubber (Silastic) as a method for prolonged systemic administrations in 1960, which was able to overcome the issues related to the oral administration of specific drugs. Inspite of significant attempts, the development and commercialization of safe implants have not matured (Kleiner *et al.*, 2014).

Localized Controlled Drug Delivery

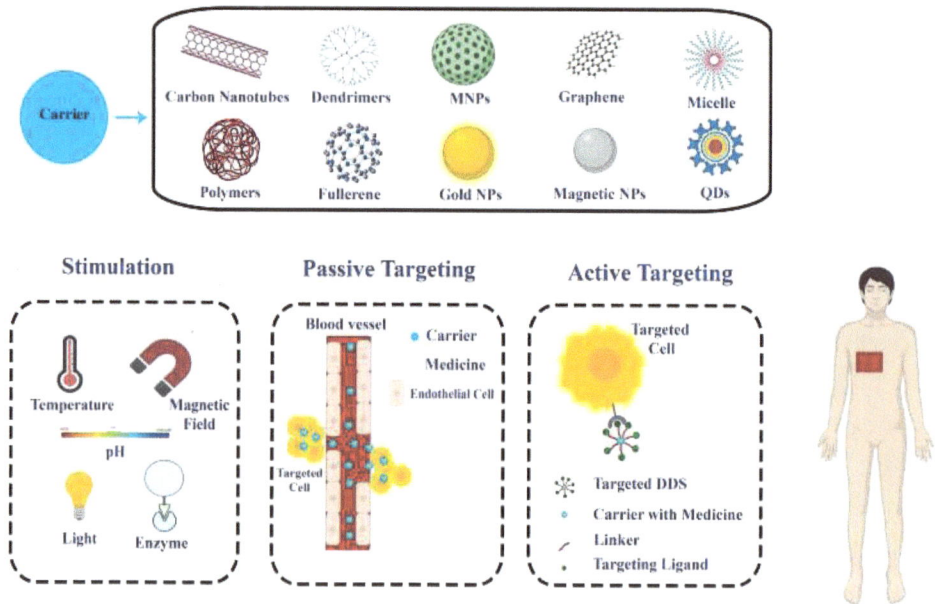

Fig. (1). Schematic illustration of localized controlled drug delivery systems.

"Localized drug delivery" refers to a particular kind of targeted drug delivery in which the movement and absorption of the drug to the bloodstream decreased, and the therapeutic agent is concentrated in a specific part of the body (Fig. (**1**). Localized delivery cuts down systemic effects on marginal organs or tissues, thereby reducing the side effects of the drug while having more control over the target site. The local effect may be achieved through injection, implantation or inhalation. In addition, systemic effects are also achievable by local administration (Rolfes *et al.*, 2012, Dhanikula and Panchagnula, 1999, Ji and Kohane, 2019). In cases where delivery is not enough to prevent the restenosis process, local drug delivery plays an important role in delivering compounds to suppress the neointimal proliferation characteristics of the restenosis lesion.

Meanwhile, anti-inflammatory agents, antiproliferative compounds, and specific antibodies may be delivered using local drug delivery. For example, the drugs used in the nonsurgical treatment process of periodontitis (a severe gum infection), have several side effects such as drug toxicity, nausea, vomiting, superimposed infections, drug interaction, and patient compliance. The aforementioned side effects have led to the enhancement of nonsurgical therapy and the introduction of local drug delivery. To develop periodontal health, controlled clinical trials were selected that measured the potential of local delivery. The clinical trials were used to demonstrate statistical and clinical data in order to investigate the results of local delivery (Ramesh *et al.*, 2016, Gill *et al.*, 2011, Lambert *et al.*, 1993, Ibsen *et al.*, 2012, Song *et al.*, 1997, Kalsi *et al.*, 2011, Szulc *et al.*, 2018, Greenstein, 2006).

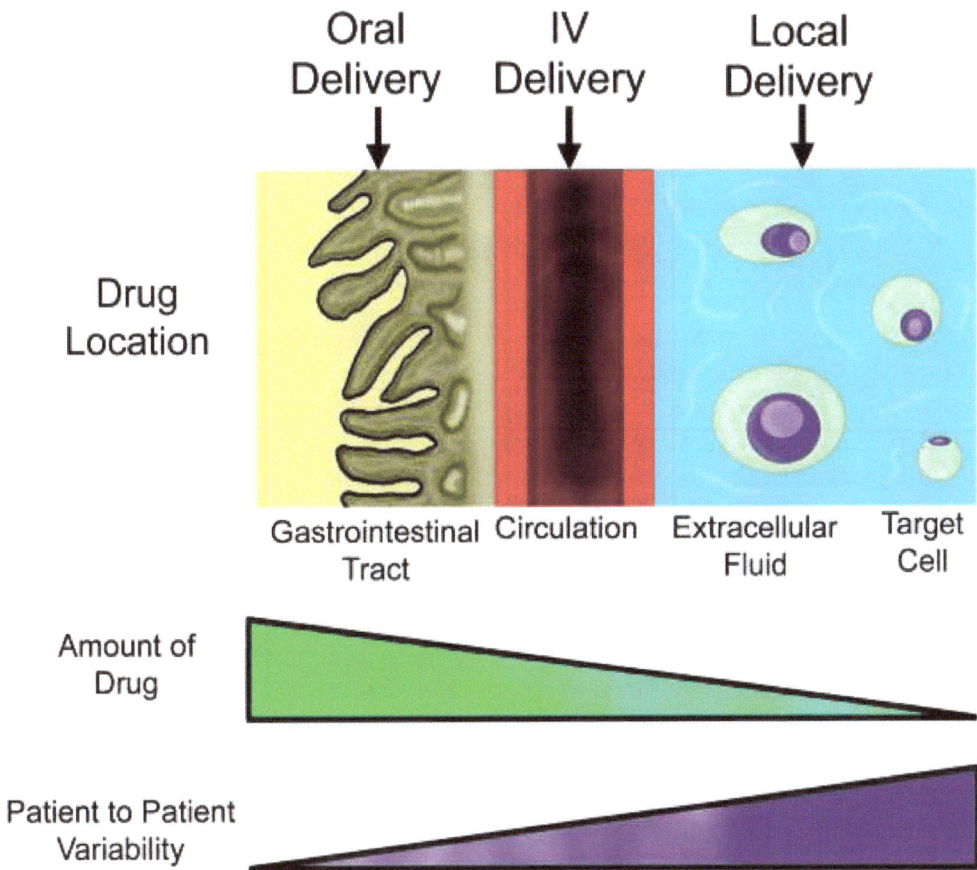

Fig. (2). Schematic of comparison between oral, intravenous and local drug delivery methods (open access) (Rolfes *et al.*, 2012).

From another point of view, there are various ways to administrate drugs in order to treat different diseases, including oral systemic drug delivery and local drug delivery (Askari *et al.*, 2021a, Askari *et al.*, 2021b). Fig. (**2**) shows a comparison between intravenous delivery and oral delivery methods. As shown in Fig. (**2**), by reducing the gastrointestinal tract, variability is decreased, and control is increased. Moreover, dependence on patient circulation for distribution in local delivery procedures has decreased, thereby increasing control and decreasing variability. In the local drug delivery method, the required effective drug amount has decreased while the treatment has increased.

Many drugs, peptides, and proteins are administrated intravenously to avoid adverse conditions, because of their short half-life. One of the challenges of intravenous administration is the short drug action time, which as a result, requires regular injections to achieve drug efficacy. Over time, injectable controlled-release delivery seems to be more commercially successful due to factors such as safety and efficacy. Topical drug administration is another path for drug delivery, but is not very effective because of the physiological character of the drugs and low impermeability of the stratum corneum. Consequently, the local drug delivery system is a safe and immune method to deliver drug to the desired site of the body, offering unique advantages over other drug delivery systems (Singh *et al.*, 2019, Aj *et al.*, 2012, Rolfes *et al.*, 2012).

When designing a biomaterial for drug delivery applications, several factors must be considered, such as biocompatibility, release rate tunability, over-elution or 'burst' release inhibition, post-drug release effects, dimensional penalties reduction, nonspecific elution reduction, material production scalability, physician and patient acceptability. Local drug delivery, or in other words, delivery of drugs to a specific area of the body, will decrease systemic drug concentration. According to this method and the drug activity protection during sequestration, numerous follow-up therapies can be lessened or even eliminated. For example, in cancer treatment, local delivery allows local and surgical administration of a therapeutic agent to the desired site, which reduces the side effects of systemic drug delivery and, at the same time, increases drug efficacy. As another example, drug-loaded nanoparticles may be used as a method for brain tumor treatment (Lam and Ho, 2009). Drug delivery systems eliminate all the off-target effects, as smaller dosages are required to achieve local therapeutic concentrations. These systems do not need to travel through the systemic circulation and are directly introduced to the inflammation site. For instance, local drug delivery systems are more useful in non-steroidal anti-inflammatory drugs (NSAID), as they do not require any extra surgery for implantation. Nanoparticles are good candidates for drug delivery due to their low viscosity and small particle size, which enables them to pass through a needle and move throughout the body easily. Localized controlled drug delivery system (LCDDS) aids the formation of periodontal pockets, which perform like a natural reservoir, meanwhile, the gingival crevicular fluid (GCF) provides a hydrated environment (leaching medium) that boosts drug distribution throughout the pocket (Haley and von Recum, 2019, Lee *et al.*, 2017, Rajeshwari *et al.*, 2019, Singh *et al.*, 2014). In the treatment of a periodontal infection, which was studied as an example before, delivering antimicrobial agents to the pocket base is necessary. Therefore, the designed drug delivery system must simplify the retention of the drug long sufficiently to guarantee drug efficacy and healing process. Some drug delivery methods, such as mouth rinse, subgingival irritation, and systemic delivery, deliver poor concentrations of drug to the activity site, but local delivery can be used in combination with all the above-mentioned items to enhance periodontal health (Greenstein and Polson, 1998).

Local drug delivery has the ability to deliver antibiotics to the target sites, and also limits both desirable and undesirable pharmacological effects to other parts of the body. In the controlled delivery method, drug access to off-target sites has decreased; drug efficacy has increased, and toxicity has decreased, which provides a safer treatment with the same effects. This method also provides constant-rate delivery of drugs, such that a smaller amount of drug is needed to treat disease for a sufficient duration. Therefore, injectable drug delivery systems are a potential route to deliver antibiotics to the action site, which noticeably decreases the cost compared to devices that require placement time and securing (Aj *et al.*, 2012, Singh *et al.*, 2009, Ji and Kohane, 2019, Singh *et al.*, 2014).

Improvement of more useful drug delivery systems is important for microorganism eradication associated with bacterial infections. To protect against infection, an operative antibiotic release must occur at concentrations above the bacteria's minimum inhibitory concentration (MIC); and the antibiotic concentration must be above the minimum bactericidal concentration (MBC) to reach the treatment point and complete the curing process. Overcoming concerns related to short half-life issues, improving pharmacokinetic and pharmacodynamic profiles, and developing localized drug delivery, are facilitated. Local delivery of antibiotics leads to lowered toxicity, decreases required dosage and prevents systemic exposure. It is noteworthy that local drug delivery can administrate drugs at high dosages, without surpassing the systemic toxicity, and can decrease side effects at the special infection sites, for example, implant-related infections. Besides, by avoiding systemic administration, patient compliance is increased, as in most cases, patients do not finish all courses of the drug, leading to bacteria resistance (Stebbins *et al.*, 2014).

Particular kinds of local delivery systems can start and continue local drug activity either by avoiding drug efflux from the arterial wall or by using delivery vehicles that will lengthen the release time. In comparison with other drug delivery systems, in local drug delivery, lower amounts of the drug are required, and thus, unfavorable effects are decreased or totally eliminated. As mentioned above, unstable biomolecules, for instance, oligonucleotides, nucleic acids and drugs with a short half-life, specifically peptides and proteins, can be delivered locally, but drug half-life is improved in localized drug delivery systems. From another point of view, localized treatment methods have minimum overlap with blood circulation and partial contact with the liver and kidneys, where drug metabolism occurs. In this case, the half-life of many drugs will increase and recover. Therefore, in local treatment, the amount of required drugs will decrease (Rolfes *et al.*, 2012, Jain *et al.*, 2005).

A standard local drug delivery system has characteristics such as simple administration, controlled drug release, biodegradability, biocompatibility, and drug concentration sustainability, meanwhile not harming other healthy tissues. Irrigating systems, gels, nanoparticles and microparticles are examples of local drug systems. Local drug delivery systems (LCDDS) have advantages compared to systemic drug delivery, which are briefly described below. One of the advantages of LCDDSs is minimized invasive effects. Moreover, LCDDSs can be applied directly to the desired site of the body, which as a result, reduces gastrointestinal concerns. Also, the drug dosage reduction, frequent drug administration and enhanced patient compliance serve as ideal means to incorporate agents which are not suitable for systemic administration, *e.g.*, Chlorhexidine (Rajeshwari *et al.*, 2019). As an example, in the delivery of metronidazole, using local drug delivery has shown minimum side effects wherein the drug is not easily adsorbed to other tissues, when prescribed in routine doses (Greenstein and Polson, 1998).

As macroscale methods for cancer treatment, LCDDS can be implanted or injected just near the solid tumors, and can present extensive therapies over the nanoscale. They can also be loaded with more drugs that are not cleared quickly. Some implantable, biodegradable polymers with the ability to release payloads after tumor removal, have been in clinical use for several years. One of the examples of these implantable, biodegradable polymers is poly (carboxyphenoxy propane-co-sebacic acid) wafers which can degrade after 3 weeks of implantation. Such biodegradable polymeric systems may be used in post-surgery treatments, to assure the complete removal of cancerous tissues. From another point of view, if drugs are loaded locally, side effects are decreased due to the avoidance of systemic circulation of chemotherapeutic drugs and healthy tissues are kept safe, and the damage to these healthy tissues is decreased. Some of the advantages of drug-loaded polymeric implants over customary systemic drug delivery methods are listed below: 1) the possibility of loading and releasing water-insoluble chemotherapeutic agents, 2) stabilization of the loaded drugs and maintenance of anti-cancer activity, 3) controlling the drug release rate and diffusing and up taking drug into the cancerous cells more precisely, 4) decreasing drug waste by the straight release of the drug at the disease site, and 5) one-time administration of the drug. Therefore, local chemotherapy of cancer has enhanced the treatment efficiency and has reduced patient morbidity (Campbell and Smeets, 2019, Wolinsky *et al.*, 2012).

Localized treatment in slow-growing tumors such as prostate, lung, cervical, and breast count as a suitable substitute for surgery. For example, brachytherapy seeds applied at the surgical resection site, have been shown to reduce the incidence of local recurrence in lung cancer patients from 19% to 2%. Moreover, adding brachytherapy to a lobectomy performed for 2–3 cm lung cancer tumors, drastically reduced recurrence rates and increased patient endurance from 44.7 months to 70 months, which represents the influences of localized therapy on decreasing localized recurrence and developing survival in patients (Wolinsky *et al.*, 2012).

Using chemotherapy is a valid, useful and effective procedure for curing localized tumors. This procedure is used as an adjuvant to surgical treatment as it eliminates or postpones metastasis. Localized chemotherapy of cancers and particularly early-stage diagnosed cancers, is more effective compared to systemic cancer therapy due to locoregional recurrence, which remains a major failure in cancer cases, and sterilization of the resection site edges with the delivery of chemotherapy agent. Also, this method decreases locoregional tumor recurrence. Moreover, a drug-eluting implant enlarges the tumor resection margins, which might penetrate the surrounding tissues, and may result in extra limited resection of diseased parenchyma. For instance, limited wedge resections of lung parenchyma can restore the current standard of care whereby the total lobe of the lung is resected if locally delivered agents could prevent locoregional recurrence (Wolinsky *et al.*, 2012, Morgan *et al.*, 2009).

1.2. SCIENTIFIC AND TECHNOLOGICAL IMPACT OF LCDDS

Due to major progress in drug delivery systems over time, new techniques such as site-specific or local controlled release have been merged, offering decreased dosage of the drug with maximum concentration at the desired site of the body. Moreover, at a specific part of the body where other usual therapies might be unsuccessful, adjunctive use of local delivery might be useful. Local drug delivery systems are utilized specifically in patients who are in the maintenance phase, in institutionalized patients, in implants that have failed at the localized refractory sites, and in patients who cannot undergo surgery. LCDDSs have also performed well in regenerative surgery and development predictability by decreasing the bacterial load (Singh *et al.*, 2009).

One of the easiest ways to gain targeted drug delivery is to place the device at the desired site where the drug must be delivered, which may be the best choice for most ocular situations. In another case, if the patient uses intravitreally injections such as antivascular endothelial growth factor (VEGF) drugs, which must be injected every 4-6 weeks and requires local and long-term delivery of a special drug, local delivery can deliver the drug for several months or years with identical procedural injection. Finally, a logical way to give local delivery is injecting a device or a matrix into the intravitreal space to have the local effect of the drug (Lavik *et al.*).

In the treatment of respiratory diseases, pulmonary drug delivery of may be a good option with advantages in comparison with other drug delivery routes. Delivering the drug agent through inhalation has the advantage of the direct delivery of the drugs inside the lungs. The local pulmonary administration of the drugs facilitates the targeted treatment of respiratory diseases such as pulmonary arterial hypertension (PAH). In this case, there is no need for extra doses, which are required in other administration routes (Gao *et al.*, 2016).

Although in the last several years, developments in the detection of cancer in early stages and progress in technology had a major effect on decreasing the rate of cancer death in patients, there are still main limitations in treatment-associated morbidity and recurrence rates. There are possible intervention points in every phase of cancer where local therapy, either curative or palliative, could complement or substitute ordinary treatments (Wolinsky *et al.*, 2012).

Nowadays, in cancer therapy, chemotherapy is still known as the most valuable approach. Chemotherapy has non-discriminating destructive effects on both normal and cancerous cells, which causes major side effects for the patient. One of the main challenges in the treatment of cancer or other diseases such as complicated sicknesses, is to release the drug within the organs and to achieve a drug delivery and release system directly at the tumor location. Hence, designing complicated plans to obtain targeted traceable drugs used for anti-cancer applications is vital (Zeng *et al.*, 2016).

Despite tremendous efforts to improve nanotherapeutic delivery agents which can penetrate the blood-brain barrier (BBB), there are no accessible clinical treatments, and the efforts are in the development stages. There are several challenges, such as the challenge of obtaining high bioavailability to the cerebral activity site, as a large number of drugs cannot penetrate the BBB; the challenge of ensuring the biocompatibility of nanoparticles; the FDA approval challenge, and the long process time challenge. Therefore, the substitute option is the application of invasive methods. Injections and infusions are frequently used methods for severe sicknesses, although there are controlled release polymeric implants applied for the treatment of brain malignant gliomas. The first polymer with FDA approval in 1995 was poly (carboxyphenoxypropane-co-sebacic acid), a biodegradable polymeric wafer, containing an anti-cancer chemotherapeutic drug naming 1,3-bis(2-chloroethyl)-1-nitrosourea (BCNU). This medication was applied to the tumor site after removing the tumor by surgery and the polymer released was eventually released after implantation and degraded after 3 weeks. After this research, several related bioresorbable implants, such as bioresorbable PLA-made microchips, were tested in clinical trials. The bioresorbable PLA-made microchips successfully decreased the size of tumors in an *in vivo* rat model *via* controlled and localized release of BCNU (Campbell and Smeets, 2019).

On the other hand, the systemic drug administration route has been utilized in curing vitreo-retinal diseases. Earlier studies have proved that a very small amount of drug was applicable to the eye, and because of the limitations caused by the blood-ocular barriers, considerable doses of the drug were required to achieve therapeutic drug amounts in the posterior segment of the eye. Therefore, these types of diseases are not easy to cure and have a long treatment time, using conventional topical or systemic drug delivery. Research has led to specialized drug delivery to the tissues of the posterior segment of the eye. Many implantable intravitreal tools used for drug delivery applications have been fabricated. However, none of the commercial products are verified to be all-comprehensive safe and simple tools. Generally, implantation methods were used to protect the tool in the posterior segment of the eye by ophthalmic surgery. The tools were entirely biodegradable and presented zero-order drug delivery in the vitreal cavity over several months or even years. As a result, several challenges need to be solved in order to devise a successful intravitreal drug delivery tool. (Choonara *et al.*, 2010).

In another case, the main cause of the incidence of periodontal disease is the growth and proliferation of pathogenic bacteria, and mainly anaerobic gram-negative bacteria, in the plaque. Antibiotics are known as a common treatment of periodontal disease, but long-term administration of antibiotic drugs is required for the treatment of chronic stage periodontal disease. Long-term administration of antibiotics may cause bacterial resistance and result in side effects, such as, gastrointestinal disorders and superinfection. Consequently, for safety concerns, oral administration of medications for curing chronic periodontal diseases is not acceptable. Hence, researchers have focused on synthetic antimicrobial drugs and local administration of antibiotics. Meanwhile, according to the reports, conventional therapies, irrigation and mouth rinses are not leading to successful results. With progressions in drug delivery systems and improvement of knowledge in local drug delivery, periodontal disease treatment has been of great interest to researchers (HIGASHI *et al.*, 1991, Yang *et al.*, 2017).

In the case of periodontal disease, local delivery of antimicrobial drugs into periodontal pockets, has been comprehensively investigated since 1979. In systemic drug delivery, the drug was restricted at a specific site and the concentration of the drug at the targeted site was high. On the other hand, local drug delivery has gained more attention, specifically in periodontology, because of lower infection and side effects risk (Nadig and Shah, 2016).

Local delivery of drugs to vasculatures assists in obtaining a high local concentration of drugs, with prolonged maintenance at a lower dosage and therefore, lower systemic toxicity. Also, drugs with lower bioavailability can reach the desired site or organ in the body without any issues. It is noteworthy that in the localized drug delivery approach, drugs with a short half-life, such as recombinant proteins and peptides, have been successfully delivered with a minimum loss, earlier than their uptake into the desired organ or tissue. But, there are challenges in systemic drug delivery, such as the variability of pharmacokinetics, specifically in oral or intravenous procedures. Challenges resulting from different dosages, often seen in animal studies and extended to human clinical trials, are also solved by local drug delivery. Some types of local drug delivery have the potential to start and continue local drug action, either by avoiding drug efflux from the arterial wall or by using delivery vehicles that will prolong the release or action duration (Kavanagh *et al.*, 2004).

For most solid tumors with locoregional lymphatic involvement in early or intermediate stages, surgical resection of the main tumor or, in some cases, nearby lymph nodes, is considered an important therapy. On the other hand, for late-stage tumors, debulking the tumor has a painkilling result, and the life quality of the patient may be improved better in some cases which depend on the tumor site. It must be considered that the advantage of eliminating cancerous tissue must be adjusted with the resulting patient morbidity (Wolinsky *et al.*, 2012).

Intermittent oral delivery is considered as a common treatment for a majority of diseases, specifically cancer. Such methods, might lead to high concentration of drug in the blood immediately after administration which may have severe side effects in patients as the level of drug in the bloodstream increases. In cancer therapy, the drugs contain high amounts of toxic molecules which harm both normal and cancerous cells. When the drug level in the bloodstream is more than

1%, some parts in the body for example, the gastrointestinal system or the kidney are disabled. Therefore local and selective drug delivery systems with the ability to remotely control the drug release in the targeted site, may be used to reduce the side effects. For this reason, many local drug delivery systems on the basis of polymers, have been investigated (Mousavi *et al.*, 2018).

Nanoparticles may be utilized as carriers for drugs and may have drug delivery applications. The prospect of designing nanoparticles over the past few years has been the enhancement of therapeutic effects of drugs and also decreasing side effects. The application of nanoparticles as drug carriers, may have advantages compared to general treatments. The first advantage of using nanoparticles as drug carriers is the uninterrupted and controlled release of the therapeutic agent, and as a result retaining the drug dosage at the required level. The second advantage of using nanoparticles as drug carriers is localized drug delivery and the supply of the drug at a special site or cell, leading to a decrease in drug dosage and, as a result improving patient compliance (Tığlı Aydın and Pulat, 2012). There are two important factors in the local delivery of nanoparticles: 1) nanoparticles are able to infuse in a slightly viscous, slightly hyperosmolar solution 2) the nanoparticle must have a negative or neutral charge (Patel *et al.*, 2012).

A group of biodegradable polymers is sensitive to changes in environmental circumstances such as temperature, pH, magnetic field and electric field. These systems are based on passive drug delivery and the drug release mechanism is often diffusion, which steadily carries out a determined dose of drug at a certain time. Administration of high levels of drugs in an organ is not feasible, as the control over drug release is decreased, and as a result, the drug release time increases. Moreover, controlled release drug delivery systems, using biodegradable polymers may have challenges such as the excessive release of drugs in the first implantation days. Consequently, the usual techniques of using polymers in drug delivery may have issues such as incomplete drug diffusion within the special site, and in some cases, unwanted interactions between the drug and deliver substances. To overcome the aforementioned issues associated with conventional drug delivery systems, smart and active drug delivery systems have been developed. Implantable chips for controlled drug release, that are known to deliver drugs on demand are an example of such systems. These systems can deliver therapeutic agents at any dosage, time, model and rate and can be externally controlled. In a specific study, a piezo-actuated silicon micropump has been investigated. The pump included a pair of check valves and a pumping membrane which directed liquid flow in the proper direction from a drug reservoir to the releasing location (Mousavi *et al.*, 2018).

Ionic polymer metal composites (IPMCs) are smart electro-active polymers (EAP) with a low power driving force of less than 8 mW, but large displacements. IPMCs have been utilized as actuators in drug delivery chips and have been of interest over the past few years. IPMCs are more flexible compared to piezoelectric actuators, and work at a lower voltage. Lee *et al.* have studied the flow rate and design calculations of IPMC actuator micropump. The studie also used a limited part analysis to optimize the electrode shape of the IPMC diaphragm and studied the stroke volume. Researchers have developed a new and different design of a chip for drug delivery applications as a single reservoir with IPMC actuator as the capping layer of the reservoir. Some of the advantages of this implantable chip may include low operational power, easy designation, simple manufacturing, biocompatibility, and external controllability. This design solved the challenge of imperfect drug release due to the incapability of the actuator to pump the entire drug content in earlier models. The IPMC can be in the interstitial water of an organ and will be in charge of dissolving the whole drug inside the reservoir. For any disease that might require smart localized drug delivery (for example, breast cancer), these chips are significantly helpful as the organ is reachable, and the device may be located in the vicinity of the cancerous cells by surgery. After the surgery, the drug release parameters such as time and dosage of the drug may be controlled by the therapist (Mousavi *et al.*, 2018).

Polymeric-based drug delivery tools that are locally administered guarantee the delivery of high dosages of anti-cancer drugs to the targeted site. However, there are several issues related to the effectiveness of the administered drug, which is influenced by the accessibility of anti-cancer drugs in the vicinity of cancerous cells. An important issue is the sufficient release of the drug to occult sites of the tumor, to avoid recurrence. For instance, lung cancer patients suffer from a 2-fold increase in locoregional recurrence following smaller "wedge" resections (17–24%) performed in the setting of limited cardiopulmonary function, as compared to a standard lobectomy resection, whereby ~50% of the entire lung affected by tumor is removed. Theoretically, local recurrence may occur, which is related to the existence of microscopic disease at or close to the surgical resection margins. The theory is confirmed by the doubling of recurrence rates following limited resections when the resection margin is less than 1 cm. According to the art, after surgical resection (curative limited resection), 39% of patients had malignant cells at the surgical margin, connecting the optimal distance of malignant negative margins to the maximum tumor diameter. Consequently, increasing the efficient curing radius of the resection margin used for local drug delivery may decrease the local recurrence possibility and increase the number of rescued patients after curative limited resection. Local drug delivery may enhance clinical results for patients in the early stage of cancer, if the targeted site receives sufficient therapeutic agents in the required time. Finally, the effectiveness of the therapy is associated with the radial diffusion profile of the embedded drug (Wolinsky *et al.*, 2012).

1.3. CHALLENGES   IN   LOCALIZED   STIMULI   RESPONSIVE MATERIALS

To overcome challenges of local drug delivery systems, more research is required about the healing and inflammatory reactions to the local accumulation of drugs and also polymers in the post-operation process. Chemotherapy is a cancer treatment method that uses agents with significant disadvantages and a wide range of side effects. The drugs are extremely cytotoxic, therefore, the dose-dependent toxicity of healthy parenchyma must be considered, and connection to nearby tissues must be avoided to prevent severe injury. Moreover, anti-filtration drugs may prevent the curing of normal tissues, after the surgery process. This issue may be caused by interrupting the infiltration of immune cells such as neutrophils and macrophages. Also, severe injury may occur at the implantation site, due to the edema, which might raise drug diffusion into the local tissue or organ. However, after implantation, the external response of body to the polymer, may result in the fabrication of a thick fibrous capsule around the implant, which would act as a diffusion obstacle for drug release. Therefore, the interactions between the local cancer treatment drug delivery and the final outcome of curing on interstitial fluid flow and tissue density must be considered, in order to verify the release of sufficient dosages of a therapeutic agent to the desired site and on a scheduled time (Wolinsky *et al.*, 2012).

Although huge advances have occurred in engineering new stimuli-responsive materials, some challenges and difficulties still remain to be addressed regarding nanomedicine applications. For instance, biodegradability and biocompatibility are two important parameters of drugs which must be ensured even before human clinical trials. As a result, there are many systems that have only been stated as an *in vitro* proof-of-concept and recorded work *in vivo*, and a few researches have reached preclinical models (Alsehli, 2020).

In general, for LSDDSs in cancer treatment by chemotherapy, the inherent toxicity of a chemotherapy agent within the body, determines the application time and dosage of the drug. *In vivo* investigations, including normal DOX administration, have solved drug resistance issues. Because of low diffusion rates and potent intracellular binding, therapeutic gradients were recognized, which have no delay after injection. The aforementioned therapeutic agents remained near blood vessels, leaving further cancerous cells removed from vessels unhurt. Moreover, the nonstop infusion administration, resulted in more gradual gradients. In case of multicellular layer models, research demonstrated that, significantly for cells away from blood vessels, gradual diffusion of specific drugs successfully increased chemotherapy efficacy. On the margins and also close to blood vessels, repeated treatments eliminate successive layers of cells. So, it can be concluded that local and permanent drug delivery can overcome issues related to drug diffusion. In the case of spheroids, due to the repeated infusion in cells located far from margins, the drug concentration was raised, which enhanced retention and therapeutic balance across the whole tumor. Nutrients diminish with durable approaches that delete subsequent layers of cells, and as a result, with the aim of reaching cancerous cells that are getting energy and therapy, which allow access to earlier elusive cells. Developed models for *in vivo* and *in vitro* investigations for drug diffusion, may have for novel ideas and approaches. Besides, developing local drug delivery systems may be significantly effective for controlling administrated dosages of a drug for a long period, with a platform for enhanced biocompatibility and versatility (Lam and Ho, 2009).

Three groups of devising an implantable tool for medical purposes, are the patient, the medical staff and the engineer. Therefore, implantable devices may be accessed by gathering information from these three groups. The progress of designing such a device depends on the requirements of patients, the doctors' decisions, and the practical possibility of the model designed by the engineer. As a general rule, patients who have temporary or permanent implants inside their body, feel uncomfortable finding something external in their body. They prefer the use of medical methods, without any pain and terminating the healing process unconsciously. Great effort is needed to overcome these issues. Due to the initiation of minimally invasive medical methods, the insertion place has become unremarkable and restoration can happen unconsciously (Joung, 2013).

From a materials viewpoint, drug delivery systems require more signs of progress in the following directions: a combination of several diverse components into one exclusive device, the need for more biocompatible and flexible external materials which are inserted into the body during implantation, and the realization of closed-looped DDSs, through the integration of multiple advanced electronic devices, such as a wireless transductors or portable batteries (Puiggalí-Jou *et al.*, 2019).

In the case of periodontal disease, presently, there is no information about the usefulness of local combinations used either together or sequentially. Theoretically, using the local and systemic drug delivery route simultaneously presents a high drug concentration at exact locations and suppresses the potential of bacterial reinfection reservoirs (*e.g.*, tonsil, tongue, mucosa and saliva). The aforementioned method may be useful as it inhibits recolonization at cured locations, though it requires more assessment. When ordinary antimicrobial agents are not helpful, specific bacteria elimination methods are required to obtain optimum local drug administration results. In this regard, local drug delivery systems may be practical. When conventional therapy is unsuccessful to achieve clinical periodontal health, clinicians should utilize bacterial and drug sensitivity testing that can be addressed by local drug delivery (Greenstein and Polson, 1998).

Biocompatibility is one of the major issues associated with the long-time use of implantable materials, and the issue may only be resolved by concerted multidisciplinary attempts. The low biocompatibility of materials may cause serious issues such as pain and discomfort in long-term implantable drug delivery, which might reduce patient acceptance. Cost/benefit ratio is another important factor that must be considered, as some local delivery systems may be costly. Another challenge is the complexity of local systems in comparison to oral routes and the required dosages for longer approval may be too expensive. Moreover, some local delivery systems need minor surgery for implants and explants, which may lower patient acceptance and raises the desire for a less invasive alternative. (Park and Park, 1996).

CONCLUSION

LCDDSs may be fabricated to establish localized controlled and triggered release by the endogenous and exogenous stimulus. LCDDSs decrease systemic cytotoxicity and enhance the efficiency of the therapeutic molecule. In specific cases, the shape/magnitude of the release profile may be manipulated for particular indications. A wide range of LCDDSs has been studied, with a specific emphasis on bio/cytocompatibility. The toxicity of the materials used in LCDDS, must be studied, especially when nanomaterials and nanostructures are used, as they may include several toxic agents that are unknown. Moreover, the therapeutic molecule/drug delivered from a LCDDS noticeably affects bio/cytocompatibility. LCDDS may manipulate the local concentration of therapeutic molecule/drug, which can result in high local toxicity in cell microenvironments and tissues. Developments in LCDDSs may require combining several fields, such as biomedicine, pharmaceutical sciences, chemical engineering, materials science, physics, chemistry and electrical engineering. The LCDDS may have closed-loop bio/nanofunctionalities so that the physiological condition may be monitored in order to manipulate the exact drug dosage online (smart LCDDSs that release the drug in response to endogenous/exogenous stimulus).

REFERENCES

Aj, M.Z., Patil, S.K., Baviskar, D.T., Jain, D.K. (2012). Implantable drug delivery system: a review. *Int. J. Pharm. Tech. Res., 4*, 280-292.

Alsehli, M. (2020). Polymeric nanocarriers as stimuli-responsive systems for targeted tumor (cancer) therapy: Recent advances in drug delivery. *Saudi Pharm. J., 28*(3), 255-265.
[http://dx.doi.org/10.1016/j.jsps.2020.01.004] [PMID: 32194326]

Askari, E., Naghib, S.M., Zahedi, A., Seyfoori, A., Zare, Y., Rhee, K.Y. (2021). Local delivery of chemotherapeutic agent in tissue engineering based on gelatin/graphene hydrogel. *J. Mater. Res. Technol., 12*, 412-422.
[http://dx.doi.org/10.1016/j.jmrt.2021.02.084]

Askari, E., Rasouli, M., Darghiasi, S.F., Naghib, S.M., Zare, Y., Rhee, K.Y. (2021). Reduced graphene oxide-grafted bovine serum albumin/bredigite nanocomposites with high mechanical properties and excellent osteogenic bioactivity for bone tissue engineering. *Biodes. Manuf., 4*(2), 243-257.
[http://dx.doi.org/10.1007/s42242-020-00113-4]

Campbell, S., Smeets, N. (2019). *Drug delivery: localized and systemic therapeutic strategies with polymer systems. Functional polymers. Polymers and polymeric composites: a reference series.*. Cham: Springer.

Choonara, Y.E., Pillay, V., Danckwerts, M.P., Carmichael, T.R., du Toit, L.C. (2010). A review of implantable intravitreal drug delivery technologies for the treatment of posterior segment eye diseases. *J. Pharm. Sci., 99*(5), 2219-2239.
[http://dx.doi.org/10.1002/jps.21987] [PMID: 19894268]

Dhanikula, A.B., Panchagnula, R. (1999). Localized paclitaxel delivery. *Int. J. Pharm., 183*(2), 85-100.
[http://dx.doi.org/10.1016/S0378-5173(99)00087-3] [PMID: 10361159]

Gao, W., Zhang, Y., Zhang, Q., Zhang, L. (2016). Nanoparticle-hydrogel: a hybrid biomaterial system for localized drug delivery. *Ann. Biomed. Eng., 44*(6), 2049-2061.
[http://dx.doi.org/10.1007/s10439-016-1583-9] [PMID: 26951462]

Gill, J. S., Bharti, V., Gupta, H., Gill, S. (2011). Non-surgical management of chronic periodontitis with two local drug delivery agents-A comparative study.
[http://dx.doi.org/10.4317/jced.3.e424]

Gooneh-Farahani, S., Naghib, S.M., Naimi-Jamal, M.R. (2020). A Novel and Inexpensive Method Based on Modified Ionic Gelation for pH-responsive Controlled Drug Release of Homogeneously Distributed Chitosan Nanoparticles with a High Encapsulation Efficiency. *Fibers Polym., 21*(9), 1917-1926.
[http://dx.doi.org/10.1007/s12221-020-1095-y]

Gooneh-Farahani, S., Naimi-Jamal, M.R., Naghib, S.M. (2019). Stimuli-responsive graphene-incorporated multifunctional chitosan for drug delivery applications: a review. *Expert Opin. Drug Deliv., 16*(1), 79-99.
[http://dx.doi.org/10.1080/17425247.2019.1556257] [PMID: 30514124]

Greenstein, G. (2006). Local drug delivery in the treatment of periodontal diseases: assessing the clinical significance of the results. *J. Periodontol., 77*(4), 565-578.
[http://dx.doi.org/10.1902/jop.2006.050140] [PMID: 16584336]

Greenstein, G., Polson, A. (1998). The role of local drug delivery in the management of periodontal diseases: a comprehensive review. *J. Periodontol., 69*(5), 507-520.
[http://dx.doi.org/10.1902/jop.1998.69.5.507] [PMID: 9623893]

Haley, R.M., von Recum, H.A. (2019). Localized and targeted delivery of NSAIDs for treatment of inflammation: A review. *Exp. Biol. Med. (Maywood), 244*(6), 433-444.
[http://dx.doi.org/10.1177/1535370218787770] [PMID: 29996674]

Higashi, K., Matsushita, M., Morisaki, K., Hayashi, S., Mayumi, T. (1991). Local drug delivery systems for the treatment of periodontal disease. *J. Pharmacobiodyn., 14*(2), 72-81.
[http://dx.doi.org/10.1248/bpb1978.14.72] [PMID: 1870076]

H R., R., Dhamecha, D., Jagwani, S., Rao, M., Jadhav, K., Shaikh, S., Puzhankara, L., Jalalpure, S. (2019). Local drug delivery systems in the management of periodontitis: A scientific review. *J. Control. Release, 307*, 393-409.
[http://dx.doi.org/10.1016/j.jconrel.2019.06.038] [PMID: 31255689]

Ibsen, S., Benchimol, M., Simberg, D., Esener, S. (2012). *Ultrasound mediated localized drug delivery. Nano-Biotechnology for Biomedical and Diagnostic Research..* Springer.

Jain, J.P., Modi, S., Domb, A.J., Kumar, N. (2005). Role of polyanhydrides as localized drug carriers. *J. Control. Release, 103*(3), 541-563.
[http://dx.doi.org/10.1016/j.jconrel.2004.12.021] [PMID: 15820403]

Ji, T., Kohane, D.S. (2019). Nanoscale systems for local drug delivery. *Nano Today, 28*, 100765.
[http://dx.doi.org/10.1016/j.nantod.2019.100765] [PMID: 32831899]

Joung, Y.H. (2013). Development of implantable medical devices: from an engineering perspective. *Int. Neurourol. J., 17*(3), 98-106.
[http://dx.doi.org/10.5213/inj.2013.17.3.98] [PMID: 24143287]

Kavanagh, C.A., Rochev, Y.A., Gallagher, W.M., Dawson, K.A., Keenan, A.K. (2004). Local drug delivery in restenosis injury: thermoresponsive co-polymers as potential drug delivery systems. *Pharmacol. Ther., 102*(1), 1-15.
[http://dx.doi.org/10.1016/j.pharmthera.2003.01.001] [PMID: 15056495]

Kleiner, L.W., Wright, J.C., Wang, Y. (2014). Evolution of implantable and insertable drug delivery systems. *J. Control. Release, 181*, 1-10.
[http://dx.doi.org/10.1016/j.jconrel.2014.02.006] [PMID: 24548479]

Lam, R., Ho, D. (2009). Nanodiamonds as vehicles for systemic and localized drug delivery. *Expert Opin. Drug Deliv., 6*(9), 883-895.
[http://dx.doi.org/10.1517/17425240903156382] [PMID: 19637985]

Lambert, C.R., Leone, J.E., Rowland, S.M. (1993). Local drug delivery catheters. *Coron. Artery Dis., 4*(5), 469-476.
[http://dx.doi.org/10.1097/00019501-199305000-00011] [PMID: 8261224]

Lavik, E. B., Kuppermann, B. D., Humayun, M. S. Section 4 translational basic science.

Lee, E.J., Huh, B.K., Kim, S.N., Lee, J.Y., Park, C.G., Mikos, A.G., Choy, Y.B. (2017). Application of materials as medical devices with localized drug delivery capabilities for enhanced wound repair. *Prog. Mater. Sci., 89*, 392-410.
[http://dx.doi.org/10.1016/j.pmatsci.2017.06.003] [PMID: 29129946]

Morgan, D., Ríos, E., DeCoursey, T.E. (2009). Dynamic measurement of the membrane potential of phagocytosing neutrophils by confocal microscopy and SEER (Shifted Excitation and Emission Ratioing) of di-8-ANEPPS. *Biophys. J., 96*(3), 687a.
[http://dx.doi.org/10.1016/j.bpj.2008.12.3627]

Nadig, P., Shah, M. (2016). Tetracycline as local drug delivery in treatment of chronic periodontitis: A systematic review and meta-analysis. *J. Indian Soc. Periodontol., 20*(6), 576-583.
[http://dx.doi.org/10.4103/jisp.jisp_97_17] [PMID: 29238136]

Park, H., Park, K. (1996). Biocompatibility issues of implantable drug delivery systems. *Pharm. Res., 13*(12), 1770-1776.
[http://dx.doi.org/10.1023/A:1016012520276] [PMID: 8987070]

Patel, T., Zhou, J., Piepmeier, J.M., Saltzman, W.M. (2012). Polymeric nanoparticles for drug delivery to the central nervous system. *Adv. Drug Deliv. Rev., 64*(7), 701-705.
[http://dx.doi.org/10.1016/j.addr.2011.12.006] [PMID: 22210134]

Puiggalí-Jou, A., del Valle, L.J., Alemán, C. (2019). Drug delivery systems based on intrinsically conducting polymers. *J. Control. Release, 309*, 244-264.

[http://dx.doi.org/10.1016/j.jconrel.2019.07.035] [PMID: 31351927]

Ramesh, A., Prakash, A. P., Thomas, B. (2016). Local drug delivery in periodontal diseases. a review. *Journal of Health and Allied Sciences NU, 6*, 074-079.

Rolfes, C., Howard, S., Goff, R., Iaizzo, P. A. (2012). Localized drug delivery for cardiothoracic surgery. *Current concepts in general thoracic surgery. InTech Open Access Chapter, 279*

Saneei Mousavi, M.S., Karami, A.H., Ghasemnejad, M., Kolahdouz, M., Manteghi, F., Ataei, F. (2018). Design of a remote-control drug delivery implantable chip for cancer local on demand therapy using ionic polymer metal composite actuator. *J. Mech. Behav. Biomed. Mater., 86*, 250-256.
[http://dx.doi.org/10.1016/j.jmbbm.2018.06.034] [PMID: 29986300]

Singh, G., Navkiran, S., Kaur, S. (2014). Local drug delivery in periodontics: a review. *J. Periodontal Med. Clin. Pract., 1*, 272-284.

Singh, P., Carrier, A., Chen, Y., Lin, S., Wang, J., Cui, S., Zhang, X. (2019). Polymeric microneedles for controlled transdermal drug delivery. *J. Control. Release, 315*, 97-113.
[http://dx.doi.org/10.1016/j.jconrel.2019.10.022] [PMID: 31644938]

Singh, S., Roy, S., Chumber, S.K. (2009). Evaluation of two local drug delivery systems as adjuncts to mechanotherapy as compared to mechanotherapy alone in management of chronic periodontitis: A clinical, microbiological, and molecular study. *J. Indian Soc. Periodontol., 13*(3), 126-132.
[http://dx.doi.org/10.4103/0972-124X.60224] [PMID: 20379409]

Song, C.X., Labhasetwar, V., Murphy, H., Qu, X., Humphrey, W.R., Shebuski, R.J., Levy, R.J. (1997). Formulation and characterization of biodegradable nanoparticles for intravascular local drug delivery. *J. Control. Release, 43*(2-3), 197-212.
[http://dx.doi.org/10.1016/S0168-3659(96)01484-8]

Stebbins, N.D., Ouimet, M.A., Uhrich, K.E. (2014). Antibiotic-containing polymers for localized, sustained drug delivery. *Adv. Drug Deliv. Rev., 78*, 77-87.
[http://dx.doi.org/10.1016/j.addr.2014.04.006] [PMID: 24751888]

Szulc, M., Zakrzewska, A., Zborowski, J. (2018). Local drug delivery in periodontitis treatment: A review of contemporary literature. *Dent. Med. Probl., 55*(3), 333-342.
[http://dx.doi.org/10.17219/dmp/94890] [PMID: 30328312]

TıĞLı AYDıN, R.S., Pulat, M. (2012). 5-Fluorouracil encapsulated chitosan nanoparticles for pH-stimulated drug delivery: evaluation of controlled release kinetics. *J. Nanomater.*

Vandana, K.L., Kalsi, R., Prakash, S. (2011). Effect of local drug delivery in chronic periodontitis patients: A meta-analysis. *J. Indian Soc. Periodontol., 15*(4), 304-309.
[http://dx.doi.org/10.4103/0972-124X.92559] [PMID: 22368351]

Wolinsky, J.B., Colson, Y.L., Grinstaff, M.W. (2012). Local drug delivery strategies for cancer treatment: Gels, nanoparticles, polymeric films, rods, and wafers. *J. Control. Release, 159*(1), 14-26.
[http://dx.doi.org/10.1016/j.jconrel.2011.11.031] [PMID: 22154931]

Yang, B., Lv, W., Deng, Y. (2017). Drug loaded poly(glycerol sebacate) as a local drug delivery system for the treatment of periodontal disease. *RSC Advances, 7*(59), 37426-37435.
[http://dx.doi.org/10.1039/C7RA02796F]

Zeinali Kalkhoran, A.H., Naghib, S.M., Vahidi, O., Rahmanian, M. (2018). Synthesis and characterization of graphene-grafted gelatin nanocomposite hydrogels as emerging drug delivery systems. *Biomed. Phys. Eng. Express, 4*(5), 055017.
[http://dx.doi.org/10.1088/2057-1976/aad745]

Zeinali Kalkhoran, A.H., Vahidi, O., Naghib, S.M. (2018). A new mathematical approach to predict the actual drug release from hydrogels. *Eur. J. Pharm. Sci., 111*, 303-310.
[http://dx.doi.org/10.1016/j.ejps.2017.09.038] [PMID: 28962856]

Zeng, Q., Shao, D., He, X., Ren, Z., Ji, W., Shan, C., Qu, S., Li, J., Chen, L., Li, Q. (2016). Carbon dots as a trackable drug delivery carrier for localized cancer therapy *in vivo*. *J. Mater. Chem. B Mater. Biol. Med.,* *4*(30), 5119-5126.
[http://dx.doi.org/10.1039/C6TB01259K] [PMID: 32263509]

CHAPTER 2

Carbon Nanostructures in Localized Controlled Drug Delivery Systems (LCDDSs)

Abstract: Nanotechnology has possible potential for developing future clinical applications. Nanoparticles may be used for biological and medical purposes due to their opportunities for multi-modal systems. Moreover, carbon nanostructures have received considerable attention in biomedicine. As an example, carbon nanomaterials have been extensively used to deliver therapeutic molecules in multi-functional controlled release systems. Carbon nanostructures may be used as nanocarriers, owing to their large surface area, privileged cumulation in tumors and excellent internalization in cancer cells. Carbon nanostructures may be used to deliver therapeutic agents preferentially to cancer tissues, to decrease side effects and cytotoxicity of drugs. However, the intrinsic cellular toxicity of carbon nanostructures remains a challenge. This chapter represents different characteristics of carbon nanostructures, resulting in their various applications in localized controlled drug delivery systems. Recent progress in methods and techniques for biofunctionalization, delivering and targeting by carbon nanostructures are presented and discussed.

Keywords: Carbon nanostructure, Cytotoxicity, Localized drug delivery, Multi-functionality, Nanotechnology , Therapeutic molecules.

2.1. INTRODUCTION

Cancer is one of the popular diseases in the 21st century. The treatment of cancer using chemotherapy methods has adverse influences and may have incomplete and different therapeutic reactions in different cases. Therefore, researchers have scrutinized various controlled release carriers to help control and target cancer drug delivery inside the lesion and potentially overcome the aforementioned issues. A variety of stimuli-responsive controlled release carriers have been explored for further progress in therapeutic efficacy. A specific group of studies has focused on the application of nanoscience and technology, for therapeutic applications, which have shown positive results in animal experiments. Stimuli-responsive drug delivery is studied to achieve controlled drug release and cell uptake in tumor region under stimulations, to further increase effectivity and reduce side effects (Yang *et al.*, 2016).

Seyed Morteza Naghib, Samin Hoseinpour & Shadi Zarshad

Carbon allotropes are the result of different chemical bondings (covalent) between carbon atoms. Each carbon allotrope owns unique physicochemical characteristics due to the exclusive spatial organization of carbon atoms. Graphite, graphene, carbon nanotube, and diamond are examples of carbon allotropes. Graphene has characteristics such as simple fabrication and modification, low cost, two external surfaces, high surface area, and non-toxicity compared to carbon nanotubes (CNTs). Therefore, graphene may be superior to CNT in many applications, such as drug delivery, due to its lower toxicity and higher biocompatibility (Bitounis *et al.*, 2013, Liu *et al.*, 2013).

In general, nanocarriers can enter the cell and interact with the cell membrane by endocytosis. In the targeted delivery of drugs to the cell nucleus, it is vital for the drug to pass the endosomal section and reach the cytosolic section. Functionalized carbon-based nanomaterials are a group of materials that can be used in stimuli-responsive drug delivery systems. Carbon-based materials, and specifically graphene, can conjugate with numerous natural polymers, such as gelatin and chitosan, for controlled release purposes. These biocompatible polymers are biodegradable, cytocompatible, and have low immunogenicity, which can be used to decrease the toxic effects of graphene (Goenka *et al.*, 2014). In the following sections, a summary of each carbon-based material is discussed.

2.2. GRAPHENE

Carbon is the most widespread element in our living ecosystems, which is biologically and environmentally safer compared to inorganic materials (Chung *et al.*, 2013). Graphene is composed of a single layer of carbon atoms with a hexagonal lattice structure. In this 2D planar structure, each carbon atom has an sp^2 hybridization and includes 4 bonds which are r and π bonds. Graphene can be synthesized using both top-down approaches such as mechanical exfoliation methods, and bottom-up approaches such as chemical vapor deposition (CVD). The electronic and crystalline properties of graphene produced *via* CVD are better compared to graphene synthesized by the graphite. Graphene has properties such as high thermal conductivity (~5000 W/m/K), high mechanical strength (Young's modulus, ~1100 Gpa), tunable bandgap, high intrinsic mobility, high electric conductivity (mobility of charge carriers, 200,000 cm^2 V^{-1} s^{-1}), and large surface area (2630 m^2/g). Graphene may be categorized as a hydrophobic material and, because of the absence of oxygen groups, counts as a hydrophobic material (Shareena *et al.*, 2018, Shen *et al.*, 2012, Rao *et al.*, 2009, Imani *et al.*, 2018).

The unique properties of graphene have resulted in the wide application of this material in different fields such as biosensors, nanoelectronic devices, drug delivery, *etc.* (Salahandish *et al.*, 2019). Moreover, the two-dimensional network of graphene decreases its toxicity in biomedical applications (Chung *et al.*, 2013, Sattari *et al.*, 2017). Some of the properties of graphene, such as bending elasticity, specific surface area, and thickness, depend on the number of layers. For example, decreasing the number of layers increases the adsorptive capability of graphene-based materials. On the other hand, increasing the number of layers increases stiffness/rigidity during cellular interactions. The lateral size of graphene-based materials may vary from nanoscale to microscale (*i.e.*, 10 nm up to >20 mm). Deformation and lateral size are vital factors of graphene in cellular uptake and a variety of biological interactions (Fig. **1**). As an example, the lateral size may affect renal clearance, and penetration of the blood-brain barrier. (McNamara and Tofail, 2015, Wick *et al.*, 2014).

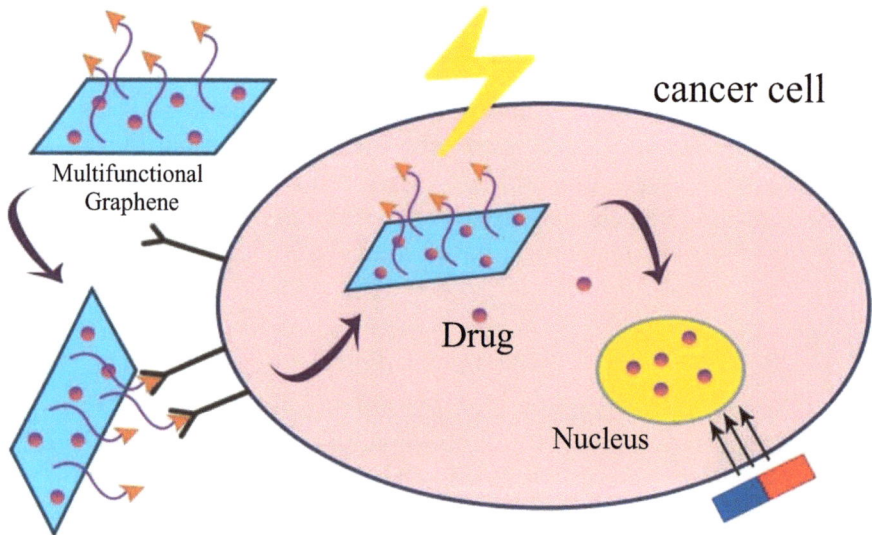

Fig. (1). Schematic of the transfer of multi-functional graphene into a tumor cell for drug delivery applications.

Graphene has a high specific surface area which can be covered with different kinds of biomolecules (Askari *et al.*, 2019, Gooneh-Farahani *et al.*, 2019, Kalkhoran *et al.*, 2018, Mamaghani *et al.*, 2018, Naghib, 2019, Naghib *et al.*, 2020). The loading ratio of graphene (the weight ratio of loaded drug to carriers), is high and can reach to 200% (Yang *et al.*, 2016, Liu *et al.*, 2013). Thus, graphene may be used in drug delivery and gene delivery applications [1].

Doxorubicin, Heparin, Camptothecin, Plasmid DNA, and siRNA are some of the drugs and molecules which can be loaded on Graphene. According to the art, planar aromatic domains, such as doxorubicin (DOX) can be loaded on graphene with a π-π bond between the graphene surface and aromatic rings which results in a steady chemical conjugation. On the other hand, the negative charge on the graphene oxide surface may have an electrostatic interaction with the positive charges on the biopolymers for example, PET (polyethyleneimine). The electrostatic interaction transfers positive charges to graphene, to produce complexes with negative molecules such as RNA or DNA for gene delivery applications (Bitounis *et al.*, 2013).

From another point of view, since most cancer treatment drugs are lipophilic in nature, the lipophilic properties of graphene may be used for cancer treatment drug delivery applications. Hydrophobic drugs can be loaded on the graphene surface as well, but hydrophobicity may cause bioavailability-related issues. Therefore, the graphene surface is usually functionalized to achieve a hydrophilic surface and to overcome the aforementioned issue. Graphene synthesized *via* the CVD approach is hydrophobic and flexible and has a critical effect on the proliferation, growth and differentiation of various cells (Chung *et al.*, 2013, Sun and Wu, 2011).

Graphene-derived structures may be categorized into single-layer graphene, bilayer graphene, and few-layer graphene (the number of layers is less than 10), despending on the chemical contents and number of layers. Graphene-based materials are not homogenous and differ in number, surface chemistry, lateral dimension, and defect density or purity. Graphene-based materials (GBMs) enhance the electrical/mechanical characteristics biomaterials, growth at biomaterials surface and enlarge cellular attachment (Shareena *et al.*, 2018, Rao *et al.*, 2009, Pinto *et al.*, 2013). Reduced graphene oxide (RGO), graphene oxide (GO) and chemically modified graphene are members of the broad family of graphene-based nanostructures (Ding *et al.*, 2015), which are discussed below.

2.3. GRAPHENE OXIDE (GO)

GO is defined as a material mostly yielded by acid-based treatment of graphite oxide after sonication. GO is different from graphene, and is a single layer of graphite oxide. The difference between graphene and GO is existence of oxygen-containing groups, including phenol, hydroxyl, carbonyl, oxygen, and epoxide groups, on the GO surface. The presence of these functional groups leads to enhanced solubility of GO in aqueous media, effortless treatment, and richer surface chemistry. GO contains both the aliphatic (sp^3) and aromatic (sp^2) domains that assist the surface interactions (Shareena *et al.*, 2018, Imani *et al.*, 2018, Reina *et al.*, 2017, Servant *et al.*, 2014, Makharza *et al.*, 2013, Askari *et al.*, 2021a).

There are approximately two dissimilar domains at each GO surface. The first one is the hydrophilic part which is composed of sp^2 carbon and the second one is the hydrophobic region where oxygen-containing groups exist. Consequently, the usual reactivity of GO comes together with the "classical" sp^2 chemistry of graphene (Diels–Alder reactions, radical reactions, 1,3-dipolar additions, etc.) with the chemistry of the oxygenated functional groups. Regularly GO increases the surface hydrophilicity of biocomposites which enhances the biocompatibility of the composite by increasing th possible adhesion sites, such as hydroxyl groups. Moreover, the presence of GO may cause a suitable circumstance in the surface topography for cell adhesion. Furthermore, the dispersibility in the cell culture media or water may improve in functionalized GO; as a result, it decreases its cytotoxicity and induces the accumulation of tissues and cells. Polyethylene glycol (PEG), chitosan, and polyethyleneimine are examples of cytocompatible biopolymers. Since many organic groups exist on the GO surface, it is necessary to consider that similar or unwanted reactions may happen, which can lead to wrong interpretations (Sun and Wu, 2011, Ding *et al.*, 2015).

It is hard to produce a single layer of graphene without any defects. Moreover, graphene has a low solubility. On the other hand, GO has outstanding aqueous processability, amphiphilicity, surface functionalization ability, and also surface-enhanced Raman scattering (SERS). These properties count as an important factor to utilize GO for biomedical purposes. The most important advantage of using GO, is the aqueous dispersibility and also colloidal constancy of GO compared to other carbon-based nanomaterials. Due to the physicochemical properties of GO, it is chemically versatile, with a high surface-to-volume ratio which may be used for cancer therapy (Bitounis *et al.*, 2013, Chung *et al.*, 2013, Imani *et al.*, 2018). GO is often used because of its easy transfer procedure, simple scalability and low-priced synthesis.

Various parameters such as shape, size, surface chemistry, and charge play an important role in the entrance and interaction of nano/microcarriers with macrophages/cells. Among these parameters, the shape is a more serious factor because of the 2D shape of graphene and GO, which is not regular in biological systems. Another important factor is rigidity. Ridity is critical for the structural integrity of drug carriers. However, the high rigidity of the carrier may be harmful to cells. Consequently, it is essential to control the rigidity of graphene and GO to optimize controlled release. Pristine graphene has characteristics such as hydrophobicity, and low dispersibility in water. Pristine graphene must be functionalized so that it can be utilized in biomedical applications. Quite the opposite, GO is dispersible in water and is hydrophilic. Regarding the synthesis procedure of graphene nanomaterials, many impurities can enter the structure, such as sulfates, nitrates, hydrazine, permanganates, peroxide residues, borohydride surfactants and some lower-molecular-weight oxidative remainders, which may result in harmful biological effects, and impact toxicity (Liu *et al.*, 2013, Chung *et al.*, 2013).

Due to the wide application of GO as a drug delivery carrier, many factors such as the production source must be considered to achieve high reproducibility. After completing the classical Hummers or a modified Hummers' technique, the reaction product includes few-layer and single-layer GO, unwanted graphite oxide, and pristine graphite that should be removed. Theoretically, to achieve high quality, GO must be divided according to its lateral dimensions, as size affects toxicity, loading ability, and adsorption/desorption kinetics (Ding *et al.*, 2015, Makharza *et al.*, 2013, Yang *et al.*, 2013).

GO used in controlled release applications is commonly 1-3 layers (1-2 nm thick), with dimensions varying from a few nanometers to several hundred nanometers. GO may be used for drug delivery purposes due to characteristics such as high specific surface area, numerous oxygen-containing groups and biocompatibility. Drugs can be loaded on the GO surface through chemical reactions or physical bondings. Various polymers and biomolecules can be chemically attached to the GO surface due to the presence of COOH and OH groups. For example, Chitosan and PEG are two molecules covalently attached to GO to change blood circulation profile and improve cytocompatibility (Shen *et al.*, 2012).

The carboxylate group produces a pH-related negative surface charge, resulting in colloidal stability. On the other hand, Hydroxyl and epoxide functional produce an uncharged but polar basic plane. It is noteworthy that unmodified graphitic domains are still hydrophobic and have π-π interactions, capable of adsorbing drugs and dry molecules. It can be concluded that GO is a hydrophilic macromolecule and can act as a surfactant at the interface or stabilize hydrophobic molecules in a solution (Goenka *et al.*, 2014, Zhu *et al.*, 2015).

In a study, a chemotherapeutic drug-1, 3-bis (2-chloroethyl)-1-nitrosourea (BCNU) with covalent interactions, which can react with esterification, was used to treat malignant brain tumors (Jaleel *et al.*, 2017, Zhang *et al.*, 2016). Photodynamic therapy (PDT) is a cancer treatment method in clinical practice, which has low toxicity and high stability in physiological circumstances. In another study, porphyrin photosensitizers-loaded sulfonic acid and folic acid linked GO were used in targeted PDT. In another study, Chlorin e6 photosensitizer-loaded GO was used to raise the accumulating photosensitizers in cancer tissue/cells. The results showed an extraordinary dose-related photodynamic impact on cancerous cells under irradiation (Shen *et al.*, 2012).

6-arm PEG functionalized GO used for delivery of hydrophobic drugs in tumor cells which enhanced cellular uptake. GO carriers may be used for photothermal therapy due to their near-NIR adsorption resulting in caspase activation, mitochondrial depolarization, oxidative stress, and finally, tumor cell necrosis and apoptosis (Chung *et al.*, 2013).

In another study, a method was used to manufacture a biocompatible, reduction-responsive and 3D nanocarrier (GON–Cy-ALG–PEG) to carry an antitumor agent (DOX). The method can be combined with photo- and chemo-thermal treatment superior to regular therapy (Shareena *et al.*, 2018).

The *in vivo* effectiveness of GO is based on passive targeting, and particularly on EPR effect, which is widespread in several cancer tissues, because of hypervascularization. Although, this method doesn't always show hopeful outcomes in *in vivo* trials. In fact, *in vivo* therapy is more complicated in comparison with *in vitro* and side effects resulting from unfavorable drug release can adversely affect the treatment process. Thus, active targeting therapy is more favorable where targeting fragments like peptides, antibodies and nucleic acids are immobilized on the GO surface. In this method, the nanosized graphene oxide can accumulate in preferred sites, to enhance therapeutic effects and decrease drug side effects of (Ding *et al.*, 2015, Reina *et al.*, 2017, Servant *et al.*, 2014).

Exogenous and endogenous drug delivery are two different approaches for delivering and releasing drugs in the body. Drug release can also accomplish in an intracellular environment. Normally drug release in the cell is because of changes in environmental situations in the cytoplasm and the ECM. So, the desorption of the drug from GO starts by decreasing the pH. For instance, DOX endures the protonation of the amino group of the sugar moiety, which destroys the interactions with the GO sheet. In external stimuli-responsive drug delivery, the efficient drug dosage increases, which improves therapeutic performance. Furthermore, local application of the drug to the target cells decreases unwanted side effects on healthy tissues. Stimulated drug release is usually activated by the photothermal effect. In other words, graphene can absorb NIR light and convert it to heat, then the temperature inside the desired cells increases and the drug is released. Although there are several safety and toxicity issues related to local heating, such as pH, blood flow rate and oxygenation alteration, that require more investigation (Ding *et al.*, 2015).

2.4. REDUCED GRAPHENE OXIDE (RGO)

The product of graphite oxide or graphene oxide during chemical/thermal reduction is called rGO which is known as a structure between the perfect graphene sheet and much oxidized GO (Askari *et al.*, 2021b). rGO has improved electrical conductivity and enhanced hydrophobicity compared to GO. During the reduction process, all or some of the oxygen-containing groups are destroyed, resulting in the production of holes and defects in the rGO structure and decreasing the surface polarity. Therefore, the adsorption of less polar drugs may be enhanced. Like GO, rGO has many applications in the biomedical field and specific drug delivery. rGO has more sp^2 carbons, and therefore has a higher NIR adsorption, which makes rGO a proper choice for photothermal and chemo-photothermal treatments (Ding *et al.*, 2015, Shim *et al.*, 2016).

Cell proliferation and attachment may be drastically reduced with oxygen content in a few-layer rGO. The amended ECM protein adsorption in few-layer rGO enhanced cell proliferation and adhesion, while highly reduced few-layer GO did not affect the cell adhesion. Cellular activities in a few-layer rGO can be changed by regulating the GO surface chemistry and reduction situation (Goenka *et al.*, 2014).

Biocompatibility is the most important factor in showing whether a nanomaterial can be utilized for biomedical applications or not. So far, none of the GO nanomaterials have been accepted for clinical trials. One more benefit of graphene-based nanomaterials over other materials is the controllable drug delivery rate for sustainable controlled release. Single layer GO/rGO has an ultra-high surface area which is suitable for effective drug loading and controlled release for local drug delivery and systemic targeting. Chemotherapy and radiation therapy are two main methods for invasive cancer therapy. Although, one of the major drawbacks of these methods is that they are not limited to cancer cells and also destroy surrounding normal cells. In addition, the high optical absorption of graphene-based nanomaterials in the NIR region, specifically GO, facilitates the application of these materials for photo-thermal therapeutic purposes. Under light irradiation, photothermal therapy (PTT) utilizes an optical-absorbing moiety to produce heat. Subsequently, tissues are subjected to a high temperature to destroy anomalous cells. GO may be a good choice for PTT applications as it can improve optical absorption in the NIR region. In an investigation, a dual drug-loaded, PEGylated GO loaded with DOX (NGO–PEG (polyethylene glycol)–DOX), was used to deliver drug and heat to the tumor cells/tissues, to combine photo- and chemo-thermal therapy in one system. High therapeutic effectivity, minimum destruction and controlled release are the properties of multimodal therapy. Multi-functional nanocomposites exhibit improved photo-thermal energy conversion coefficient and NIR-triggered drug release or targeting characteristics with real-time imaging guidance (Shareena *et al.*, 2018).

The cytotoxicity of GBN has been assessed in many cells, for example, cancer cells, neuronal cells, lung epithelial cells, fibroblasts and animal models. Apoptosis and necrosis are two kinds of cell death. Apoptosis is caused by plasma membrane damage and necrosis is triggered by reactive oxygen species (ROS). Cytocompatible GBN may be used to decrease the cytotoxicity of graphene. Cytocompatible GBN may be derived from plant extracts, microbes, and cytocompatible biopolymers to manufacture graphene-based nanostructures. Cytotoxicity depends on many aspects, including stiffness, lateral size, hydrophobicity, dosage, surface functionalization and layer number. Implantation, injection, dermal penetration, ingestion and inhalation are the defined procedures to insert any nanomaterial into the human body for biomedical purposes. In addition, the entrance route, dosage and length of the nanomaterial have an important impact on toxicity (Shareena *et al.*, 2018).

As mentioned above, GO is soluble, while the main disadvantage of graphene is weak solubility in an aqueous medium. To solve this issue, PNIPAM is embedded into graphene to form GO/PNIPAM composites. These nanocomposites are dispersible and also thermo-responsive, which are great candidates for drug delivery. The pH- and thermo-sensitive GO interpenetrating networks of PNIPAM hydrogel are prepared by covalent bonding between PNIPAM and GO. NIR laser irradiation therapy has both cytocompatibility and deep tissue penetration (*e.g.*, NIR light travels at least 10 cm through breast tissue). The rGO/PNIPAM nanocomposite is mostly affected by temperature when a small amount of rGO is used. Quite the opposite, the thermal therapy does not considerably affect the nanocomposites with large contents of rGO, signifying that this thermo- photo-sensitive trait of rGO/PNIPAM nanocomposite can be practical for controlled drug release. Nanocomposites, which are composed of graphene-based materials and PNIPAM, can be used for photo-/chemo-thermal therapy purposes as they can reduce damages, side effects and non-specific drug delivery (Seo *et al.*, 2016).

In conclusion, graphene contains a defect-free structure and approximately no oxygen-containing group leading to outstanding electrical and optical conductivity, whereas, GO has oxygen-containing groups and weak electrical and optical conductivity. The electrical conductivity of graphene is more than rGO and GO. Water-solubility of GO is more than rGO and graphene (rGO> graphene) owing to the various oxygen-containing groups in their structures. Therefore, graphene is a hydrophobic substance, whereas GO has a hydrophilic nature. The reactivity of GO is more than rGO and graphene (rGO> graphene) (Zhang *et al.*, 2016).

2.5. ENDOGENOUS STIMULI-RESPONSIVE LOCALIZED DRUG DELIVERY WITH GRAPHENE

2.5.1. pH-responsive Localized Drug Delivery With Graphene

In the past few years, charge-reversal nano-carriers such as pH-sensitive systems have gained attention (Fig. **2**). Charge-reversal nano-carriers switch the surface charge from negative to positive under specific conditions. pH-sensitive systems are based on the unusual changes of pH: in the diseased locations, including cancer cells, infection, inflammation, and ischemia (Gooneh-Farahani *et al.*, 2020). In comparison to normal cells, cancerous cells are more acidic, which is the main concept of pH-sensitive drug delivery systems., hydrophobic drugs such as DOX (an anthracycline antibiotic) are protonated in acidic circumstances, which weakens hydrophobic interactions and the π-π stacking of drug molecules resulting in drug release. In the chemotherapy intravenous administration method, DOX distribution in cancerous sites is limited because of the cellular barriers, but the issue may be solved by using nanocarriers especially GO. There is a strong bond between the GO surface and DOX molecules which is because of the π-π interactions with quainine (hydrophobic part of DOX). Drugs with small size molecules and pH-dependent solubility are extensively utilized for pH-sensitive drug delivery systems, especially when used with GO nanocarriers. For instance, DOX-GO complexes exhibit pH-sensitive drug release mechanism because of the solubility of DOX at low pH conditions. Anti-inflammatory drugs with various hydrophilicity (ibuprofen and 5-fluorouracil) can be delivered by using a CS-GO complex with a pH-responsive release (Yang *et al.*, 2016, Liu *et al.*, 2013, Chung *et al.*, 2013).

2.5.2. Redox-responsive Localized Drug Delivery with Graphene

It is identified that the cellular redox environment is controlled by glutathione intensity (GSH). GSH is a thiol compound with a high concentration (5–10 mM) in the cytoplasm of mammalian cells. Lack of GSH levels for all-time results in improved susceptibility to oxidative stress, while excess amounts of GSH usually raise oxidative stress resistance and antioxidant capacity. Consequently, intracellular GSH might serve as a stimulant to trigger drug release from DDSs. For example, GO-Ag composites loaded with DOX with disulfide bonds are detached by the intracellular GSH to trigger the drug release. In another experiment, the application of GSH and light multi-responsive GO-BPEI-PEG nano-carrier showed a considerable increase in cancer cell destruction. Finally, it can be concluded that redox-responsive drug delivery can offer innovative methods for cancer treatment (Fig. **2**) (Yang *et al.*, 2016).

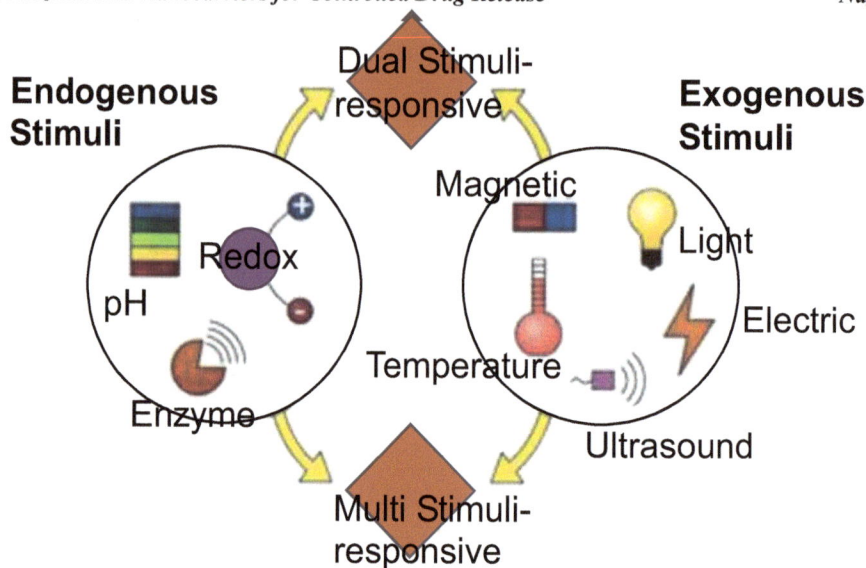

Fig. (2). Various methods of stimuli-responsive drug delivery for different biomedical applications (Pham *et al.*, 2020).

2.6. GRAPHENE-BASED DRUG DELIVERY SYSTEMS RESPONSIVE TO EXTERNAL PHYSICAL STIMULI

2.6.1. Light-responsive Drug Delivery Systems with Graphene

As mentioned before, the destruction in cancer chemotherapy and radiotherapy methods is not limited to tumor cells, leading to unfavorable side effects on healthy organs. PDT and PPT are two effective procedures with the ability to kill cancer cells under certain light irradiation (Fig. **2**). These two approaches selectively destroy cancer cells in tumor sites without harming healthy surrounding cells. Photodynamic therapy (PDT) is based on reactive oxygen species (ROS) created from photosensitizer (PS) molecules, which perform under appropriate light irradiation (Liu *et al.*, 2013).

Photothermal therapy (PTT) mechanisms produce heat *via* optical-absorbing nano-agents under NIR irradiation, which is utilized to destroy cancerous cells. Nano-graphene is an example of a photothermal agent for photothermal ablation of cancer cells. Direct photothermal ablation is used in high temperatures (*e.g.*, above 50 °C), while mild photo-thermal methods elevate the cancer tissues to a temperature of 43-45 °C (Sun *et al.*, 2008, Liu *et al.*, 2008c, Feng *et al.*, 2011).

In an experiment, chlorine 6 (Ce6) was loaded onto GO-PEG surface with hydrophobic interactions and π–π stacking. It was discovered that mild photothermal heating induced by 808nm laser irradiation might considerably boost the cellular uptake of Ce6 with no noticeable toxicity, and enhance the performance PDT against tumor cells. Nano graphene is a material with intrinsic photothermal conversion under NIR laser irradiation to release therapeutic agents from the nanocarrier, and can be used in photothermal-sensitive triggered drug delivery. Thus, graphene and its derivatives may be used in light-responsive drug delivery applications. In addition, mild photothermal heating induced by NIR laser irradiation improves the cellular uptake of drugs with nanographene. This method can be used for controlled drug release to decrease damage to healthy organs. Therefore, NIR induced photothermal method may be used for external stimuli-responsive applications (Yang *et al.*, 2016).

2.6.2. Temperature-responsive Drug Delivery Systems with Graphene

In addition to light, other stimuli such as heat may also be used for thermal responsive drug delivery based on temperature-responsive polymers and graphene (Fig. **2**). One of the recognized temperature-responsive polymers is PNIPAM (Poly (N-isopropylacrylamide)) with adjustable critical solution temperature (LCST) in water. PNIPAM has been utilized as a thermo-responsive polymer for controlled drug release applications. PNIPAM functionalizes nanographene so that it can be loaded with drugs such as ibuprofen (IBU) or CPT, which have shown temperature-sensitive drug delivery profiles. These systems respond to temperature variations which can be tempted by direct heating (water) or indirect heating (hyperthermia effect), such as magnetic and photothermal hyperthermia (Yang *et al.*, 2016).

2.7. TOXICITY AND BIOCOMPATIBILITY OF GRAPHENE MATERIALS

Toxicity is an undeniable issue of any biomaterial in biomedical applications, which must be considered before clinical application. Graphene-based materials have diverse surface chemistry, which can result in different interactions with cells, organs, and biomolecules. Toxicity is directly related to the production of ROS, which is regularly concentration-dependent and time-dependent. Researchers have revealed that the toxicity of graphene-based materials depends on their concentration or surface chemistry (Zhang *et al.*, 2016).

With the growing application of graphene in different fields, the importance of *in vitro* and *in vivo* toxicological evaluation is increasing as well. Therefore, *in vitro* adherence of mammalian cells to graphene was examined with rat pheochromocytoma cells (PC12). Although, graphene may cause cell proliferation, MTT assays showed 40% cell death. This confirmed the health issue of graphene-based materials. The *in vitro* toxicity of hydrophobic graphene has been determined after dispersion. While there is not much information about the dispersion quality, a group of scientists demonstrated that for concentrations of over 10 µg/ml of graphene, there is a slow increase in cellular toxicity and a decrease in dose- and time-related metabolic bioactivity. The impact of graphene on human red blood cells (RBC) shows that GO sheets which are small in size, have higher hemolytic in comparison with aggregated sheets. Although, chitosan improves the dispersion of GO, it reduces the hemolytic activity as well. While there are a few *in vivo* investigations, it is obvious that different graphene-derived substances have diverse toxicites. Unfavorable exposure reactions rely on many parameters which require cautious monitoring and thorough examination before the results can be achieved. Surface modification and sheet lateral size of graphene are factors that must be considered. It is known that ROS leads to oxidative stress in target cells, which is a type of toxicity. It is assumed that oxidative stress might be noticeable toxicity because of the chemical similarity with carbon nanotubes (CNTs). In fact, graphene leads to high oxidative stress because of the generation of reactive oxygen species in a time and concentration-dependent way. It was discovered that shape also plays an important role in toxicity. It is worth mentioning that the toxicity and safety of graphene-based materials have not been totally determined, and the biocompatibility and toxicity of these materials must be studied carefully. Many investigations have reported the potential of graphene and GO and their hybrids for drug delivery applications due to their low toxicity, although the present experimental results do not show the same (Bitounis *et al.*, 2013, Goenka *et al.*, 2014, Liu *et al.*, 2013).

Intrinsic physical-chemical characteristics affect the biocompatibility of graphene-based materials. These Intrinsic physical-chemical characteristics are related to the production process and the used materials [13]. Graphene-based materials are used for antimicrobial applications owing to their bactericidal activity. Another significant parameter is size, which influences the distribution of GO after intravenous administration. Researches have shown that micro-sized GO is trapped in the lungs after administration, however, submicron-sized GO can easily pass through the vascular tissue and accumulate in the liver. GO sheets include a large number of hydrophilic groups, like carboxyl, hydroxyl and epoxy groups, on their edge or basal planes, which considerably increase their hydrophilic nature, results in higher biocompatibility in comparison with graphene. Although, rGO and carboxylated graphene are less toxic than pure graphene or GO. Surface modification of graphene and GO would decrease their toxicity and increase biocompatibility (Liu *et al.*, 2013, Goenka *et al.*, 2014, Chung *et al.*, 2013, Zhu *et al.*, 2015, Chai *et al.*, 2017).

Graphene and its derivatives, cause strong lung cytotoxicity due to their size, since they are nondegradable. Researchers employed hydrogen peroxide and horseradish peroxidase (HRP) to degrade GO. Accordingly, this can be a future approach to degrade graphene-derived substances and decrease health and environmental risks (Zhang *et al.*, 2016, Kotchey *et al.*, 2011).

2.8. CARBON NANOTUBE (CNT)

The progress of novel and effective DDSs is a basic factor to develop the pharmacological profiles of several kinds of drugs. Various kinds of DDSs are available nowadays. CNT has potential applications for biomedical purposes. It is a tubular and novel option for carrying drug and therapeutic molecules. CNTs can be used in many fields such as diagnosis, thermal ablation, and drug delivery in cancer due to their unique properties (Bianco *et al.*, 2005, Prato *et al.*, 2008, Deng *et al.*, 2007).

CNTs can be synthesized through different methods such as chemical vapor deposition, laser ablation and electric arc discharge. These methods include high temperature and pressure and also the use of reaction catalysts, which result in fine-structured CNTs. Some methods may include impurities such as graphitic debris and catalytic particles in the products. High thermal and electrical conductivity, ultralight weight, hollow structure, high surface area, high aspect ratio, and well-ordered and great tensile strength are unique properties of CNTs that have turned this nanomaterial into a promising choice for biomedical applications and especially drug delivery. CNT seems to be more dynamic than other nanomaterials. Normally, single-walled (SWCNT) or multiwalled (MWCNT) are two kinds of CNT structures which will be discussed in the next sections (Prakash *et al.*, 2011, Madani *et al.*, 2011, Rosen and Elman, 2009, Wu *et al.*, 2011, Meng *et al.*, 2012).

CNTs have a hydrophobic nature and are insoluble in all solvents, which restricts their application in biomedicine. CNTs can be functionalized with many agents such as drugs, nucleic acids, proteins and peptides *via* different methods, including covalent bonding, electrostatic interaction and adsorption. In addition, functionalized CNTs have low toxicity and are not immunogenic, and can be utilized in nanobiotechnology and nanomedicine. By rolling up a single layer of graphene, single-wall carbon nanotubes (SWCNT) are produced, and by concentrically rolling up more than one layer, multi-wall carbon nanotubes (MWNT) are produced (Bianco *et al.*, 2005, Prakash *et al.*, 2011, Liu *et al.*, 2008a, Tans *et al.*, 1997, Kong *et al.*, 1998, Bethune *et al.*, 1993).

CNTs can be oxidized with strong acids, leading to length reduction while generating carboxylic groups and improving dispersibility in aqueous solutions. Adding functional groups to the external walls or tips of the CNT result in solubility, which is a key factor for biocompatibility. Functionalized CNTs (f-CNT) can be conjugated with a wide range of active molecules such as peptides, proteins, and nucleic acids. Functionalized CNTs can penetrate into cells easily. Therefore, they can be used for the delivery of small molecules. As an example, ammonium-containing CNTs are highly water-soluble and are utilized for drug delivery applications. Moreover, hollow monolithic structure, nanoneedle shape, and their capability of reaching preferred functional groups on their outer layers have made CNTs applicable for the delivery of therapeutic agents. Antibiotics linked to CNT can simply enter mammalian cells without any toxic results in comparison to the antibiotic alone. In another study, single-wall carbon nanotube have been functionalized with alternative carborane cages to produce a novel delivery system for boron neutron capture treatment. These kinds of water-soluble CNT, were used for the ellimination of cancer cells. The study showed that some particular tissues included carborane following intravenous administration of the CNT conjugate and, more fascinatingly, that carborane was concentrated mostly at the tumor site (Bianco *et al.*, 2005, Prato *et al.*, 2008, Allen and Cullis, 2004, Sahoo *et al.*, 2011).

Functional groups, including amines and carboxylates, can be modified by therapeutic agents to produce CNT conjugates with pharmacological activity. Nanotubes, with the ability to carry therapeutic agents and magnetic, optical, or other probes for imaging, can be used to cure cancer or other complicated diseases requiring taking action at specific parts of the body (Prato *et al.*, 2008).

CNTs have magnificent properties such as mechanical properties leading to highly stable *in vivo* activity, and the ability to simply surpass biological barriers, resulting in new biocompatible delivery systems with low-cost bulk production, which can deliver drugs directly to the cancer site. But CNTs also have limitations and disadvantages such as non-biodegradability, large surface area for protein opsonization, strong aggregation tendency, and high carbon nanotube variety which impede standardization. Intravenous administration is another advantage of CNTs, but it may also block blood vessels if the size of the drug is large, which results in toxicity. In order to recover, the CNTs can react with strong acids, leading to the production of carboxylic groups on the surface, which enhance the hydrophilic nature of CNTs and increase their dispersibility in aqueous solutions (Madani *et al.*, 2011, Rosen and Elman, 2009).

There are different ways to attach drugs to the CNTs. The drugs may be attached to the surface throughout functional groups, which is called wrapping, or may be loaded inside the CNTs, called filling modes. Wrapping may be achieved through covalent or non-covalent approaches, and may be used for anti-cancer drugs. Covalent functionalization is the reaction of carbon atoms on the CNT wall with a therapeutic molecule. In the non-covalent approach, the drug is physically attached to the walls with π–π stackings, hydrophobic interactions, or electrostatic adsorption. Covalent conjugation of drugs, such as 10-hydroxycamptothecin, cisplatin and methotrexate, might change the chemical structure of the drug, specifically, if they are covalently conjugated by nonbiodegradable linkages, which may lead to lower drug effectiveness and adverse side effects. Thus, physical drug adsorption to CNTs is more favorable since there is no change in the chemical entities. The non-covalent approach has been utilized for surfactants, natural polymers, synthetic polyelectrolytes, and amphiphilic block polymers or polymeric micelles. One of the major drawbacks of non-covalent conjugation is the lack of proficient attachment, consequently releasing the drug before reaching the targeted site. A CNT with a diameter of 80nm can keep up to 5 million drug molecules (Prakash *et al.*, 2011, Madani *et al.*, 2011, Wu *et al.*, 2011, Kostarelos *et al.*, 2007).

There are various ways of delivering drugs to the desired site with the help of CNTs. Different experiments have exhibited that when the therapeutic agent is loaded inside a CNT, it will exit the tube and enter the cell environment, but there is no precise description of the amount of the therapeutic agent. To overcome the issue, the CNT is loaded with the drug, and then the two ends of the CNT are covered with drug molecules that can cleave intracellularly. In another method, the drug may be attached *via* a linker, for example, disulfide, to the CNT that can cleave under specific situations such as reducing agents, heat and pH changes. Using CNTs in conjugation with radiofrequency and laser therapy, specifically in tumor treatment, is favorable. Thermal ablation can be used for cancer therapy as it is non-invasive and harmless to healthy tissues. Normally, thermal ablations heat cells up to 55°C leading to protein denaturation and coagulative necrosis of the cells, which consequently stops the function of targeted cells. Contact with NIR causes cell death by damaging plasma membrane or protein denaturation, which is a successful method for cancer therapy and lung, liver and prostate malignancies. Two different laser beam transmission methods exist, which are short and long laser nanosecond exposure. Nanosecond exposure is typically utilized for the ablation of metastatic cancer cells. The temperature in this mode reaches a maximum of 300°C with minimum damage to the surrounding medium. In the second procedure, which is used for the ablation of primary tumor cells which have a large size, a few minutes of exposure at a temperature of 45°C–65°C is required, which may damage normal cells as well. To solve this problem, laser beams that produce a higher temperature in the range of 80°C–95°C have been created. This temperature is sufficient to destroy cancer cells, however, it has a negligible impact on surrounding normal tissues, because of the smaller exposure time. CNTs are able to absorb NIR light and convert it to heat. This nano-scale material which has high thermal conductivity, can transmit heat to the surrounding, generating high-frequency ultrasound waves (Madani *et al.*, 2011, Meng *et al.*, 2012).

Many factors such as surface chemistry, size, morphology, dosage and chemical components impact the toxicity of CNT. It is obvious that the cytotoxicity level of CNTs must be kept at a specific stage. The reduction in particle size, and increase in surface area, increase the space for chemical interactions, which will increase toxicity as well. CNTs can cause toxicity, including oxidative stress, physical membrane damage causing rupture, blockage of intracellular metabolic pathways, and generation of reactive oxygen species. The toxicity of CNTs is time- and dose-dependent. Unfunctionalized CNTs can enter the cytoplasm and the cell nucleus resulting in cell death. Functionalization increases the biocompatibility of CNTs and decreases their toxicity. The number of nanoparticles entering the body also affects cytotoxicity (Madani *et al.*, 2011, Rosen and Elman, 2009, Meng *et al.*, 2012).

2.8.1. Multi-Wall Carbon Nanotube (MWCNT)

Several concentric CNTs with an inner diameter of 1-3 nm and outer 2-100 nm produce a multiwall carbon nanotube (MWCNT). According to the arrangements of graphite sheets, two types of MWCNTs exist. One is a "Russian-doll"-like structure where the graphite sheets are ordered in concentric layers, and the other is a "parchment-like" type where a single sheet of graphite is rolled around itself. In comparison with SWCNTs, MWCNTs are recognized to be more practical for thermal cancer therapy, because MWCNTs release considerable vibrational energy after NIR exposure which leads to localized heating in the tissue, which can destroy cancerous cells. MWCNTs have more electrons per particle and hold more metallic tubes leading to their tendency to absorb NIR light (Madani *et al.*, 2011, Rosen and Elman, 2009).

2.8.2. Single Wall Carbon Nanotube (SWCNT)

The definition of a single-wall carbon nanotube (SWCNT) is a single cylindrical carbon layer with a diameter of 0.4–2 nm, and a length of up to a few micrometers depending on the synthesis temperature. Higher growth temperatures result in a larger diameter. Armchair, zigzag, chiral, and helical are the existing arrangements of SWCNTs. This structure is useful in drug delivery since its one-dimensional structure, and ultrahigh surface lead to a high capacity for loading drugs. SWCNTs can absorb NIR light which may be utilized for the optical stimulation of nanotubes inside the living cells, while keeping biological systems transparent to NIR radiation safe. Quite the opposite, blood and biological tissues are transmitting, which help CNTs target specific cells in drug delivery applications. Due to properties, CNTs can absorb NIR light and release heat and target tumor cells. This results in localized hyperthermia and the destruction of tumor cells. SWCNTs have significant properties such as targeting *via* EPR effect, and facile penetration into cells which causes the possibility of delivering various drugs for therapy. SWCNTs have sp^2-hybridized carbon surfaces and a high surface area. Therefore, drugs, biomolecules and specific targeting molecules may be conjugated to their surface *via* covalent or non-covalent interactions. It has been proven that a complex composed of SWCNT and the anti-cancer agent has more blood circulation time compared with anti-cancer drugs on their own, resulting in sustainable uptake of drugs by tumor cells with EPR effect. Reports have shown that after the entrance and release of drug by SWCNT, the SWCNT slowly egresses *via* the biliary route, which makes SWCNT an appropriate choice for drug delivery applications. Generally, the medium influences loading, for example, DOX is an anticancer drug with condensed aromatic molecules, which is loadable with π-π stacking. This loading is pH-dependent, offering further control for tumor cell targeting. It is noteworthy that loading at normal blood pH is more than acidic pH environment. Moreover, lysosomes, endosomes of rapidly growing tissues in the tumor origin and parasitically or virally infected cells have an acidic pH. SWCNTs are capable of delivering small interfering RNAs (siRNAs) through non-covalent interactions. A recent investigation studied cationic SWNTs and their potential to shape stable complexes with siRNAs to stop the expression of telomerase reverse transcriptase (TERT) and prevent cell proliferation both *in vitro* and *in vivo* in tumor models (Madani *et al.*, 2011, Meng *et al.*, 2012, Rosen and Elman, 2009, Liu *et al.*, 2008b, Krajcik *et al.*, 2008, Zhang *et al.*, 2006).

Single-walled CNTs (SWCNTs) show considerable cytotoxicity in human and animal cells, but Multi-walled CNTs (MWCNTs) have mild impacts on human and animal cells. As an example, a large amount of *E. coli* cells were not activated after straight contact with highly purified SWCNTs. The SWCNTs were deposited without any culture medium. Although, the process mechanism is still uncertain. Investigations have exhibited that between characterized SWCNT and MWCNT, a single wall CNT is more toxic to bacteria and has the ability to be utilized as a substitute agent to destroy microbial infections which are resistant to conventional antibiotic treatments. Singh *et al.* studied tissue distribution and also blood clearance rates of CNTs. The study included significant results about the toxicity CNTs. Urine excretion of both single-wall and multi-wall CNTs and electron microscopy results were analysed, which revealed that both MWCNTs and SWCNTs exited body *via* renal excretion (Rosen and Elman, 2009).

2.9. FULLERENE

Fullerene family materials, mainly C$_{60}$, with outstanding properties such as photochemical, electrochemical, physical, and low systemic toxicity, are nanoscaled materials that with numerous applications. C$_{60}$ has a diameter of 0.7

nanometers; its derivatives are water-soluble and, therefore, may be applicable in a broad diversity of applications, such as biological and biomedical fields. The unique spherical structure and strong apolar character of fullerenes help the construction of lipid-like systems, and make fullerenes capable of passing through the cellular membrane. Fullerenes may act as scaffolds in drug delivery, as they can be functionalized and absorb drugs. Also, the great properties of fullerene have led to its application in PDT. The absorption of visible light, with a useful intersystem crossing to a long-lived triplet state, stimulates fullerenes to generate ROS upon illumination and make fullerenes PS. In some cases, fullerene has very low solubility in common organic solvents, which leads to a decrease in its biomedical efficacy and usefulness. Covalent modification of the aromatic structure and partial masking of the apolar fullerene surface are potential solutions to overcome the aforementioned issue. In the partial masking approach, several methods have been effectively applied, such as 1) co-solvation with polyvinylpyrrolidone in organic solvents; 2) incorporation in artificial lipid membranes; 3) fullerene complexation with cyclodextrins or calixarenes; and 4) inclusion into suspensions. These approaches have resulted in hopeful consequences. However, maintaining the intrinsic hydrophobicity of fullerene is of great interest. Fullerene covalent modification resulted in highly stable derivatives. A suitable way to get water-soluble C_{60} derivatives is to conjugate them with amino acids or sugars wherein fullerene substituted phenylalanine derivatives, dipeptides from a fullerene amino acid or multi-fullerene peptides are the most known examples. In a study, researchers have designed a novel pH-responsive drug carrier including fullerene and 6-amino-c-cyclodextrin (ACD) for PDT. In this study, fullerene was quickly released from its complex at a pH of 6.7 with ACD owing to electrostatic repulsion between ammonium groups, and followed by rapid C_{60} release at some acidic cancer cell surfaces. Fullerene also can deliver bioactive molecules like warfarin. Warfarin is a coumarin anticoagulant drug that can cause thrombosis due to rapid discontinuation (Montellano *et al.*, 2011, Shi *et al.*, 2014, Shi *et al.*, 2013, Partha and Conyers, 2009, Nobusawa *et al.*, 2012).

2.10. OTHER CARBON NANOSTRUCTURES:

Cancer is the most known disease which leads to the death of many people every year. Thus, designing an effective method for the treatment of cancer is important. Conventional sole-modal therapy methods have several drawbacks, such as impaired target specificity, poor bioavailability, and systematic-, organ- toxicity. Therefore, combined therapies may be a potential approach to overcome the aforementioned limitations. Combined therapies may have higher effectiveness and a lower risk of recurrence. A group of combined therapies includes lipid- and polymer-based nanocapsules holding two or three drugs. However, the efficacy depends on the loading ability of different drugs. Many studies have focused on the progression of 2D nanocarriers for multimodal therapies. 2D nanomaterials such as graphene, Bi2Se3, MoOx, WS2, and MoS2 have unique properties that can exhibit amazing efficiency in cancer therapy. Meanwhile, the development of methods to generate multi-functional 2D nanomaterials with higher loading ability for synergistic combination therapy is still a major challenge (Partha and Conyers, 2009).

2.11. BLACK PHOSPHORUS (BP)

Black phosphorus (BP) which is also known as phosphorene, is a nanoscale sheet with a variety of biomedical applications. BP is a 2D planar material with a honeycomb lattice of phosphorus atoms, in which each phosphorus atom is linked to three other neighboring phosphorus atoms *via* a single bond (Li *et al.*, 2017).

In comparison with other 2D materials such as graphene, BP is stable at room temperature and under normal pressure. On the other hand, BP can degrade and cause fluorescence in some conditions (Tatullo *et al.*, 2019).

BP is a metal-free layered semiconductor with a thickness-dependent gap adjustable from about 0.3 eV for bulk to 2.0 eV for a single layer. BP has a high surface-to-volume ratio due to its planar lattice configuration, leading to a higher drug loading capacity. BP may be used as a photosensitizer for PDT due to its electronic structure. Additionally, both BP nanoparticles and BP quantum dots demonstrate wide absorptions across the whole visible light region. Therefore, these materials may be synthesized to achieve near-infrared (NIR) photothermal characteristics, making them applicable for the photothermal treatment (PTT). However, the application of BP in drug delivery has not been investigated. BP has a negative charge in water, with an interlayer distance of ~5.24 Å. Therefore, electrostatic interactions can load positive charge molecules and small drugs into the interlayer spaces. Phosphorus is one of the major components of nucleic acid, so it is necessary for maintaining human health. BP has been utilized as a biosensing material for the discovery of target analytes (*e.g.*, immunoglobulin G (IgG) and myoglobin (Mb)) because of its inherent electrochemical characteristics (Li *et al.*, 2017, Chen *et al.*, 2017, Choi *et al.*, 2018, Zhang *et al.*, 2015, Lee *et al.*, 2016, Sun *et al.*, 2016, Sun *et al.*, 2015).

BP has high drug loading efficiency and can hold high amounts of DOX on its surface (950% in weight) for pH-/photo responsive drug release. The high drug capacity shows the capability of BP to eliminate tumor cells, profiting from the synergistic mixture of chemotherapy, photothermal therapy and photodynamic therapy. Since the toxicity is material-, size- and concentration-dependent, BP has lower toxicity in comparison with graphene, but it is more toxic than MoS_2 and WSe_2. Small-sized BP has less toxicity compared to large-sized BP, has higher reactivity with water and oxygen, and simply degrades in an aqueous medium. BP has higher *in vivo* biodegradability and a lower tendency to release nanoparticles in the human body, in comparison with other nanomaterials. BP makes nontoxic intermediates, such as phosphate, and other PxOy products, upon exposure to water and oxygen. Therefore, it can be safely utilized for *in vivo* purposes (Chen *et al.*, 2017, Lee *et al.*, 2016, Tatullo *et al.*, 2019, Sun *et al.*, 2016).

CONCLUSION

The findings of this chapter emphasize the potential application of carbon nanomaterials as nanocarriers for multi-functional therapies and advanced DDSs. Therapeutic molecules may be attached to carbon nanomaterials to produce a matrix to selectively deliver a precise amount of drug to a specific target, owing to the strong biofunctionalization potential of carbon-based nanomaterials. An ideal nano-scaled system should respond to a precise stimulus *via* the particular targeting functional groups. Carbon nanomaterials may be applicable in other biological and biomedical fields, such as biosensors, tissue regeneration scaffolds, neurological tissue stimulation and biofabrication.

REFERENCES

Allen, T.M., Cullis, P.R. (2004). Drug delivery systems: entering the mainstream. *Science, 303*(5665), 1818-1822.
[http://dx.doi.org/10.1126/science.1095833] [PMID: 15031496]

Askari, E., Naghib, S.M., Seyfoori, A., Maleki, A., Rahmanian, M. (2019). Ultrasonic-assisted synthesis and *in vitro* biological assessments of a novel herceptin-stabilized graphene using three dimensional cell spheroid. *Ultrason. Sonochem., 58*, 104615.
[http://dx.doi.org/10.1016/j.ultsonch.2019.104615] [PMID: 31450294]

Askari, E., Naghib, S.M., Zahedi, A., Seyfoori, A., Zare, Y., Rhee, K.Y. (2021). Local delivery of chemotherapeutic agent in tissue engineering based on gelatin/graphene hydrogel. *J. Mater. Res. Technol., 12*, 412-422.
[http://dx.doi.org/10.1016/j.jmrt.2021.02.084]

Askari, E., Rasouli, M., Darghiasi, S.F., Naghib, S.M., Zare, Y., Rhee, K.Y. (2021). Reduced graphene oxide-grafted bovine serum albumin/bredigite nanocomposites with high mechanical properties and excellent osteogenic bioactivity for bone tissue engineering. *Biodes. Manuf., 4*(2), 243-257.
[http://dx.doi.org/10.1007/s42242-020-00113-4]

Bethune, D.S., Kiang, C.H., de Vries, M.S., Gorman, G., Savoy, R., Vazquez, J., Beyers, R. (1993). Cobalt-catalysed growth of carbon nanotubes with single-atomic-layer walls. *Nature, 363*(6430), 605-607.
[http://dx.doi.org/10.1038/363605a0]

Bianco, A., Kostarelos, K., Prato, M. (2005). Applications of carbon nanotubes in drug delivery. *Curr. Opin. Chem. Biol., 9*(6), 674-679.
[http://dx.doi.org/10.1016/j.cbpa.2005.10.005] [PMID: 16233988]

Bitounis, D., Ali-Boucetta, H., Hong, B.H., Min, D.H., Kostarelos, K. (2013). Prospects and challenges of

graphene in biomedical applications. *Adv. Mater.,* *25*(16), 2258-2268.
[http://dx.doi.org/10.1002/adma.201203700] [PMID: 23494834]

Chai, Q., Jiao, Y., Yu, X. (2017). Hydrogels for biomedical applications: their characteristics and the mechanisms behind them. *Gels,* *3*(1), 6.
[http://dx.doi.org/10.3390/gels3010006] [PMID: 30920503]

Chen, W., Ouyang, J., Liu, H., Chen, M., Zeng, K., Sheng, J., Liu, Z., Han, Y., Wang, L., Li, J., Deng, L., Liu, Y.N., Guo, S. (2017). Black phosphorus nanosheet-based drug delivery system for synergistic photodynamic/photothermal/chemotherapy of cancer. *Adv. Mater.,* *29*(5), 1603864.
[http://dx.doi.org/10.1002/adma.201603864] [PMID: 27882622]

Choi, J.R., Yong, K.W., Choi, J.Y., Nilghaz, A., Lin, Y., Xu, J., Lu, X. (2018). Black phosphorus and its biomedical applications. *Theranostics,* *8*(4), 1005-1026.
[http://dx.doi.org/10.7150/thno.22573] [PMID: 29463996]

Chung, C., Kim, Y.K., Shin, D., Ryoo, S.R., Hong, B.H., Min, D.H. (2013). Biomedical applications of graphene and graphene oxide. *Acc. Chem. Res.,* *46*(10), 2211-2224.
[http://dx.doi.org/10.1021/ar300159f] [PMID: 23480658]

Deng, X., Jia, G., Wang, H., Sun, H., Wang, X., Yang, S., Wang, T., Liu, Y. (2007). Translocation and fate of multi-walled carbon nanotubes *in vivo. Carbon,* *45*(7), 1419-1424.
[http://dx.doi.org/10.1016/j.carbon.2007.03.035]

Ding, X., Liu, H., Fan, Y. (2015). Graphene-based materials in regenerative medicine. *Adv. Healthc. Mater.,* *4*(10), 1451-1468.
[http://dx.doi.org/10.1002/adhm.201500203] [PMID: 26037920]

Feng, L., Zhang, S., Liu, Z. (2011). Graphene based gene transfection. *Nanoscale,* *3*(3), 1252-1257.
[http://dx.doi.org/10.1039/c0nr00680g] [PMID: 21270989]

Goenka, S., Sant, V., Sant, S. (2014). Graphene-based nanomaterials for drug delivery and tissue engineering. *J. Control. Release,* *173*, 75-88.
[http://dx.doi.org/10.1016/j.jconrel.2013.10.017] [PMID: 24161530]

Gooneh-Farahani, S., Naghib, S.M., Naimi-Jamal, M.R. (2020). A novel and inexpensive method based on modified ionic gelation for pH-responsive controlled drug release of homogeneously distributed chitosan nanoparticles with a high encapsulation efficiency. *Fibers Polym.,* *21*(9), 1917-1926.
[http://dx.doi.org/10.1007/s12221-020-1095-y]

Gooneh-Farahani, S., Naimi-Jamal, M.R., Naghib, S.M. (2019). Stimuli-responsive graphene-incorporated multifunctional chitosan for drug delivery applications: a review. *Expert Opin. Drug Deliv.,* *16*(1), 79-99.
[http://dx.doi.org/10.1080/17425247.2019.1556257] [PMID: 30514124]

Imani, R., Mohabatpour, F., Mostafavi, F. (2018). Graphene-based Nano-Carrier modifications for gene delivery applications. *Carbon,* *140*, 569-591.
[http://dx.doi.org/10.1016/j.carbon.2018.09.019]

Jaleel, J.A., Sruthi, S., Pramod, K. (2017). Reinforcing nanomedicine using graphene family nanomaterials. *J. Control. Release,* *255*, 218-230.
[http://dx.doi.org/10.1016/j.jconrel.2017.04.041] [PMID: 28461100]

Kong, J., Soh, H.T., Cassell, A.M., Quate, C.F., Dai, H. (1998). Synthesis of individual single-walled carbon nanotubes on patterned silicon wafers. *Nature,* *395*(6705), 878-881.
[http://dx.doi.org/10.1038/27632]

Kostarelos, K., Lacerda, L., Pastorin, G., Wu, W., Wieckowski, S., Luangsivilay, J., Godefroy, S., Pantarotto, D., Briand, J.P., Muller, S., Prato, M., Bianco, A. (2007). Cellular uptake of functionalized carbon nanotubes is independent of functional group and cell type. *Nat. Nanotechnol.,* *2*(2), 108-113.
[http://dx.doi.org/10.1038/nnano.2006.209] [PMID: 18654229]

Kotchey, G.P., Allen, B.L., Vedala, H., Yanamala, N., Kapralov, A.A., Tyurina, Y.Y., Klein-Seetharaman, J., Kagan, V.E., Star, A. (2011). The enzymatic oxidation of graphene oxide. *ACS Nano,* *5*(3), 2098-2108.

[http://dx.doi.org/10.1021/nn103265h] [PMID: 21344859]

Krajcik, R., Jung, A., Hirsch, A., Neuhuber, W., Zolk, O. (2008). Functionalization of carbon nanotubes enables non-covalent binding and intracellular delivery of small interfering RNA for efficient knock-down of genes. *Biochem. Biophys. Res. Commun., 369*(2), 595-602.
[http://dx.doi.org/10.1016/j.bbrc.2008.02.072] [PMID: 18298946]

Lee, H.U., Park, S.Y., Lee, S.C., Choi, S., Seo, S., Kim, H., Won, J., Choi, K., Kang, K.S., Park, H.G., Kim, H.S., An, H.R., Jeong, K.H., Lee, Y.C., Lee, J. (2016). Black phosphorus (BP) nanodots for potential biomedical applications. *Small, 12*(2), 214-219.
[http://dx.doi.org/10.1002/smll.201502756] [PMID: 26584654]

Li, Y., Liu, Z., Hou, Y., Yang, G., Fei, X., Zhao, H., Guo, Y., Su, C., Wang, Z., Zhong, H., Zhuang, Z., Guo, Z. (2017). Multi-functional nanoplatform based on black phosphorus quantum dots for bioimaging and photodynamic/photothermal synergistic cancer therapy. *ACS Appl. Mater. Interfaces, 9*(30), 25098-25106.
[http://dx.doi.org/10.1021/acsami.7b05824] [PMID: 28671452]

Liu, J., Cui, L., Losic, D. (2013). Graphene and graphene oxide as new nanocarriers for drug delivery applications. *Acta Biomater., 9*(12), 9243-9257.
[http://dx.doi.org/10.1016/j.actbio.2013.08.016] [PMID: 23958782]

Liu, Z., Chen, K., Davis, C., Sherlock, S., Cao, Q., Chen, X., Dai, H. (2008). Drug delivery with carbon nanotubes for *in vivo* cancer treatment. *Cancer Res., 68*(16), 6652-6660.
[http://dx.doi.org/10.1158/0008-5472.CAN-08-1468] [PMID: 18701489]

Liu, Z., Davis, C., Cai, W., He, L., Chen, X., Dai, H. (2008). Circulation and long-term fate of functionalized, biocompatible single-walled carbon nanotubes in mice probed by Raman spectroscopy. *Proc. Natl. Acad. Sci. USA, 105*(5), 1410-1415.
[http://dx.doi.org/10.1073/pnas.0707654105] [PMID: 18230737]

Liu, Z., Robinson, J.T., Sun, X., Dai, H. (2008). PEGylated nanographene oxide for delivery of water-insoluble cancer drugs. *J. Am. Chem. Soc., 130*(33), 10876-10877.
[http://dx.doi.org/10.1021/ja803688x] [PMID: 18661992]

Madani, S.Y., Naderi, N., Dissanayake, O., Tan, A., Seifalian, A.M. (2011). A new era of cancer treatment: carbon nanotubes as drug delivery tools. *Int. J. Nanomedicine, 6*, 2963-2979.
[PMID: 22162655]

Makharza, S., Cirillo, G., Bachmatiuk, A., Ibrahim, I., Ioannides, N., Trzebicka, B., Hampel, S., Rümmeli, M.H. (2013). Graphene oxide-based drug delivery vehicles: functionalization, characterization, and cytotoxicity evaluation. *J. Nanopart. Res., 15*(12), 2099.
[http://dx.doi.org/10.1007/s11051-013-2099-y]

McNamara, K., Tofail, S.A.M. (2015). Nanosystems: the use of nanoalloys, metallic, bimetallic, and magnetic nanoparticles in biomedical applications. *Phys. Chem. Chem. Phys., 17*(42), 27981-27995.
[http://dx.doi.org/10.1039/C5CP00831J] [PMID: 26024211]

Meng, L., Zhang, X., Lu, Q., Fei, Z., Dyson, P.J. (2012). Single walled carbon nanotubes as drug delivery vehicles: Targeting doxorubicin to tumors. *Biomaterials, 33*(6), 1689-1698.
[http://dx.doi.org/10.1016/j.biomaterials.2011.11.004] [PMID: 22137127]

Montellano, A., Da Ros, T., Bianco, A., Prato, M. (2011). Fullerene C^{60} as a multifunctional system for drug and gene delivery. *Nanoscale, 3*(10), 4035-4041.
[http://dx.doi.org/10.1039/c1nr10783f] [PMID: 21897967]

Naghib, S.M. (2019). Two-dimensional functionalised methacrylated graphene oxide nanosheets as simple and inexpensive electrodes for biosensing applications. *Micro & Nano Lett., 14*(4), 462-465.
[http://dx.doi.org/10.1049/mnl.2018.5320]

Naghib, S.M., Zare, Y., Rhee, K.Y. (2020). A facile and simple approach to synthesis and characterization of methacrylated graphene oxide nanostructured polyaniline nanocomposites. *Nanotechnol. Rev., 9*(1), 53-60.
[http://dx.doi.org/10.1515/ntrev-2020-0005]

Nobusawa, K., Akiyama, M., Ikeda, A., Naito, M. (2012). pH responsive smart carrier of [60] fullerene with 6-amino-cyclodextrin inclusion complex for photodynamic therapy. *J. Mater. Chem., 22*(42), 22610-22613. [http://dx.doi.org/10.1039/c2jm34791a]

Partha, R., Conyers, J.L. (2009). Biomedical applications of functionalized fullerene-based nanomaterials. *Int. J. Nanomedicine, 4*, 261-275. [PMID: 20011243]

Pham, S.H., Choi, Y., Choi, J. (2020). Stimuli-responsive nanomaterials for application in antitumor therapy and drug delivery. *Pharmaceutics, 12*(7), 630. [http://dx.doi.org/10.3390/pharmaceutics12070630] [PMID: 32635539]

Pinto, A.M., Gonçalves, I.C., Magalhães, F.D. (2013). Graphene-based materials biocompatibility: A review. *Colloids Surf. B Biointerfaces, 111*, 188-202. [http://dx.doi.org/10.1016/j.colsurfb.2013.05.022] [PMID: 23810824]

Prakash, S., Malhotra, M., Shao, W., Tomaro-Duchesneau, C., Abbasi, S. (2011). Polymeric nanohybrids and functionalized carbon nanotubes as drug delivery carriers for cancer therapy. *Adv. Drug Deliv. Rev., 63*(14-15), 1340-1351. [http://dx.doi.org/10.1016/j.addr.2011.06.013] [PMID: 21756952]

Prato, M., Kostarelos, K., Bianco, A. (2008). Functionalized carbon nanotubes in drug design and discovery. *Acc. Chem. Res., 41*(1), 60-68. [http://dx.doi.org/10.1021/ar700089b] [PMID: 17867649]

Rahimi Mamaghani, K., Naghib, S.M., Zahedi, A., Zeinali Kalkhoran, A.H., Rahmanian, M. (2018). Fast synthesis of methacrylated graphene oxide: a graphene-functionalised nanostructure. *Micro & Nano Lett., 13*(2), 195-197. [http://dx.doi.org/10.1049/mnl.2017.0461]

Rao, C.N.R., Sood, A.K., Subrahmanyam, K.S., Govindaraj, A. (2009). Graphene: the new two-dimensional nanomaterial. *Angew. Chem. Int. Ed., 48*(42), 7752-7777. [http://dx.doi.org/10.1002/anie.200901678] [PMID: 19784976]

Reina, G., González-Domínguez, J.M., Criado, A., Vázquez, E., Bianco, A., Prato, M. (2017). Promises, facts and challenges for graphene in biomedical applications. *Chem. Soc. Rev., 46*(15), 4400-4416. [http://dx.doi.org/10.1039/C7CS00363C] [PMID: 28722038]

Rosen, Y., Elman, N.M. (2009). Carbon nanotubes in drug delivery: focus on infectious diseases. *Expert Opin. Drug Deliv., 6*(5), 517-530. [http://dx.doi.org/10.1517/17425240902865579] [PMID: 19413459]

Sahoo, N.G., Bao, H., Pan, Y., Pal, M., Kakran, M., Cheng, H.K.F., Li, L., Tan, L.P. (2011). Functionalized carbon nanomaterials as nanocarriers for loading and delivery of a poorly water-soluble anticancer drug: a comparative study. *Chem. Commun. (Camb.), 47*(18), 5235-5237. [http://dx.doi.org/10.1039/c1cc00075f] [PMID: 21451845]

Salahandish, R., Ghaffarinejad, A., Naghib, S.M., Niyazi, A., Majidzadeh-A, K., Janmaleki, M., Sanati-Nezhad, A. (2019). Sandwich-structured nanoparticles-grafted functionalized graphene based 3D nanocomposites for high-performance biosensors to detect ascorbic acid biomolecule. *Sci. Rep., 9*(1), 1226. [http://dx.doi.org/10.1038/s41598-018-37573-9] [PMID: 30718545]

Sattari, M., Fathi, M., Daei, M., Erfan-Niya, H., Barar, J., Entezami, A.A. (2017). Thermoresponsive graphene oxide – starch micro/nanohydrogel composite as biocompatible drug delivery system. *Bioimpacts, 7*(3), 167-175. [http://dx.doi.org/10.15171/bi.2017.20] [PMID: 29159144]

Seo, H.I., Cheon, Y.A., Chung, B.G. (2016). Graphene and thermo-responsive polymeric nanocomposites for therapeutic applications. *Biomed. Eng. Lett., 6*(1), 10-15. [http://dx.doi.org/10.1007/s13534-016-0214-6]

Servant, A., Bianco, A., Prato, M., Kostarelos, K. (2014). Graphene for multi-functional synthetic biology:

The last 'zeitgeist' in nanomedicine. *Bioorg. Med. Chem. Lett., 24*(7), 1638-1649.
[http://dx.doi.org/10.1016/j.bmcl.2014.01.051] [PMID: 24594351]

Shareena, T.P.D., Mcshan, D., Dasmahapatra, A.K., Tchounwou, P.B. (2018). A review on graphene-based nanomaterials in biomedical applications and risks in environment and health. *Nano-Micro Lett., 10*, 1-34.

Shen, H., Zhang, L., Liu, M., Zhang, Z. (2012). Biomedical applications of graphene. *Theranostics, 2*(3), 283-294.
[http://dx.doi.org/10.7150/thno.3642] [PMID: 22448195]

Shi, J., Liu, Y., Wang, L., Gao, J., Zhang, J., Yu, X., Ma, R., Liu, R., Zhang, Z. (2014). A tumoral acidic pH-responsive drug delivery system based on a novel photosensitizer (fullerene) for *in vitro* and *in vivo* chemo-photodynamic therapy. *Acta Biomater., 10*(3), 1280-1291.
[http://dx.doi.org/10.1016/j.actbio.2013.10.037] [PMID: 24211343]

Shi, J., Zhang, H., Wang, L., Li, L., Wang, H., Wang, Z., Li, Z., Chen, C., Hou, L., Zhang, C., Zhang, Z. (2013). PEI-derivatized fullerene drug delivery using folate as a homing device targeting to tumor. *Biomaterials, 34*(1), 251-261.
[http://dx.doi.org/10.1016/j.biomaterials.2012.09.039] [PMID: 23069706]

Shim, G., Kim, M.G., Park, J.Y., Oh, Y.K. (2016). Graphene-based nanosheets for delivery of chemotherapeutics and biological drugs. *Adv. Drug Deliv. Rev., 105*(Pt B), 205-227.
[http://dx.doi.org/10.1016/j.addr.2016.04.004] [PMID: 27085467]

Sun, C., Wen, L., Zeng, J., Wang, Y., Sun, Q., Deng, L., Zhao, C., Li, Z. (2016). One-pot solventless preparation of PEGylated black phosphorus nanoparticles for photoacoustic imaging and photothermal therapy of cancer. *Biomaterials, 91*, 81-89.
[http://dx.doi.org/10.1016/j.biomaterials.2016.03.022] [PMID: 27017578]

Sun, S., Wu, P. (2011). A one-step strategy for thermal- and pH-responsive graphene oxide interpenetrating polymer hydrogel networks. *J. Mater. Chem., 21*(12), 4095-4097.
[http://dx.doi.org/10.1039/c1jm10276a]

Sun, X., Liu, Z., Welsher, K., Robinson, J.T., Goodwin, A., Zaric, S., Dai, H. (2008). Nano-graphene oxide for cellular imaging and drug delivery. *Nano Res., 1*(3), 203-212.
[http://dx.doi.org/10.1007/s12274-008-8021-8] [PMID: 20216934]

Sun, Z., Xie, H., Tang, S., Yu, X.F., Guo, Z., Shao, J., Zhang, H., Huang, H., Wang, H., Chu, P.K. (2015). Ultrasmall black phosphorus quantum dots: synthesis and use as photothermal agents. *Angew. Chem. Int. Ed., 54*(39), 11526-11530.
[http://dx.doi.org/10.1002/anie.201506154] [PMID: 26296530]

Tans, S.J., Devoret, M.H., Dai, H., Thess, A., Smalley, R.E., Geerligs, L.J., Dekker, C. (1997). Individual single-wall carbon nanotubes as quantum wires. *Nature, 386*(6624), 474-477.
[http://dx.doi.org/10.1038/386474a0]

Tatullo, M., Genovese, F., Aiello, E., Amantea, M., Makeeva, I., Zavan, B., Rengo, S., Fortunato, L. (2019). Phosphorene is the new graphene in biomedical applications. *Materials (Basel), 12*(14), 2301.
[http://dx.doi.org/10.3390/ma12142301] [PMID: 31323844]

Wick, P., Louw-Gaume, A.E., Kucki, M., Krug, H.F., Kostarelos, K., Fadeel, B., Dawson, K.A., Salvati, A., Vázquez, E., Ballerini, L., Tretiach, M., Benfenati, F., Flahaut, E., Gauthier, L., Prato, M., Bianco, A. (2014). Classification framework for graphene-based materials. *Angew. Chem. Int. Ed., 53*(30), 7714-7718.
[http://dx.doi.org/10.1002/anie.201403335] [PMID: 24917379]

Wu, H., Liu, G., Wang, X., Zhang, J., Chen, Y., Shi, J., Yang, H., Hu, H., Yang, S. (2011). Solvothermal synthesis of cobalt ferrite nanoparticles loaded on multiwalled carbon nanotubes for magnetic resonance imaging and drug delivery. *Acta Biomater., 7*(9), 3496-3504.
[http://dx.doi.org/10.1016/j.actbio.2011.05.031] [PMID: 21664499]

Yang, K., Feng, L., Liu, Z. (2016). Stimuli responsive drug delivery systems based on nano-graphene for cancer therapy. *Adv. Drug Deliv. Rev., 105*(Pt B), 228-241.

[http://dx.doi.org/10.1016/j.addr.2016.05.015] [PMID: 27233212]

Yang, K., Feng, L., Shi, X., Liu, Z. (2013). Nano-graphene in biomedicine: theranostic applications. *Chem. Soc. Rev., 42*(2), 530-547.
[http://dx.doi.org/10.1039/C2CS35342C] [PMID: 23059655]

Zeinali Kalkhoran, A.H., Naghib, S.M., Vahidi, O., Rahmanian, M. (2018). Synthesis and characterization of graphene-grafted gelatin nanocomposite hydrogels as emerging drug delivery systems. *Biomed. Phys. Eng. Express, 4*(5), 055017.
[http://dx.doi.org/10.1088/2057-1976/aad745]

Zhang, B., Wang, Y., Zhai, G. (2016). Biomedical applications of the graphene-based materials. *Mater. Sci. Eng. C, 61*, 953-964.
[http://dx.doi.org/10.1016/j.msec.2015.12.073] [PMID: 26838925]

Zhang, X., Xie, H., Liu, Z., Tan, C., Luo, Z., Li, H., Lin, J., Sun, L., Chen, W., Xu, Z., Xie, L., Huang, W., Zhang, H. (2015). Black phosphorus quantum dots. *Angew. Chem. Int. Ed., 54*(12), 3653-3657.
[http://dx.doi.org/10.1002/anie.201409400] [PMID: 25649505]

Zhang, Z., Yang, X., Zhang, Y., Zeng, B., Wang, S., Zhu, T., Roden, R.B.S., Chen, Y., Yang, R. (2006). Delivery of telomerase reverse transcriptase small interfering RNA in complex with positively charged single-walled carbon nanotubes suppresses tumor growth. *Clin. Cancer Res., 12*(16), 4933-4939.
[http://dx.doi.org/10.1158/1078-0432.CCR-05-2831] [PMID: 16914582]

Zhu, C., Du, D., Lin, Y. (2015). Graphene and graphene-like 2D materials for optical biosensing and bioimaging: A review. *2D Materials, 2*, 032004.

CHAPTER 3

Polymers in Localized Controlled Drug Delivery Systems (LCDDSs)

Abstract: Polymeric and biopolymeric materials and nanostructures have been extensively used in drug delivery, and especially in the development of localized controlled drug delivery systems (LCDDS). Stimuli-sensitive biopolymeric materials are achieving remarkable consideration as smart multipurpose systems that exhibit superb potential in several applications. LCDDS allow high delivery levels at the target area, low cytotoxicity, excellent biocompatibility and prolonged drug exposure that can be helpful for targeted cellular therapeutic molecules. This chapter focuses on synthetic and natural degradable biopolymeric materials for LCDDS, focusing on their advantages, challenges, and clinical applicability. Recent progress in typical and stimuli-sensitive biopolymeric materials has also been reviewed. The features of biodegradable polymers and biopolymers for various purposes are discussed, and the advantages of these materials and biomaterials are highlighted. Moreover, different emerging functions of these polymers in a drug delivery system are discussed.

Keywords: Biocompatibility, Biodegradable, Biopolymer, Localized controlled drug delivery, Polymer, Stimuli-sensitive.

3.1. INTRODUCTION

The origin of the word ''polymer'' refers to the Greek language, which is the combination of ''many'' and ''parts''. Polymers have specific properties such as high molecular mass; every molecule includes several structural units arranged in a consistent manner. The term ''monomer'' defines small molecules which shape a polymer *via* polymerization reaction. Polymers have various applications in many biomedical fields, such as binders in tablets to gain viscosity, emulsions, and suspensions, to improve drug stability. Moreover, solid polymers can be utilized as systems for drug targeting and controlled release in drug delivery. Polymers can also be used as film coatings to reduce the undesired taste of drugs. Polymers are categorized into two groups; biodegradable and non-biodegradable. Non-biodegradable polymers accumulate in the body and cause high toxicity. It has been reported that polymer characteristics may affect their drug delivery

Seyed Morteza Naghib, Samin Hoseinpour & Shadi Zarshad

characteristics (Prajapati *et al.*, 2019, Luliński, 2017, Davis *et al.*, 1996, Raizada *et al.*, 2010). Passive or active methods are two accessible methods for drug delivery implants. In the passive method, polymer depots are more regular, which can remain at a stable drug diffusion rate. Another form of polymers is degraded inside the body at a specific rate; thus, the drug is released at a determined rate (Aj *et al.*, 2012).

Polymers have a structural and functional role in localized drug delivery (Askari *et al.*, 2021a, Askari *et al.*, 2021b). However, there are still serious concerns such as high-production cost of polymers used for drug delivery, biodegradability, toxicity, implant procedure pain, and the drug delivery system insertion route (Gooneh-Farahani *et al.*, 2020, Gooneh-Farahani *et al.*, 2019, Kalkhoran *et al.*, 2018, Zeinali Kalkhoran *et al.*, 2018). In other words, several important issues such as duration, pulses, reproducibility, lack of dose dumping, erodibility, lack of irritation and carcinogenicity must be considered when using implants in drug delivery. Polymers are inert materials that can be used as carriers in drug delivery, to release drugs at the desired site of action (Danckwerts and Fassihi, 1991, Sur *et al.*, 2019, Jain *et al.*, 2005). Polymers used as drug delivery carriers are biocompatible, flexible, and soluble. Moreover, the biological and physicochemical properties of polymers may be manipulated, so they can be used as matrices in drug delivery (Kazemi *et al.*, 2020a, Kazemi *et al.*, 2020b, Rahimzadeh *et al.*, 2020, Rahmanian *et al.*, 2019). It is noteworthy that polymeric drug carriers are promising in the field of drug discovery due to their ability to localize drug effects and stabilize drugs to extend therapeutic effectiveness. Nanoparticles (NPs), microparticles, and hydrogels are common shapes of polymeric carriers utilized in intravenous administration, oral delivery, and subcutaneous and localized delivery, respectively (Huang *et al.*, 2019, Sponchioni *et al.*, 2019).

Using polymers for passive drug delivery has advantages such as increased circulation time, lower toxicity, immunogenicity, and degradability. Polymers used for this reason must be non-toxic, water-soluble, non-immunogenic and must not cause health issues before and after drug release. In other words, they must be safe at every phase and have a harmless excretion. Polymers must undergo transport phases, such as circulation in the bloodstream, cell binding, cell internalization, and intracellular delivery, and pass a variety of biological obstacles to reach the desired site (Puoci *et al.*, 2008, Schmaljohann, 2006, Fu *et al.*, 2018).

Cancer is defined as the abnormal growth of unhealthy cells wherein the growth is uncontrollable, and the cells can expand to other sections of the body (Salahandish *et al.*, 2018a, Salahandish *et al.*, 2018b). Chemotherapy is a cancer treatment method. A variety of effective chemotherapeutic drugs, such as paclitaxel, and doxorubicin, eliminate tumor cells by damaging their DNA or RNA. Even though many methods for chemotherapeutic delivery of anticancer drugs have been known in the art, local drug delivery has been of more interest, among others. In local drug delivery, specific anticancer drugs are delivered to cancer cells with high accuracy. Since 85% of solid tumors are composed of cancer cells, this approach can deliver and release drugs more effectively (Fig. **1**). Polymers have numerous applications, but the most important challenge is related to their biocompatibility (Alsehli, 2020, De Souza *et al.*, 2010, Ju *et al.*, 2018).

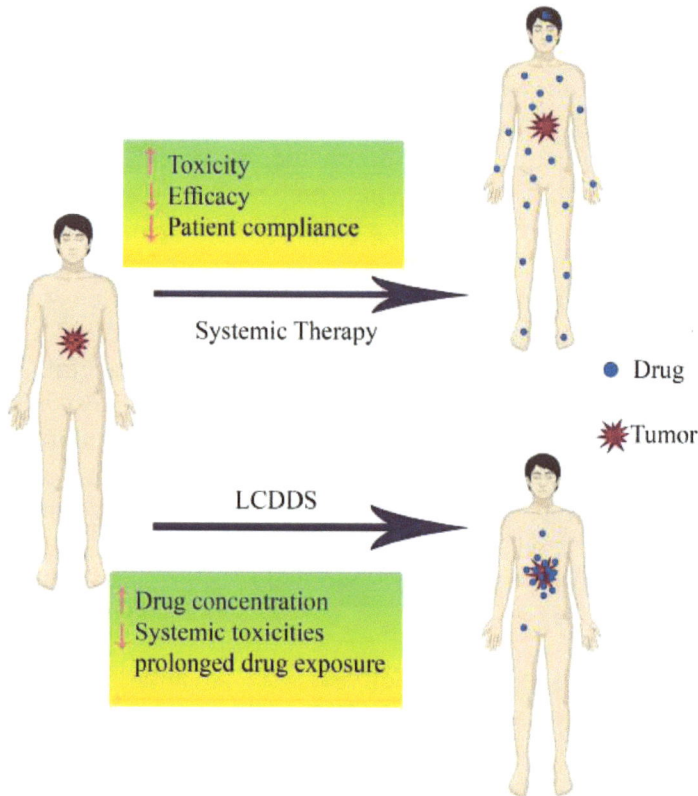

Fig. (1). Advantageous of localized chemotherapy in comparison with systemic drug delivery.

The major concern about anti-cancer drugs is their cytotoxicity. The main cause of cytotoxicity is that the anti-cancer drugs are not delivered precisely to the cancerous cells and damage healthy neighbor cells. Therefore, nanotechnology-based drug delivery systems can increase the therapeutic effects of anticancer drugs meanwhile reducing side effects. Different types of drug delivery systems with different characteristics have been investigated. Liposomes, carbon nanotubes, polymeric micelles, and dendrimers are examples that have been widely utilized in cancer treatment. Polymeric carriers have an adjustable core-shell structure. Drugs may be chemically attached to polymeric carriers, or may be physically encapsulated in the core, wherein physical encapsulation has been greatly used in the art (Alsehli, 2020, Kavand *et al.*, 2020).

Ligand-based nanoparticles, PEGylated nanoparticles, dendrimers, and polymeric micelles are different kinds of Polymer-based nanoparticles that have advantages such as low toxicity, controlled size distribution, simple preparation, good retention and protection of the drug, enhanced therapeutic effectiveness and high stability in the biological environment (Sur *et al.*, 2019).

NPs refer to particles with a size less than 100nm, however, the size of NPs used for drug delivery applications may vary from 100 to 1000 nm, which is due to the structure of drug delivery systems. Drug delivery systems are composed of two parts, including a carrier and an active pharmaceutical ingredient. In addition, the size and surface charge of polymeric nanoparticles must be studied as well. Size is an important factor for nanoparticles to penetrate several biological barriers and reach the desired site. The surface charge of the nanoparticles may result in the interaction of nanoparticles with the cell membrane or keep them in the systemic flow. Molecular weight plays a vital role in the drug release mechanism of nanoparticles. The high molecular weight of polymer results in a high retention time of the drug. Therefore, high molecular weight biodegradable polymers (HMWBP) are appropriate carriers for therapeutic agents, DNA, proteins, *etc.* Dextran, heparin, pullulan, and hyaluronic acid are examples of HMWBP. Meanwhile, the main challenge about HMWBPs, is their slow *in vivo* degradation rate, which may cause them to accumulate in tissues. Thus, low-weight biodegradable polymers are better candidates for drug delivery systems due to their high solubility and permeability (George *et al.*, 2019, Hasçiçek *et al.*, 2017).

Polymer-based nanoparticles are capable of transferring DNA, protein, or drug to various organs in the body. Therapeutic agents can be attached, dissolved, entrapped to the matrix, or encapsulated, depending on the preparation process. Nanospheres and nanocapsules are two popular shapes of polymeric nanoparticles. The drug may be embedded into a nanosphere or encapsulated inside a nanocapsule (Sur *et al.*, 2019). Polymeric nanoparticles can release the drug at a specific rate which is beneficial in many disease treatments. Polymers used in biological applications must be less than 40 KDa so that they can be cleaned by the kidney. Large-size polymers are difficult to deliver and may cause immunogenicity and long-term toxicity as they remain in the body for a long time which would restrict their application. Small-size polymeric nanoparticles can easily enter smaller parts of the body and, various functional groups can conjugate to their surface due to their large surface area (Sur *et al.*, 2019, Fu *et al.*, 2018).

When using non-biodegradable polymers for drug delivery purposes, the size of the polymer must be smaller than the renal threshold so that they will not accumulate in the body. On the other hand, the immune response or toxicity must be studied for biodegradable polymers. Biodegradable polymers, such as poly(lactic acid) (PLA) and PLGA, go through non-enzymatical or enzymatical *in vivo* biodegradation, which results in safe and biocompatible by-products. In comparison with non-biodegradable polymers, biodegradable polymers are non-allergetic and non-immunogenic, have lower toxicity, and do not require removal from the body (Schmaljohann, 2006, Prajapati *et al.*, 2019, Ji and Kohane, 2019, Puiggalí-Jou *et al.*, 2019).

Erosion and degradation can happen in both bulk and surface. When surface degradation occurs, even though the polymer volume fraction is still unaffected, the polymer matrix is gradually eliminated from the surface. In opposition, in bulk degradation, no variation in physical size occurs until it is completely eroded or degraded. But, the amount of polymer remaining in the carrier is eventually reduced. Insecurity about the safety of the by-products of degradation is a big challenge for biodegradable polymers. After degradation, a vast distribution of fragment sizes remains. Therefore, it is hard to experimentally report the toxicity of the remainders. Preferably, parenterally administered polymers are degraded into metabolic and smaller compounds which will not cause toxicity and are cleared naturally (De Souza *et al.*, 2010).

It is noteworthy that the drug release rate of microspheres highly relies on the location of the drug. If the encapsulated drug is on the surface, a first burst release happen (Davis *et al.*, 1996).

In cancer therapy, the treatment type depends on cancer form, diagnosis phase, and patient tolerance. In fact, tumor, node, and distant metastasis (TNM) staging system is the method for the classification of tumors. TNM expresses the tumor expansion rate inside the body. Moreover, cancer staging has been categorized into early, intermediate, or late-stage. In early-stage cancer, there is no obvious spreading sign, and the tumor is located in the anatomical site. In the intermediate stage, there are signs of lymph node involvement or a bigger tumor mass. In late-stage cancer, the tumor has metastasized to other parts of the body. Available drug delivery systems may be categorized by the method of action or administration route.

The first category, is systemic drug delivery which includes nanosized materials such as dendrimers and polymeric nanoparticles. These carriers are placed on the tumor site *via* conjugations with the chemical section depending on the unique cell marker, such as monoclonal antibody, which is called "active targeting"; or the carriers are placed on the tumor with passive diffusion through tumor vasculatures which are called "passive targeting". Another approach is stimuli-responsive delivery of drugs with the aid of pH changes, and electric or magnetic field changes. Although nanomaterials used for intravenous administration can eliminate tumorous cells, the main challenge is the localization of these materials so that they can be removed *via* the reticuloendothelial system.

The second category is the application of biodegradable polymeric carriers for controlled release delivery to implant intratumorally or in the vicinity of abnormal cells. In this category, there is no need for a second surgery to eliminate the implant. Synthetic and natural polymers are two types of polymers used in biomedical fields which will be discussed in the next section. Conventional cancer treatment therapies have serious drawbacks as they damage healthy cells. Therefore, local drug delivery is used to achieve targeted and sustainable drug delivery systems and decrease the side effects of conventional therapies. Each polymer has benefits and drawbacks. For instance, sodium alginate sodium carboxymethyl cellulose (Na-CMC) has a higher encapsulation efficiency (EE) compared to sodium alginate-hydroxypropyl methylcellulose (HPMC) and sodium alginate-carbopol 934P. In most cases, synthetic polymers have further versatile functionalities. They have a longer degradation time, and can be simply combined with new delivery systems such as inorganic nanoparticles and natural polymers (Wolinsky *et al.*, 2012, Deng *et al.*, 2019, Wang *et al.*, 2019).

BUP and LID have been utilized successfully as local anesthetics, which have several drawbacks. Some of the drawbacks of BUP and LID are health problems, such as neurotoxicity and also short effectivity time. To solve these problems, polymeric-based nanoparticles have been investigated to lower side effects and time effect (Kohrs *et al.*, 2019).

Another major challenge is hard manufacturing process of dry powdered polymeric nanoparticles. High levels of exposure through dermal absorption and inhalation may cause health issues for workers. Although, fundamental safety regulations and wearing suitable equipment may lower the risk. In addition, some specific polymer nanoparticles are toxic and hazardous for living species and the environment, may contaminate groundwater, and also threaten human food chain (Sur *et al.*, 2019).

In conclusion, biodegradable polymers with biomedical applications may be categorized as natural and synthetic biopolymers based on their source (George *et al.*, 2019).

3.2. SYNTHETIC POLYMERS

Polymers have been widely utilized in drug delivery systems. Implantable and injectable local anesthetic drug delivery systems have significantly decrease the toxicity of anesthetic impacts and also increased their effective time. Although, external delivery tools have drawbacks such as low accuracy, which restricts the clinical applications of DDS. Therefore, nanoparticles may be used to produce drug delivery systems for perioperative anesthesia therapy. LID and BUP are the most used anesthetics (Kohrs *et al.*, 2019).

One of the most important properties of synthetic polymers is their customizability which result in the application-specific design of local implants with customized mechanical properties, elastic modulus, drug release, and degradation. Several materials have been produced for the design of a drug delivery system. Polyanhydrides based on adipic and sebacic acid, polyesters based on glycolide, lactide, caprolactone, and also polycarbonates, and phosphate-based polymers are a few examples of materials used in drug delivery systems. In addition, synthetic polymers, which have a hydrophobic nature, and cause a minimum infection, are less immunogenic and less toxic. Therefore, synthetic polymers can be used for the long-term delivery and stabilization of water-insoluble drugs. But synthetic polymers also have negative aspects, such as accumulation of acidic degradation products, which may cause inflammation at the implant site. However, this effect can be reduced by changing the degradation profile and chemical composition (Wolinsky *et al.*, 2012, Wang *et al.*, 2019).

3.2.1. Polyesters

Polyester-based polymers, especially PLGA (poly(lactic acid-co-glycolic acid)), are biocompatible and biodegradable, and have been extensively utilized for drug delivery purposes. Most commercialized implants are made up of PLGA. However, polyester-based polymers have problems related to acidic degradation products, which may result in the unstability of the drug. These polymers can be simply prepared by condensation or ring-opening polymerization and mostly degrade through ester bonds. Poly(glycolic acid) (PGA), poly(e-caprolactone) (PCL), poly(D,L-lactic acid) (PLA) and poly(D,L-lactic-co-glycolic acid) (PLGA) are examples of polyester-based polymers (Ju *et al.*, 2018, Kohrs *et al.*, 2019).

3.2.1.1. Polylactic Acid (PLA) and Polyglycolic Acid (PGA)

PLA has been polymerized from lactic acid, which is biocompatible, biodegradable, and non-toxic. This polymer is hydrophobic in nature and can be used in lipid polymer-based hybrid nanoparticles. Moreover, PLA may be used for controlled release in drug delivery applications due to its high mechanical strength. The existence of methyl group in PLA results in higher hydrophobicity, and stability against hydrolysis compared to PGA. PLA was initially utilized for a drug delivery system composed of BUP polyester microspheres to extend the percutaneous blockade of peripheral nerves. Further, the main formulation factors were manipulated to outstand release profiles of BZC or BUP from diverse types of biodegradable drug delivery tools in PLA solutions. For instance, in a study, LID-coated poly (L-lactide) (PLLA) microneedle arrays were fabricated. In this study, LID was coated just at the needle tips and therefore released into the PBS occurred faster, which considerably lowered drug loss. PLLA microneedles are also suitable for fast transdermal delivery of drugs with minimum pain. Generally, PLA and PEG can be copolymerized to create adjustable micelles, wherein modifying the PEG and PLA ratio will result in improved drug incorporation effectiveness (Sur *et al.*, 2019, Kohrs *et al.*, 2019).

In another example, PLA nanoparticles loaded with breviscapine easily penetrate the blood-brain barrier (BBB) through a systematical administration route. This drug delivery highly depends on the size of nanoparticles, meaning that particles with larger sizes (~300 nm) can carry more drugs in comparison with smaller-sized particles (Patel *et al.*, 2012).

Sensorineural hearing loss (SNHL) is a widespread incapacity in industrial countries. One of the challenges of SNHL is difficult delivery of drugs to the inner part of the ear, which is related to the restricted blood flow in the inner ear. For clinical situations, the main therapy is introduced as systemic steroids. But studies have demonstrated that only restricted amounts of drug could reach the targeted site. PEG-PLA nanoparticles have been used to overcome the mentioned limitation and improve delivery efficacy. Local application can enhance drug delivery to the inner ear. A one-time injection into the tympanic cavity is not able to deliver a sufficient amount of drugs to the inner ear, where drug-delivery systems are capable of delivering higher amounts of drugs for sustained periods (Nakagawa and Ito, 2011).

Poly (glycolic acid) (PGA) is a non-toxic, biodegradable and biocompatible polymer, with suitable mechanical properties. PGA can increase the efficiency of drug formulations for controlled release drug delivery purposes. The degradation process of PGA is based on the unspecific breakup of the ester backbone under physiological situations. Ester is degraded into glycine inside the body and can leave the body with urine or may be transformed into carbon dioxide and water (Prajapati *et al.*, 2019).

3.2.1.2. Poly Lactic-co-glycolic Acid (PLGA)

Ring-opening copolymerization of cyclic dimers (1, 4-dioxane-2,5- diones) of glycolic acid and lactic acid (PLA and PGA) is called PLGA. PLGA can be utilized in biomedical applications such as drug delivery and surgical devices due to suitable mechanical properties, non-immunogenicity, biodegradability, bioavailability, biocompatibility and nontoxicity. PLGA is a smart FDA-approved polymer which is soluble in many solvents, and therefore can be used for controlled/ sustained drug release. Tg of this polymer ranges from 45° C to 55°C; therefore, it may be subjected to hydrolysis inside the body. Injectable microspheres of PLGA, are regularly used to carry drugs such as, anesthetics, anti-inflammatory agents, *etc.* PLGA is compatible with both hydrophobic and hydrophilic small molecules. Intravascular administered nanoparticles are a great way for local administration of therapeutic agents such as nucleic acids, proteins, and drugs. One of the major drawbacks of using PLGA carriers is associated with their bulk erosion which leads to sporadic dumping of drug and, consequently, suboptimal tissue contact profile and toxicity (Prajapati *et al.*, 2019, Kohrs *et al.*, 2019, Wang *et al.*, 2002, Bhardwaj *et al.*, 2008, Sur *et al.*, 2019, Song *et al.*, 1997).

The molecular weight of PLGA may vary from 10,000 to more than 100,000 Da. PLGAs with lower molecular weight have a higher polymer degradation speed, and thus faster drug release. The polymer molecular weight depends on the viscosity of the organic phase and is connected to the drug diffusion and particle size. PLGA microparticles may have positive, neutral, or negative electrical charges. The manufacturing process of the negative surface charge is uncapped (carrying free carboxylic groups) meanwhile, the manufacturing process of the neutral surface charge is capped (steric). A mixture of PLGA and PLGA-g-poly(L-lysine) block copolymer is applied to produce PLGAs with positive surface charge (Molavi *et al.*, 2020).

The blood-brain barrier (BBB) has an important role in modifying the microenvironment of the brain. The microenvironment of the brain is composed of endothelial cells with tight junctions surrounded by perivascular parts. The tight complicated junctions make a physical barrier and restrict paracellular transfer through the BBB. BBB acts as a metabolic barrier to drug release. In an investigation, it was demonstrated that camptothecin-loaded PLGA nanoparticles could easily pass through BBB to treat intracranial tumor models. Also, parameters such as surface charge, coating, and size may be manipulated to increase the efficiency of the drug delivery system. For example, coating paclitaxel loaded PLGA nanoparticles coated with glutathione can enhance BBB penetration, while coating PLGA with poloxamer and polysorbate can enhance central nervous penetration (Patel *et al.*, 2012).

In another study, it was shown that PLGA microsphere/PVA hydrogel-based composite can be used as an external drug-eluting coating for implantable tools. According to the results of the present study, the drug release profile could simply change by combining various kinds of PLGA microspheres. It is possible to load and release more than one drug at the same time in a composite *via* embedding various drugs in the microspheres (Bhardwaj *et al.*, 2008).

The degradation mechanism is another important factor affecting the application of polymers in drug release. Chain degradation of PLGA occurs at a steady rate but, biodegradation of the PLGA matrix occurs at random rate on swollen polymers. Normally, factors such as the polymer molecular weight, existence of ester or carboxyl groups, Tg, crystallinity, and lactide to glycolide (L/G) ratio would affect PLGA degradation time. In addition, the absence of methyl groups on the glycolide side, results in crystallinity. Thus, amorphous, crystalline or quite amorphous (PLA) structures may be achieved by changing the L/G ratio. Moreover, Lactide has a more hydrophobic nature compared to glycolide. Therefore, reducing the lactide share will result in quicker drug release which is due to higher hydrolytic degradation speed. Among PLGA copolymers available in the market, copolymers with 50/50 L/G ratios have a higher degradation speed (Wang *et al.*, 2019).

Drug-loaded matrices are implanted inside the cavities to prevent recurrence and extend survival in post-surgery and prime tumor resection stages of cancer treatment. Drug-loaded PLGA can be used for this reason because of its promising drug release profile and customizable shape and size. As an example, paclitaxel-loaded PLGA can control the release of a drug within 80 days *in vitro* (Meinel *et al.*, 2012). In this regard, Cao *et al.* developed a liposomal doxorubicin-loaded PLGA-PEG-PLGA based thermo-sensitive biogel for LCDDS. This biogel was used for cancer treatment. In this study, the drug release rate was kept stable for up to 11 days without remarkable burst release. The results showed higher anticancer productivity and reduced side effects, in comparison with the doxorubicin-loaded hydrogel (Fig. **2**).

3.2.1.3. Polycaprolactones (PCL)

Polycaprolactone (PCL) is a biodegradable, biocompatible, non-toxic, and aliphatic semicrystalline polyester. This polymer is highly permeable and is soluble in a variety of organic solvents, with a Tg around -60°C, and melting temperature ranging from 55° C to 60° C and PCL can produce composites with bioerodible polymers. PCL is hydrolyzed at neutral pH, and the degradation speed is increased when copolymerized with lactide or glycolide. Subcutaneous administration of PCL is useful for the systemic and local delivery of drugs owing to its biocompatibility and biodegradability (Nakagawa and Ito, 2011, Prajapati *et al.*, 2019, Wang *et al.*, 2019).

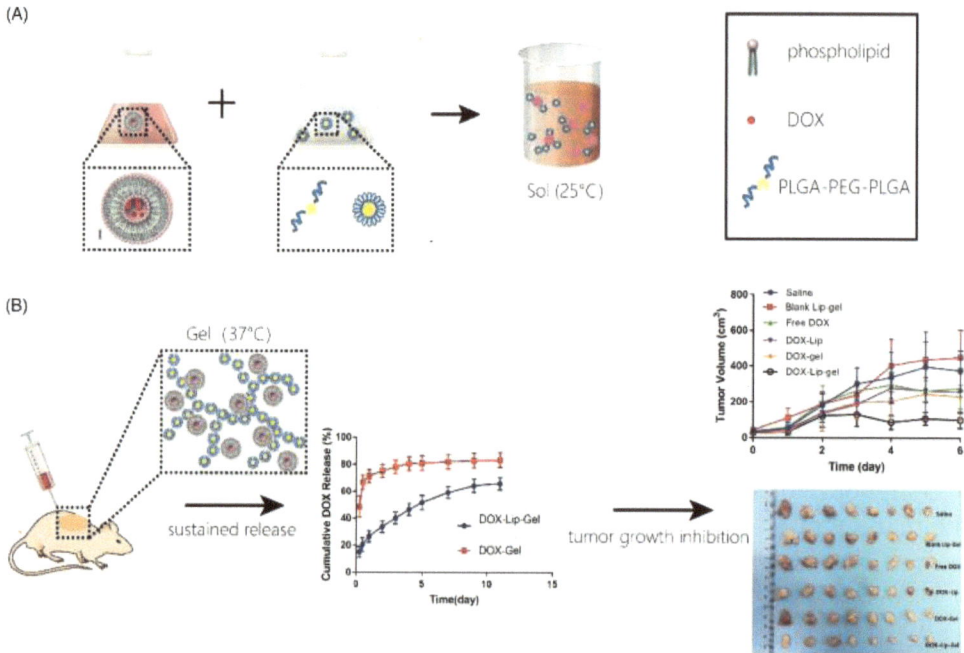

Fig. (2). Schematic representation of (a) liposomal doxorubicin (DOX) was dissolved in PLGA-PEG-PLGA copolymer suspension to form DOX-liposome (Lip)-Gel (25 °C). (b) DOX-Lip-Gel was injected and transformed into a solid gel in situ at 37 °C, facilitating the controlled release of the drug and meaningful inhibitory effect on tumor progression (open access) (Cao *et al.*, 2019).

A copolymer composed of PCL/PEG was studied for local and specifically injectable systems. The copolymer was biocompatible and non-toxic and had FDA approval. This copolymer may be transformed into a hydrogel due to its powder morphology to enhance drug loading. The gelation temperature highly depends on the MW and PCL length. Thus, the designation of a PEG/PCL hydrogel not only requires the appropriate gelation temperature, but also the MW should be controlled. In local drug delivery systems, an injectable hydrogel with thermoresponsive properties is favorable. The powdery form of the copolymer is accessible at room temperature leading to technical ease. Liquid state at room temperature, low viscosity, miscibility of the drug, and the simple transformation to hydrogel, low invasivity of targeted delivery, gelation/solidification at body temperature are some required properties of an injectable hydrogel. A major challenge of PEG/PCL hydrogels is that they are formed at temperatures higher than LCST, which may lead to the degradation of thermolabile drugs. Moreover, high hydrophobicity and crystallinity of PCL hinder drug release. Therefore, slow drug release and slow degradation have reduced the application of PCL in drug delivery (Lu and Chen, 2004, Davis *et al.*, 1996).

3.2.1.4. Poly(Alkyl Cyanoacrylates) (PACA)

Polymers such as PLA and PLGA are biodegradable and biocompatible and have FDA approval. PACA has been used in CNS but is not approved by FDA for clinical trials.

3.2.3. Poly(Ortho Esters)

This polymer was investigated as a bioerodible polymer in the 1970s. It is known as a pH-responsive polymer in which the orthoester bonds lead to an acceptable degradation rate. The presence of suberic acid in the polymer may increase the degradation rate. However, basic and neutral excipients are used to keep the degradation rate constant as acidic derivatives are produced during hydrolysis (Wang *et al.*, 2002, Heller and Barr, 2004).

Poly(ortho esters) are divided into four groups, including POE I, POE II, POE III, and POE IV. POE IV is bioerodible and has all the required commercialization features. Reproducible and easy production, favored thermal and mechanical properties, and also preferred drug release and erosion rates are some of the properties of POE IV. The thermal and mechanical properties of POE IV may be adjusted by choice of diols utilized in the synthesis. The drug release rate of POE IV may be adjusted from days to months. The erosion rate depends on the diol to latent acid diol ratio. In anhydrous situation, erosion happens from the surface and is stable at room temperature. Surface erosion results in controlled release, and the pH remains neutral inside the polymer matrix as the acidic products of hydrolysis diffuse away. Solid materials and injectable semi-solid materials are two groups of these material. Solid materials can be in different forms, including strands, microspheres, and wafers. In semi-solid materials, the drug is easily mixed with the material at room temperature without a solvent. The degradation mechanism of polyorthoester is based on the hydrolysis of ester backbone, wherein simultaneous diols are produced and the acidic levels are considerably lower than PLGA. As mentioned before polyorthoesters are pH-sensitive and are stable in physiological pH, and the degradation initiates at a pH of 5, with negligible levels of autohydrolysis. Since tumors have an acidic pH tumor-targeted drug delivery may be accomplished using polyorthoesters (Heller *et al.*, 2002, Einmahl *et al.*, 2001, Jenkins, 2007).

Although PLGA undergoes bulk erosion, the hydrolysis of POEs occurs on the surface due to hydrophobic hydrocarbon–ether ring and also zero-order release kinetics of drug release. POEs are mostly utilized for biodegradable hydrophobic implants. Polyorthoester and polyethylene glycol are highly suitable for tumor-targeting drug delivery. Other investigations have studied the healing of postsurgery pain, osteoarthritis, and eye diseases (Pandey *et al.*, 2019, Kolawole *et al.*, 2007).

3.2.4. Poly(Anhydrides)

Polyanhydride is a biodegradability synthetic polymer with 2 carbonyl groups conjugated with an ether bond. Polyanhydride has numerous applications in drug delivery, including oral, injectable delivery, anticoagulants neuroactive drugs, local anesthetics, and vaccines. Significantly, eye disorders are treated with controlled drug release using polyanhydrides. This polymer is hydrophobic and is degraded *via* surface erosion. Therefore, when a drug is loaded inside the polymer, the drug is shielded inside the polymer until surface erosion occurs. The degradation of polyanhydrides highly depends on MW, pH, and crystallinity. For example, in a basic pH, the degradation rate is high, however, in an acidic pH the degradation rate is low (Prajapati *et al.*, 2019, Davis *et al.*, 1996).

Linear degradation, hydrophobicity, low Tm, flexibility, stability, and solubility in organic solutions are important factors for any polymer used in drug delivery. Accordingly, polyanhydride counts as a suitable polymer for drug delivery due to its non-inflammatory and non-toxic by-products. Moreover, the hydrolytic reactivity of polymer linkages may control degradation. Different kinds of monomers and their ratio would result in synthesis feasibility and designation of surface erosion polymers. Long-chain fatty acid terminals can affect polymer degradation rate and hydrophobicity, while adding amino acids to polyanhydrides, can enhance mechanical properties (Jain *et al.*, 2005).

Polyanhydride disks can carry and release chemotherapeutic agents such as carmustine or BCNU, to the residual cavity resulting from tumor resection surgery. These disks, which have a diameter of 1.45 cm and a thickness of 1.0 mm are implantable, and up to 8 disks can be implanted in a cavity, wherein each disk can deliver a defined dose of drug. The commercial name of this polymer is polifeprosan. It is composed of poly[bis(p-carboxyphenoxy)propane: sebacic acid] in a 20:80 molar ratio and has been utilized for local delivery of carmustine (Kleiner *et al.*, 2014).

3.2.5. Poly(amides)

The outcome of polycondensation of like 1,2-bis(3-aminopropyl amine) ethane and diacid chloride is called polyamide. Polyamide is thermoplastic and semicrystalline with amide groups divided by alkane. Polyamide is categorized by the number of carbon atoms separating the N atoms and also alkane parts. Polyamides containing amide groups divided by alkane parts, and carbons separating the nitrogen describe a significant kind of nylon. Nylon is a well-known polyamide with high tensile strength which has been widely utilized in catheters and balloons for angiography. The hydrogen bonds can keep the molecular chains in a controlled and solid phase before and even after the alkane part has melted. The synthesis procedure and the polyamide type, highly affect the strength and length of the hydrogen bonds (Pandey *et al.*, 2019, Kolawole *et al.*, 2007).

The exclusive characteristics of polyamides originate from the intramolecular structures within the linear chains in the polymer, and the intermolecular structures between the linear chains in the polymer hydrogen bond with carbonyl and amide. Polyaminoacid is the most well-known polyamide. The hydrolytic cleavage stability of polyamide is more than polyanhydrides and polyesters, due to the amide linkage. The degradation mechanism of this polymer is based on enzymes and is tunable by changing the hydrophilicity of the amino acids (Kolawole *et al.*, 2007, Wang *et al.*, 2002).

3.2.6. Poly(Ester Amides)

Polyesters like PLGA have been widely used in drug delivery applications. However, such polymers have serious drawbacks, such as bulk degradation of PLGA, which results in the accumulation of acidic byproducts and therefore, tissue inflammation and toxicity. Moreover, coupling bioactive agents are required to fulfill the weak mechanical properties, which have limited the use of these polymers. Poly(ester amide)s (PEAs) have shown processability, biodegradability, biocompatibility, and cell-material interaction with favorable thermal and mechanical characteristics which is due to the presence of both ester and amide bonds in their chemical backbone. The degradation route of PEAs is enzymatic and hydrolytic which releases non-toxic diols, amino acids, and dicarboxylic acids. The improved cellular response of PEAs is due to the buffering impact owing to the existence of amide bonds similar to proteins (Moustafa, 2014, Natarajan *et al.*, 2017).

3.2.7. Poly(Phosphoesters)

In the 1970s, polyphosphoester (PPE) was investigated as analog of nucleic acid, which is an inorganic polymer and synthesized by ring-opening polymerization and polycondensation. This polymer has 2 substitution sections called R and R′ (Zhao *et al.*, 2003). The polymer type is defined based on the R′ changes, including R′=H, which is called polyphosphites; R′ = alkoxy or aryloxy group, which is called polyphosphate and R′ = alkyl or aryl group, which is known as polyphosphonate. In addition, it is biodegradable and has low toxicity. The degradation of phosphate bonds through enzymatic cleavage or/and hydrolysis leads to the production of alcohol, diol, and phosphate. Moreover, the biocompatibility maybe adjusted by replacing the R and R′ side groups of homopolymers. Biocompatibility is one of the main challenges of using polymers for drug delivery. This challenge may be solved by the organocatalyzed ROP synthesis procedure, as the remaining by-products are completely and easily eliminated. Biodegradability and biocompatibility of water-insoluble polyphosphoesters have made this polymer an appropriate choice for drug carriers, significantly drugs with low MW, weak solubility, DNA plasmids and proteins. The structural flexibility of polyphosphoesters is due to the valence layer of the phosphorus atom. The reactive side chain in polyphosphate and polyphosphonate cases allows the conjugation of bioactive molecules (Jenkins, 2007, Wang *et al.*, 2009, Yilmaz and Jérôme, 2016, Zhao *et al.*, 2003).

PPEs can be synthesized in a controlled manner resulting in diverse macromolecular structures. In addition, they can form nanostructures with different functionalities and a wide range of properties. There are several challenges associated with PPEs. For instance, the chemical structure, thermoresponsivity, *in vivo* cell adhesion and proliferation must be further studied (Zhao *et al.*, 2003).

3.3. NATURALLY-DERIVED POLYMERS

Natural polymers are originated from microbes, animals and plants, which have been widely utilized in gene and drug delivery owing to their biocompatibility, bioavailability and biodegradability and lower toxicity in comparison with synthetic polymers (Prajapati *et al.*, 2019, Sur *et al.*, 2019).

3.3.1. Polysaccharides-Based Polymers

Polysaccharides made of monosaccharide units which are attached by ether bond O-glycosidic linkages, have been widely used for drug delivery purposes, due to their simple functionalizing, nontoxicity, stability, biodegradability, and biocompatibility. Polysaccharide-based polymers are low-cost as they exist in large quantities in nature. These polymers are found in pectin, guar gum, in microbes such as dextran, xanthan gum, in algals such as alginate, and in animals. The hydrophilic nature of these polymers results in bioadhesion with body tissues and improves retention of therapeutic agents in tissues for example cancerous tumors. Chitosan, Hyaluronic acid are examples of these polymers (Prajapati *et al.*, 2019, Ju *et al.*, 2018).

3.3.1.1. Chitosan

Chitosan is a natural, linear cationic polysaccharide, and one of the most existing polysaccharides in biomass. Chitosan is produced by deacetylation of chitin, which affects the gelation temperature of aqueous chitosan solutions, and originated from shells of crustaceans such as shrimps and crabs. Two hydroxyl and one carboxyl groups exist in the repeating glucosidic residue of chitosan. It can be produced in different forms including powders, threads, fiber meshes, beads, matrixes, films (for cancer therapy), membranes, nanoparticles, and hydrogels based on their applications. Chitosan is biodegradable and biocompatible. It has low toxicity and low immunogenicity. Therefore, it has many biomedical applications, such as targeted drug delivery or materials for sutures and wound healing, *etc.* The characteristics of chitosan are similar to ECM; therefore, it can be used for cell growth, and in tissue formation and facilitates the penetration of drugs through biological barriers. The major challenge of chitosan is its low solubility. Chitosan only dissolves in acidic solutions. *In vitro* studies have demonstrated that enzymes such as chitosanase, papain, and lysozyme affect chitosan degradation, and the crystallinity degree influences the biodegradability rate (Wolinsky *et al.*, 2012, Prajapati *et al.*, 2019, Davis *et al.*, 1996, Sur *et al.*, 2019, Kohrs *et al.*, 2019, Peers *et al.*, 2020, Sung and Kim, 2020, Bhattarai *et al.*, 2010, Zhang *et al.*, 2014).

The synthesis of chitosan nanoparticles is facile, and are stable. In addition, chitosan nanoparticles can be administered with different methods. Consequently, they are a good candidate for controlled release targeted delivery. Moreover, because of the presence of amine groups, they can be swiftly uptaken by cells. Protonation of amines on chitosan glucosamine monomers is easy in an acidic medium (pH less than 6.5) so chitosan would have cationic characteristics that facilitate its interaction with anionic elements, for instance, nucleic acids. But its solubility in solutions with a pH of more than 6.5 is weak. Chitosan and its derivatives have various applications in biomedical field. For instance, amphiphilic chitosan is used in insulin delivery and vaccine delivery. Moreover, trimethyl chitosan is widely utilized as well. Graphene-chitosan hybrids are used in stimuli-sensitive drug delivery systems. Also, chitosan-based delivery, such as chitosan hydrogels integrated with radioactive agent 131I-norcholesterol (131I-NC) has been used as a substitute for treatment of local recurrence and growth of tumors in cancer chemotherapy. Moreover, the surface of chitosan may be modified to have a diversity of ligands to cross BBB, such as transferrin receptor antibodies (Hasçiçek *et al.*, 2017, Ansari *et al.*, 2020, Patel *et al.*, 2012).

Glycol chitosan is a popular chitosan derivative with outstanding properties such as water solubility in different physiological states and biodegradability, and therefore has been extensively utilized for core-shell drug delivery. When this polymer is dissolved in an aqueous medium, self-assembly occurs. Self-assembly is influenced by the hydrophobic substitution of polymer, ionic strength, MW, and the type hydrophobicity. Also, hydrophobic compounds may be used to form spherical nanoparticles, in order to encapsulate lipophilic drugs for controlled release (Prajapati *et al.*, 2019).

Chemical hydrogels degrade slower than physical chitosan hydrogels, due to their weak mechanical properties. Stimuli-responsive chitosan hydrogels can be produced by in situ gelations at body temperature or at the desired location, which are mostly injectable. For this reason, 3 approaches exist, including:

1. application of enzymes such as tyrosinase which assist in crosslinking,
2. the employment of crosslinking below useful control of crosslinking kinetics,
3. physical crosslinking of chitosan chains *via* modification of environmental factors such as pH or temperature.

Drug delivery with pH-sensitive carriers may be used for cancer therapy. pH locally rises in the tumor environment and the therapeutic agent can be released in the acidic environment with no destructive effect on normal cells. Although chitosan has an anti-tumor activity, chitosan-based localized delivery systems are not reached clinical trials yet. The major limitation of chitosan-based localized delivery systems is achieving a high degree of purity, as unreacted cross-linking agents or contaminants may influence its safety profile (Bhattarai *et al.*, 2010, Ju *et al.*, 2018).

3.3.1.2. Hyaluronic Acid-based Polymers

Hyaluronic acid is a viscoelastic, biodegradable, biocompatible, and nonimmunogenic natural mucopolysaccharide, present in ECM, heart valves, synovial fluid, and vitreous of the eye. It has been utilized in wound healing and drug delivery. One important feature of this polymer is its simple elimination through digestion with hyaluronidase if it causes any trouble inside the body. HA holds the richness of functional reactive location for the cross-linking, conjugation of ligands, which makes them a perfect choice for therapeutic purposes. The MW of macro scale HA may vary from thousands to millions of Daltons depending on the polymer chain length. Nanocarriers and nanomicelles of hyaluronic acid are harmless for drug delivery and also are compatible with blood and are able to target tumor cells (Kohrs *et al.*, 2019, Gao *et al.*, 2016, Prajapati *et al.*, 2019).

The major application of HA is for BUP delivery. In a study, BUP was conjugated with a derivative of HA (Hylan B). *In vitro* studies demonstrate the prolonged duration of BUP, more than 16 hours, which is considerable in comparison with BUP-free (0.4 hours). In addition, *in vivo* studies showed, that the time was 5 times more than free BUP, meaning that HA is useful in increasing local anesthesia time. Also, HA composites may be used for biomedical applications owing to their significant compatibility. For instance, multi-targeted carrageenan composite (CARR)/HA-based wafers loaded with LID and silver nanoparticles (AgNPs) can successfully kill bacteria. Hardness is also adjustable by altering the content of HA for chronic leg ulcer treatment. Therefore, this composite has several advantages, including quick drug release, efficient antimicrobial activity and application in chronic leg ulcer healing (Gianolio *et al.*, 2005, Lombardo *et al.*, 2019, Kohrs *et al.*, 2019).

3.3.2. Polypeptides-Based Polymers

Polymer-based treatments and diagnoses have led to the development of polypeptide-based constructs. Polypeptides are a broad family of macromolecules with two synthesis approaches, including synthetic techniques and recombinant DNA techniques, which are also referred to as genetically encoded techniques. The first approach includes ring-opening polymerization of α-amino-*N*-carboxyanhydrides (NCAs) (for designing hybrid materials), stepwise solid-phase polypeptide synthesis (SPPS) or native chemical ligation (NCL), which are based on amino acids and their derivatives as monomers and is practical in designing hybrids and combine sequences of peptidic and non-peptidic nature. Current synthetic methods have resulted in new polymer structures with significant abilities. In other words, they have multivalent surfaces to make steady tracing agents or drugs with a higher ability to load drugs, and multiple ways for cellular trafficking because of dissimilarities in conformation and sizes. The important drawbacks are stereochemistry and controlling chain length (Duro-Castano *et al.*, 2014, Shao *et al.*, 2019, Chow *et al.*, 2008).

3.3.2.1. Collagen-based Polymers & Gelatin-based Polymers

Many natural and synthetic biodegradable materials can deliver agents with low MW for instance steroids. On the other hand, polymers like alginate and gelatin are capable of sustained delivery of proteins, peptides, neurotrophins and growth factors. Both neurotrophins and growth factors have protecting impact on inner ear cells. Gelatin is a natural polymer of collagen derivatives which is broadly utilized for hemostasis in clinics. Gelatin-based controlled release drug delivery systems, which have modifiable isoelectric points, have been investigated. These systems are used to produce a positively charged basic gelatin or a negatively charged acidic gelatin which results in electrostatic interactions of charged therapeutic molecules and gelatin with another charge to for form polyion complexes. It has been shown that gelatin polymers are useful for sustained delivery to the inner ear of brain-derived neurotrophic factor (BDNF) in animals. Additionally, *in vivo* studies revealed that the local use of BDNF keeps SGNs against aminoglycoside toxicity (Song *et al.*, 1997).

There are drawbacks associated with using collagen in local chemotherapy, including weak mechanical properties and early initiation of degradation after implantation, wherein cross-linking approaches can be a considerable solution. In 1995, Davidson *et al.* developed a matrix of collagen for local delivery of cisplatin after tumor resection in order to avoid tumor recurrence in animal experiments. The matrix was capable of holding high amounts of drugs for up to 7 days, resulting in long time local contact of drugs while sparing healthy tissues. Also, recently, a new gelatin hydrogel has been developed for cisplatin local delivery, which is injected straight under the tumor. Results demonstrate that the release of the drug during 14 days had anti-tumor impact and increased endurance and reduced unwanted side effects related to the systemic administration (Ju *et al.*, 2018).

3.3.2.1.1. Gelatin

Gelatin is a water-soluble derivative of animal tissues such as mineral salts and proteins. Gelatin is the main connective component of tissue, bone, skin and consists of both basic and acidic functional groups, which is achievable by controlled hydrolysis of insoluble protein, collagen, and *etc.* Collagen has wide applications in the food and pharmaceutical industries. It shapes a triple-stranded helical structure in solutions at low temperatures. Generally, two kinds of gelatin exist, type A and type B. The first kind is achievable by acid treatment of collagen and the second one is obtainable by treatment of alkaline with the isoelectric point of 9 and 5, respectively. Many functional groups in this polymer lead to its high functionality. There are several opportunities for chemical modification and covalent drug attachment due to the initial structure of gelatin. The drugs may be attached straight on their surface or inside the matrix of particles. Gelatin is useful in ocular drug delivery since it is a derivative of native protein collagen existing in the eye, especially in the stroma of the middle cell layer of the cornea. Gelatin is known as a denature material of collagen, which regularly alters its structure in gelation depending on temperature, concentration and energy. In addition, hydrogen bonds in the side chains of amino acids help gelatin formation and enhance the complexity of hydrophobic interactions between gelatin and the drugs. So, attempts must be made to have a standard gelatin-based drug delivery system (Sur *et al.*, 2019, Hasçiçek *et al.*, 2017, Kohrs *et al.*, 2019).

3.3.2.1.2. GelMA

Gelatin methacryloyl (GelMA) is a hydrogel mostly used for controlled release drug delivery. It has a low production cost and is made of gelatin. GelMA has properties such as biocompatibility, biodegradability, low immunogenicity and tenability. GelMA may be used for the sustainable and local drug release. It imitates the physiochemical properties of ECM, as it can be classified as an artificial ECM material, and can control the fate of stem cells. Additionally, cells are easily the proliferated on its surface. GelMA is capable of delivering antitumor agents, growth factors, antimicrobial agents, and siRNA. GelMA drug carriers are able to interact with drugs *via* covalent linking and physisorption, in which chemical modification, physical properties and hydrophobicity may affect the interactions. The stiffness of GelMA hydrogels is influenced by synthesis factors, including the degree of functionalization (DoF), crosslinking parameters such as curing time, and hydrogel concentration (Shao *et al.*, 2019, Miri *et al.*, 2018, Vigata *et al.*, 2020).

CONCLUSION

Polymers and biopolymers with special characteristics (degradability, cytocompatibility, bioactivity, low toxicity, stimuli sensitivity *etc.*) and advantages (low production cost, extensive functions, environmentally friendliness, easy production, *etc.*) are promising substances and biomaterials in different applications, especially LCDDS. Here, we described the characteristics, benefits and application of polymers and biopolymers in typical and stimuli-sensitive systems.

REFERENCES

Aj, M.Z., Patil, S.K., Baviskar, D.T., Jain, D.K. (2012). Implantable drug delivery system: a review. *Int. J. Pharm. Tech. Res., 4*, 280-292.

Alsehli, M. (2020). Polymeric nanocarriers as stimuli-responsive systems for targeted tumor (cancer) therapy:

Recent advances in drug delivery. *Saudi Pharm. J., 28*(3), 255-265.
[http://dx.doi.org/10.1016/j.jsps.2020.01.004] [PMID: 32194326]

Ansari, R., Sadati, S.M., Mozafari, N., Ashrafi, H., Azadi, A. (2020). Carbohydrate polymer-based nanoparticle application in drug delivery for CNS-related disorders. *Eur. Polym. J., 128*, 109607.
[http://dx.doi.org/10.1016/j.eurpolymj.2020.109607]

Askari, E., Naghib, S.M., Zahedi, A., Seyfoori, A., Zare, Y., Rhee, K.Y. (2021). Local delivery of chemotherapeutic agent in tissue engineering based on gelatin/graphene hydrogel. *J. Mater. Res. Technol., 12*, 412-422.
[http://dx.doi.org/10.1016/j.jmrt.2021.02.084]

Askari, E., Rasouli, M., Darghiasi, S.F., Naghib, S.M., Zare, Y., Rhee, K.Y. (2021). Reduced graphene oxide-grafted bovine serum albumin/bredigite nanocomposites with high mechanical properties and excellent osteogenic bioactivity for bone tissue engineering. *Biodes. Manuf., 4*(2), 243-257.
[http://dx.doi.org/10.1007/s42242-020-00113-4]

Bhardwaj, U., Papadimitrakopoulos, F., Burgess, D.J. (2008). A review of the development of a vehicle for localized and controlled drug delivery for implantable biosensors. *J. Diabetes Sci. Technol., 2*(6), 1016-1029.
[http://dx.doi.org/10.1177/193229680800200611] [PMID: 19885291]

Bhattarai, N., Gunn, J., Zhang, M. (2010). Chitosan-based hydrogels for controlled, localized drug delivery. *Adv. Drug Deliv. Rev., 62*(1), 83-99.
[http://dx.doi.org/10.1016/j.addr.2009.07.019] [PMID: 19799949]

Cao, D., Zhang, X., Akabar, M., Luo, Y., Wu, H., Ke, X., Ci, T. (2019). Liposomal doxorubicin loaded PLGA-PEG-PLGA based thermogel for sustained local drug delivery for the treatment of breast cancer. *Artif. Cells Nanomed. Biotechnol., 47*(1), 181-191.
[http://dx.doi.org/10.1080/21691401.2018.1548470] [PMID: 30686051]

Chow, D., Nunalee, M.L., Lim, D.W., Simnick, A.J., Chilkoti, A. (2008). Peptide-based biopolymers in biomedicine and biotechnology. *Mater. Sci. Eng. Rep., 62*(4), 125-155.
[http://dx.doi.org/10.1016/j.mser.2008.04.004] [PMID: 19122836]

Danckwerts, M., Fassihi, A. (1991). Implantable controlled release drug delivery systems: a review. *Drug Dev. Ind. Pharm., 17*(11), 1465-1502.
[http://dx.doi.org/10.3109/03639049109026629]

Davis, S.S., Illum, L., Stolnik, S. (1996). Polymers in drug delivery. *Curr. Opin. Colloid Interface Sci., 1*(5), 660-666.
[http://dx.doi.org/10.1016/S1359-0294(96)80105-1]

De Souza, R., Zahedi, P., Allen, C.J., Piquette-Miller, M. (2010). Polymeric drug delivery systems for localized cancer chemotherapy. *Drug Deliv., 17*(6), 365-375.
[http://dx.doi.org/10.3109/10717541003762854] [PMID: 20429844]

Deng, H., Dong, A., Song, J., Chen, X. (2019). Injectable thermosensitive hydrogel systems based on functional PEG/PCL block polymer for local drug delivery. *J. Control. Release, 297*, 60-70.
[http://dx.doi.org/10.1016/j.jconrel.2019.01.026] [PMID: 30684513]

Duro-Castano, A., Conejos-Sánchez, I., Vicent, M. (2014). Peptide-based polymer therapeutics. *Polymers (Basel), 6*(2), 515-551.
[http://dx.doi.org/10.3390/polym6020515]

Einmahl, S., Behar-Cohen, F., D'Hermies, F., Rudaz, S., Tabatabay, C., Renard, G., Gurny, R. (2001). A new poly(ortho ester)-based drug delivery system as an adjunct treatment in filtering surgery. *Invest. Ophthalmol. Vis. Sci., 42*(3), 695-700.
[PMID: 11222529]

Fu, X., Hosta-Rigau, L., Chandrawati, R., Cui, J. (2018). Multi-stimuli-responsive polymer particles, films, and hydrogels for drug delivery. *Chem, 4*(9), 2084-2107.
[http://dx.doi.org/10.1016/j.chempr.2018.07.002]

Gao, W., Zhang, Y., Zhang, Q., Zhang, L. (2016). Nanoparticle-hydrogel: a hybrid biomaterial system for localized drug delivery. *Ann. Biomed. Eng., 44*(6), 2049-2061.
[http://dx.doi.org/10.1007/s10439-016-1583-9] [PMID: 26951462]

George, A., Shah, P.A., Shrivastav, P.S. (2019). Natural biodegradable polymers based nano-formulations for drug delivery: A review. *Int. J. Pharm., 561*, 244-264.
[http://dx.doi.org/10.1016/j.ijpharm.2019.03.011] [PMID: 30851391]

Gianolio, D.A., Philbrook, M., Avila, L.Z., MacGregor, H., Duan, S.X., Bernasconi, R., Slavsky, M., Dethlefsen, S., Jarrett, P.K., Miller, R.J. (2005). Synthesis and evaluation of hydrolyzable hyaluronan-tethered bupivacaine delivery systems. *Bioconjug. Chem., 16*(6), 1512-1518.
[http://dx.doi.org/10.1021/bc050239a] [PMID: 16287249]

Gooneh-Farahani, S., Naghib, S.M., Naimi-Jamal, M.R. (2020). A Novel and Inexpensive Method Based on Modified Ionic Gelation for pH-responsive Controlled Drug Release of Homogeneously Distributed Chitosan Nanoparticles with a High Encapsulation Efficiency. *Fibers Polym., 21*(9), 1917-1926.
[http://dx.doi.org/10.1007/s12221-020-1095-y]

Gooneh-Farahani, S., Naimi-Jamal, M.R., Naghib, S.M. (2019). Stimuli-responsive graphene-incorporated multifunctional chitosan for drug delivery applications: a review. *Expert Opin. Drug Deliv., 16*(1), 79-99.
[http://dx.doi.org/10.1080/17425247.2019.1556257] [PMID: 30514124]

Hasçiçek, C., Sengel-Turk, C.T., Gumustas, M., Ozkan, A.S., Bakar, F., Das-Evcimen, N., Savaser, A., Ozkan, Y. (2017). Fulvestrant-loaded polymer-based nanoparticles for local drug delivery: Preparation and *in vitro* characterization. *J. Drug Deliv. Sci. Technol., 40*, 73-82.
[http://dx.doi.org/10.1016/j.jddst.2017.06.001]

Heller, J., Barr, J. (2004). Poly(ortho esters)--from concept to reality. *Biomacromolecules, 5*(5), 1625-1632.
[http://dx.doi.org/10.1021/bm040049n] [PMID: 15360265]

Heller, J., Barr, J., Ng, S.Y., Abdellauoi, K.S., Gurny, R. (2002). Poly(ortho esters): synthesis, characterization, properties and uses. *Adv. Drug Deliv. Rev., 54*(7), 1015-1039.
[http://dx.doi.org/10.1016/S0169-409X(02)00055-8] [PMID: 12384319]

Huang, D., Deng, M., Kuang, S. (2019). Polymeric carriers for controlled drug delivery in obesity treatment. *Trends Endocrinol. Metab., 30*(12), 974-989.
[http://dx.doi.org/10.1016/j.tem.2019.09.004] [PMID: 31668904]

Jain, J.P., Modi, S., Domb, A.J., Kumar, N. (2005). Role of polyanhydrides as localized drug carriers. *J. Control. Release, 103*(3), 541-563.
[http://dx.doi.org/10.1016/j.jconrel.2004.12.021] [PMID: 15820403]

Jenkins, M. (2007). *Biomedical polymers.*. Elsevier.

Ji, T., Kohane, D.S. (2019). Nanoscale systems for local drug delivery. *Nano Today, 28*, 100765.
[http://dx.doi.org/10.1016/j.nantod.2019.100765] [PMID: 32831899]

Ju, P., Hu, J., Li, F., Cao, Y., Li, L., Shi, D., Hao, Y., Zhang, M., He, J., Ni, P. (2018). A biodegradable polyphosphoester-functionalized poly(disulfide) nanocarrier for reduction-triggered intracellular drug delivery. *J. Mater. Chem. B Mater. Biol. Med., 6*(44), 7263-7273.
[http://dx.doi.org/10.1039/C8TB01566J] [PMID: 32254638]

Zeinali Kalkhoran, A.H., Naghib, S.M., Vahidi, O., Rahmanian, M. (2018). Synthesis and characterization of graphene-grafted gelatin nanocomposite hydrogels as emerging drug delivery systems. *Biomed. Phys. Eng. Express, 4*(5), 055017.
[http://dx.doi.org/10.1088/2057-1976/aad745]

Kavand, A., Anton, N., Vandamme, T., Serra, C.A., Chan-Seng, D. (2020). Synthesis and functionalization of hyperbranched polymers for targeted drug delivery. *J. Control. Release, 321*, 285-311.
[http://dx.doi.org/10.1016/j.jconrel.2020.02.019] [PMID: 32057990]

Kazemi, F., Naghib, S.M., Mohammadpour, Z. (2020). Multifunctional micro-/nanoscaled structures based

on polyaniline: an overview of modern emerging devices. *Mater. Today Chem., 16*, 100249.
[http://dx.doi.org/10.1016/j.mtchem.2020.100249]

Kazemi, F., Naghib, S.M., Zare, Y., Rhee, K.Y. (2020). Biosensing Applications of Polyaniline (PANI)-Based Nanocomposites: A Review. *Polym. Rev. (Phila. Pa.),* 1-45.

Kleiner, L.W., Wright, J.C., Wang, Y. (2014). Evolution of implantable and insertable drug delivery systems. *J. Control. Release, 181*, 1-10.
[http://dx.doi.org/10.1016/j.jconrel.2014.02.006] [PMID: 24548479]

Kohrs, N. J., Liyanage, T., Venkatesan, N., Najarzadeh, A., Puleo, D. A. (2019). Drug delivery systems and controlled release.
[http://dx.doi.org/10.1016/B978-0-12-801238-3.11037-2]

Kolawole, O.A., Pillay, V., Choonara, Y.E. (2007). Novel polyamide 6, 10 variants synthesized by modified interfacial polymerization for application as a rate-modulated monolithic drug delivery system. *J. Bioact. Compat. Polym., 22*(3), 281-313.
[http://dx.doi.org/10.1177/0883911507078269]

Lombardo, D., Kiselev, M.A., Caccamo, M.T. (2019). Smart nanoparticles for drug delivery application: development of versatile nanocarrier platforms in biotechnology and nanomedicine. *J. Nanomater., 2019*, 1-26.
[http://dx.doi.org/10.1155/2019/3702518]

Lu, Y., Chen, S.C. (2004). Micro and nano-fabrication of biodegradable polymers for drug delivery. *Adv. Drug Deliv. Rev., 56*(11), 1621-1633.
[http://dx.doi.org/10.1016/j.addr.2004.05.002] [PMID: 15350292]

Luliński, P. (2017). Molecularly imprinted polymers based drug delivery devices: a way to application in modern pharmacotherapy. A review. *Mater. Sci. Eng. C, 76*, 1344-1353.
[http://dx.doi.org/10.1016/j.msec.2017.02.138] [PMID: 28482502]

Meinel, A.J., Germershaus, O., Luhmann, T., Merkle, H.P., Meinel, L. (2012). Electrospun matrices for localized drug delivery: Current technologies and selected biomedical applications. *Eur. J. Pharm. Biopharm., 81*(1), 1-13.
[http://dx.doi.org/10.1016/j.ejpb.2012.01.016] [PMID: 22342778]

Miri, A.K., Hosseinabadi, H.G., Cecen, B., Hassan, S., Zhang, Y.S. (2018). Permeability mapping of gelatin methacryloyl hydrogels. *Acta Biomater., 77*, 38-47.
[http://dx.doi.org/10.1016/j.actbio.2018.07.006] [PMID: 30126593]

Molavi, F., Barzegar-Jalali, M., Hamishehkar, H. (2020). Polyester based polymeric nano and microparticles for pharmaceutical purposes: A review on formulation approaches. *J. Control. Release, 320*, 265-282.
[http://dx.doi.org/10.1016/j.jconrel.2020.01.028] [PMID: 31962095]

Moustafa, A.M. (2014). *Poly (Ester Amide) and Poly (Ethyl Glyoxylate).* Nanoparticles for Controlled Drug Release.

Nakagawa, T., Ito, J. (2011). Local drug delivery to the inner ear using biodegradable materials. *Ther. Deliv., 2*(6), 807-814.
[http://dx.doi.org/10.4155/tde.11.43] [PMID: 22822510]

Natarajan, J., Madras, G., Chatterjee, K. (2017). Poly(ester amide)s from Poly(ethylene terephthalate) Waste for Enhancing Bone Regeneration and Controlled Release. *ACS Appl. Mater. Interfaces, 9*(34), 28281-28297.
[http://dx.doi.org/10.1021/acsami.7b09299] [PMID: 28766935]

Pandey, S.P., Shukla, T., Dhote, V.K., Mishra, D.K., Maheshwari, R., Tekade, R.K. (2019). Use of polymers in controlled release of active agents. *Basic Fundamentals of Drug Delivery.*. Elsevier.

Patel, T., Zhou, J., Piepmeier, J.M., Saltzman, W.M. (2012). Polymeric nanoparticles for drug delivery to the central nervous system. *Adv. Drug Deliv. Rev., 64*(7), 701-705.

[http://dx.doi.org/10.1016/j.addr.2011.12.006] [PMID: 22210134]

Peers, S., Montembault, A., Ladavière, C. (2020). Chitosan hydrogels for sustained drug delivery. *J. Control. Release, 326*, 150-163.
[http://dx.doi.org/10.1016/j.jconrel.2020.06.012] [PMID: 32562854]

Prajapati, S.K., Jain, A., Jain, A., Jain, S. (2019). Biodegradable polymers and constructs: A novel approach in drug delivery. *Eur. Polym. J., 120*, 109191.
[http://dx.doi.org/10.1016/j.eurpolymj.2019.08.018]

Puiggalí-Jou, A., del Valle, L.J., Alemán, C. (2019). Drug delivery systems based on intrinsically conducting polymers. *J. Control. Release, 309*, 244-264.
[http://dx.doi.org/10.1016/j.jconrel.2019.07.035] [PMID: 31351927]

Puoci, F., Iemma, F., Picci, N. (2008). Stimuli-responsive molecularly imprinted polymers for drug delivery: a review. *Curr. Drug Deliv., 5*(2), 85-96.
[http://dx.doi.org/10.2174/156720108783954888] [PMID: 18393809]

Rahimzadeh, Z., Naghib, S.M., Zare, Y., Rhee, K.Y. (2020). An overview on the synthesis and recent applications of conducting poly(3,4-ethylenedioxythiophene) (PEDOT) in industry and biomedicine. *J. Mater. Sci., 55*(18), 7575-7611.
[http://dx.doi.org/10.1007/s10853-020-04561-2]

Rahmanian, M., seyfoori, A., Dehghan, M.M., Eini, L., Naghib, S.M., Gholami, H., Farzad Mohajeri, S., Mamaghani, K.R., Majidzadeh-A, K. (2019). Multifunctional gelatin–tricalcium phosphate porous nanocomposite scaffolds for tissue engineering and local drug delivery: *In vitro* and *in vivo* studies. *J. Taiwan Inst. Chem. Eng., 101*, 214-220.
[http://dx.doi.org/10.1016/j.jtice.2019.04.028]

Raizada, A., Bandari, A., Kumar, B. (2010). Polymers in drug delivery: a review. *Int. J. Pharm. Res. Dev, 2*, 9-20.

Salahandish, R., Ghaffarinejad, A., Naghib, S.M., Majidzadeh-A, K., Zargartalebi, H., Sanati-Nezhad, A. (2018). Nano-biosensor for highly sensitive detection of HER2 positive breast cancer. *Biosens. Bioelectron., 117*, 104-111.
[http://dx.doi.org/10.1016/j.bios.2018.05.043] [PMID: 29890392]

Salahandish, R., Ghaffarinejad, A., Omidinia, E., Zargartalebi, H., Majidzadeh-A, K., Naghib, S.M., Sanati-Nezhad, A. (2018). Label-free ultrasensitive detection of breast cancer miRNA-21 biomarker employing electrochemical nano-genosensor based on sandwiched AgNPs in PANI and N-doped graphene. *Biosens. Bioelectron., 120*, 129-136.
[http://dx.doi.org/10.1016/j.bios.2018.08.025] [PMID: 30172235]

Schmaljohann, D. (2006). Thermo- and pH-responsive polymers in drug delivery. *Adv. Drug Deliv. Rev., 58*(15), 1655-1670.
[http://dx.doi.org/10.1016/j.addr.2006.09.020] [PMID: 17125884]

Shao, Y., You, D., Lou, Y., Li, J., Ying, B., Cheng, K., Weng, W., Wang, H., Yu, M., Dong, L. (2019). Controlled Release of Naringin in GelMA-Incorporated Rutile Nanorod Films to Regulate Osteogenic Differentiation of Mesenchymal Stem Cells. *ACS Omega, 4*(21), 19350-19357.
[http://dx.doi.org/10.1021/acsomega.9b02751] [PMID: 31763559]

Song, C.X., Labhasetwar, V., Murphy, H., Qu, X., Humphrey, W.R., Shebuski, R.J., Levy, R.J. (1997). Formulation and characterization of biodegradable nanoparticles for intravascular local drug delivery. *J. Control. Release, 43*(2-3), 197-212.
[http://dx.doi.org/10.1016/S0168-3659(96)01484-8]

Sponchioni, M., Capasso Palmiero, U., Moscatelli, D. (2019). Thermo-responsive polymers: Applications of smart materials in drug delivery and tissue engineering. *Mater. Sci. Eng. C, 102*, 589-605.
[http://dx.doi.org/10.1016/j.msec.2019.04.069] [PMID: 31147031]

Sung, Y.K., Kim, S.W. (2020). Recent advances in polymeric drug delivery systems. *Biomater. Res., 24*(1),

12.
[http://dx.doi.org/10.1186/s40824-020-00190-7] [PMID: 32537239]

Sur, S., Rathore, A., Dave, V., Reddy, K.R., Chouhan, R.S., Sadhu, V. (2019). Recent developments in functionalized polymer nanoparticles for efficient drug delivery system. *Nano-Structures & Nano-Objects, 20*, 100397.
[http://dx.doi.org/10.1016/j.nanoso.2019.100397]

Vigata, M., Meinert, C., Pahoff, S., Bock, N., Hutmacher, D.W. (2020). Gelatin methacryloyl hydrogels control the localized delivery of albumin-bound paclitaxel. *Polymers (Basel), 12*(2), 501.
[http://dx.doi.org/10.3390/polym12020501] [PMID: 32102478]

Wang, B., Wang, S., Zhang, Q., Deng, Y., Li, X., Peng, L., Zuo, X., Piao, M., Kuang, X., Sheng, S., Yu, Y. (2019). Recent advances in polymer-based drug delivery systems for local anesthetics. *Acta Biomater., 96*, 55-67.
[http://dx.doi.org/10.1016/j.actbio.2019.05.044] [PMID: 31152941]

Wang, P.P., Frazier, J., Brem, H. (2002). Local drug delivery to the brain. *Adv. Drug Deliv. Rev., 54*(7), 987-1013.
[http://dx.doi.org/10.1016/S0169-409X(02)00054-6] [PMID: 12384318]

Wang, Y.C., Yuan, Y.Y., Du, J.Z., Yang, X.Z., Wang, J. (2009). Recent progress in polyphosphoesters: from controlled synthesis to biomedical applications. *Macromol. Biosci., 9*(12), 1154-1164.
[http://dx.doi.org/10.1002/mabi.200900253] [PMID: 19924681]

Wolinsky, J.B., Colson, Y.L., Grinstaff, M.W. (2012). Local drug delivery strategies for cancer treatment: Gels, nanoparticles, polymeric films, rods, and wafers. *J. Control. Release, 159*(1), 14-26.
[http://dx.doi.org/10.1016/j.jconrel.2011.11.031] [PMID: 22154931]

Yilmaz, Z.E., Jérôme, C. (2016). Polyphosphoesters: New trends in synthesis and drug delivery applications. *Macromol. Biosci., 16*(12), 1745-1761.
[http://dx.doi.org/10.1002/mabi.201600269] [PMID: 27654308]

Zeinali Kalkhoran, A.H., Vahidi, O., Naghib, S.M. (2018). A new mathematical approach to predict the actual drug release from hydrogels. *Eur. J. Pharm. Sci., 111*, 303-310.
[http://dx.doi.org/10.1016/j.ejps.2017.09.038] [PMID: 28962856]

Zhang, L., Wang, L., Guo, B., Ma, P.X. (2014). Cytocompatible injectable carboxymethyl chitosan/N-isopropylacrylamide hydrogels for localized drug delivery. *Carbohydr. Polym., 103*, 110-118.
[http://dx.doi.org/10.1016/j.carbpol.2013.12.017] [PMID: 24528707]

Zhao, Z., Wang, J., Mao, H.Q., Leong, K.W. (2003). Polyphosphoesters in drug and gene delivery. *Adv. Drug Deliv. Rev., 55*(4), 483-499.
[http://dx.doi.org/10.1016/S0169-409X(03)00040-1] [PMID: 12706047]

CHAPTER 4

Carbon Nanostructure/polymer Composites Processing and Characteristics in Localized Controlled Drug Delivery System (LCDDSs)

Abstract: Carbon nanostructures such as carbon nanotubes, graphene, graphene oxide and their derivatives, have been recognized in biomedicine and drug delivery, due to their outstanding optical, mechanical, thermal, and electrical characteristics. Carbon nanostructures/ polymer composites with various active and functional groups provide many binding sites for inorganic/organic species and biomolecules and are described as favorable candidates to label and drag different drugs, genes, proteins and therapeutic molecules. This chapter focuses on studies about the deployment of nanostructures/ polymer composites, for efficient drug delivery, especially localized controlled drug/gene delivery systems (LCDDS). Effects of various parameters and features, including composite microstructures, hydrophobicity and hydrophilicity of composites, glass transition and polymer matrix molecular weight, on LCDDS are fully examined and discussed.

Keywords: Carbon nanostructure, Carbon nanotube, Composite, Graphene, Polymer, Local drug delivery.

4.1. INTRODUCTION

Nanoscale composites are called nanocomposites, as the filler has a nanoscale size of less than 100 nanometers. Polymeric nanocomposites are organic-inorganic materials which can be synthesized through various routes, such as *in situ* polymerization intercalation, template synthesis, melt intercalation, and exfoliation adsorption (Fawaz and Mittal, 2015). Stimuli-responsive polymer-based nanocomposites have attracted great attention in drug delivery and industry (Kazemi and Naghib, 2020, Naghib and Kazemi, 2020). The used materials and synthesis methods reveal the type of the microstructure. Exfoliated (nanocomposite or delaminated), intercalated (nanocomposite and/or flocculated), and unintercalated (phase separated or microcomposite) materials are 3 types of microstructures (Fawaz and Mittal, 2015).

Seyed Morteza Naghib, Samin Hoseinpour & Shadi Zarshad

Biopolymers have been used to improve targeting biological and functioning reactions (Gooneh-Farahani *et al.*, 2020, Gooneh-Farahani *et al.*, 2019). Various components are added to biopolymers to enhance their ultimate properties for biomedical applications (Rahmanian *et al.*, 2019). Carbon based nanomaterials such as graphene and carbon nanotubes are appropriate choices due to their mechanical, physical, chemical and biological properties (Gooneh-Farahani *et al.*, 2019, Kalkhoran *et al.*, 2018a, Kalkhoran *et al.*, 2018b). Other additives include metal nanoparticles, bioactive glasses, and inorganic particles such as apatite, which have been widely used to enhance the properties of biopolymers. Carbon-based nanocomposites are applicable in biomedical applications, especially drug delivery and tissue engineering, as they have the characteristics of carbon materials and the biocompatibility and biodegradability of polymers simultaneously (Aram and Mehdipour-Ataei, 2020).

Theoretically, a composite is a mixture of a plurality of separable elements, wherein each element has distinctive mechanical and chemical properties. As a general rule, there are two parts in a composite, which are referred to as the matrix and the reinforcement, wherein reinforcement has been distributed in the matrix. Composites are lightweight materials with enhanced mechanical properties. The mechanical properties of composites may be controlled by the interaction between reinforcement and matrix in the inter-phase area and microstructure. Carbon fibers may be used to fabricate lighter weight composites owing to their elevated strength to weight ratio. Carbon fibers must include a plurality of carbon atoms, an increased crystal plane orientation degree along the fiber axis, and a lengthened chain with a high molecular weight (MW) in order to obtain the required functions. Simple processing, low-cost production, and productivity are some of the advantages of polymeric materials (Das *et al.*, 2019).

One approach to categorize nanofillers is based on their dimension, wherein nanowires and nanotubes are categorized as one-dimensional, graphene is categorized as two-dimensional; nanoclays and spherical nanoparticles are categorized as three-dimensional nanofillers. Since graphene and CNTs have a high aspect ratio and improved mechanical strength, they have been extensively used as nanofillers to reinforce polymers. Graphene has a planar structure with an average thickness of less than 5 nanometers. Carbon-based nanomaterials, including CNTs, fullerene, graphene, nanodiamonds and other carbon derivatives have been widely used due to their unique mechanical properties, high electrical and thermal conductivity, and large surface area. These materials include a large number of atoms on their surface, which can enhance their interaction with the polymeric matrix. The combination of polymeric matrices with carbon nanomaterials results in novel nanocomposites with enhanced properties, with a variety of applications due to their enhanced properties. The properties and interactions of polymers and nanomaterials in a nanocomposite, and the properties of the nanocomposite depend on the synthesis method. In order to improve the interfacial interactions and dispersion of carbon-nanocomposites, covalent and non-covalent surface modification methods have been investigated. The covalent approach is based on the patterning of a chemical bond between the nanomaterial and polymer. This results in a powerful interfacial interaction that disrupts the nanomaterials conjugation systems and modifies its characteristics. The non-covalent approach relies on the existence of intermolecular interactions on the surface of the nanomaterial surface through wrapping or physical adsorption. Although normally, this interaction is not strong and limits useful stress transport. This method includes 1) *in situ* polymerization 2) melt blending in intense shearing circumstance and 3) solution mixing.

In *in situ* polymerization, carbon nanomaterials are filled with monomers, and then the polymerization starts by adding an initiator, such as heat or irradiation. In melt blending in intense shearing circumstances, the nanomaterial is blended into a molted polymeric matrix. In solution mixing, an appropriate solution is needed in order to disperse the polymer and carbon nanomaterials. Consequently, new approaches for surface modification of these materials are required to enhance the properties of nanocomposites. Graphene oxide (GO) has suitable properties for biomedical applications due to its biocompatibility, amphiphilicity, and processability which is capable of interacting with biological cells. Due to the great number of carboxyl acid and oxygen containing groups (carbonyl, epoxide and hydroxyl) in the edges and basal planes, GO is stably dispersed in water. However, insolubility of GO in polar and non-polar solvents has limited its application. For this reason, various functionalization methods have been reported. Some of these methods include, the reaction of GO and hexamethylene diisocyanate called HDI which is mixed with a conductive polymer like poly(3,4-ethylenedioxythiophene):poly(styrenesulfonate)   (PEDOT:PSS),   polyaniline (PANI), and polypyrrole-3-carboxylic acid (PPy-COOH) with diverse weight percentages through an effortless solution casting method. The products were further analyzed with various methods to study the effect of percentage and functionalization on the nanocomposite. The results demonstrated that the range of 2-5 weight percent, which is also widely utilized in fuel cells and batteries, had the optimum properties. Some studies have shown that by adding only small amounts of 2dimensional material (<1–5 wt%), such as graphene to the polymeric matrix, the mechanical properties are enhanced by up to 200% compared to pure samples (Díez-Pascual, 2020, Bhattacharya, 2016, Liu *et al.*, 2019).

In spite of conventional composites, optimum properties of nanocomposites are achieved when very low amounts of nanofillers (2 vol%) are added. This is due to the improvement in dispersion, interface chemistry, intrinsic properties of the nanofiller and nanoscale properties of fillers. Consequently, low volume fractions of nanofillers lead to a high interfacial area that can enhance the performance of the polymeric matrix and optimize its mechanical and thermal characteristics. Normally, reinforcement characteristics depend on the aspect ratio of nanomaterials. The size of the nanomaterials and the interface properties of the nanofiller and the matrix affect the features of the reinforced polymer. A variety of nanocomposites may be fabricated depending on the synthesis method and properties of the nanofiller (Ramanathan *et al.*, 2008, Alubaidy *et al.*, 2013).

Nanocomposites reinforced with carbon nanotubes or graphene-based materials have been utilized greatly in engineering applications due to their unique properties such as exclusive morphology and low mass density. For example, polymer matrixes reinforced with CNTs can have a 10 to 150 GPa tensile strength, a 1TPa tensile modulus and a defectless structure. Efficient interfacial interaction between the nanofiller and the polymeric matrix, which is required for better mechanical properties, and homogeneous dispersion of the nanofiller in the matrix are parameters that may affect the properties of the nanocomposite. For example, in a CNT/polymer nanocomposite, pristine structure, dispersion, interfacial interaction with polymeric matrix and orientation of the filler and matrix molecules may affect the microstructural progress (Fig. **1**) (Papageorgiou *et al.*, 2020, Song *et al.*, 2013).

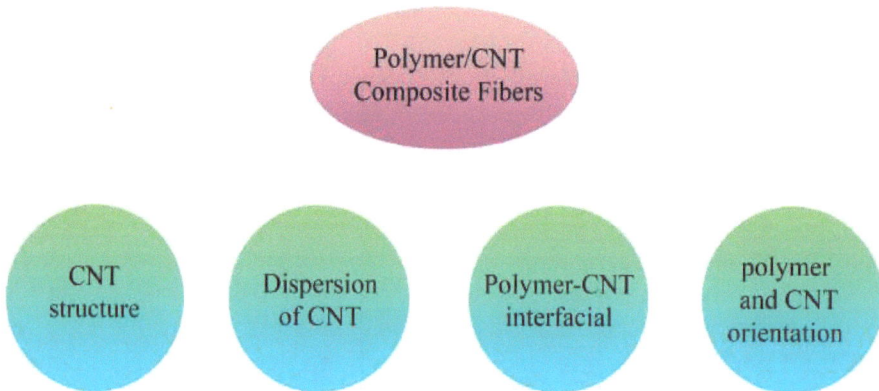

Fig. (1). 4 main parameters influencing microstructural progress of CNTs/polymer nanocomposite fiber in processing

Graphene materials may be modified through covalent and non-covalent approaches. In the covalent approach, the modifier and graphene have strong interactions in the composite. This approach leads to the destruction of graphene structure and consequently, weakens its mechanical and electrical properties. In the non-covalent approach, the graphene structure is preserved. However, this approach may not be utilized in some applications which require strong interactions. The interactions of this approach are electrostatic, van der Waals, π-π, and H bonding, which are weaker compared to covalent interactions.

Natural and synthetic polymeric fibers such as cotton (natural) and polyester (synthetic) have been widely used in packaging, and biomedical applications due to their chemical stability, low density, abrasion resistance, high strength, toughness, thermostable properties, and durability. Therefore, the combination of nanofillers with these fibers can enhance the properties of composites. It is noteworthy that CNTs were first used as nanofillers before graphene-based materials. Although aggregation and high production costs limit the application of CNTs in polymeric nanocomposites. Graphene-based materials have solved the aforementioned issues. It has been shown that, the combination of a polymer chain affects the structural progress of the fiber that forms the composite. Composite fibers including aromatic polymeric matrixes have weaker mechanical properties compared to flexible polymeric matrixes. The properties of composites are enhanced by adding CNT fillers to aromatic polymeric chains. Several studies have demonstrated that carbon-based nanofillers used in polymeric composites affect the morphology of the polymer. Parameters such as crystallization, orientation and nucleation in low amounts of fillers (<1 wt %) have considerable effects on the properties of the nanocomposite (Ji *et al.*, 2016, Liu *et al.*, 2019, Song *et al.*, 2013, Said *et al.*, 2020). In many applications, toughness of the material is a critical feature which is defined as the amount of required stress to spread a preexisting flaw. Therefore, the properties pf carbon composites may be enhanced by considering the processing-structure-property relationships of carbon fiber fracture toughness. There is a straight correlation between the reinforcing carbon fiber fracture toughness and the fracture resistance of the carbon fiber composite (Newcomb, 2016).

In some cases, such as low impedance, high electrical conductivity, and flawless integration of biomolecules with an electrode-tissue interface; intrinsically conducting polymers (ICPs) have been utilized due to their suitable biocompatibility. However, they have limitations such as low stability and low mechanical strength. To solve this issue, the surface of the polymer may be modified with physiologically active species, or blended with a non-conductive polymer with required mechanical properties such as chitosan. Physical or chemical surface treatments have also been used to solve the aforementioned issue. In this regard, nanoparticles may be used to produce nanostructure conducting polymer (Liu *et al.*, 2020).

In a study, a drug delivery system composed of SWNT–PEDOT (poly(3,4-ethylenedioxythiophene)) has been studied to investigate the drug release profile and electrochemical functioning. SWNTs are conductive, which could reduce the resistance of PEDOT and consequently, increase the electrical conductivity of the system. According to the nanoscale size of the filler and increase of the specific surface area of the composite, the charge capacity and release profile were increased by using SWCNT in an implantable drug delivery system (Xiao *et al.*, 2012). Askari *et al.* fabricated a stimuli-responsive implantable protein-integrated graphene/gelatin for localized delivery of chemotherapeutic agent to a tissue engineering substitute. The drug release rate was controlled by the concentration of protein-integrated graphene in the composite to inhibit cancer cell growth after surgery. Fig. (**2**) shows the schematic representation of synthesis of modified graphene with ultrasonic technique and the interaction between nanosheets of protein-integrated graphene and gelatin chains (Askari *et al.*, 2021).

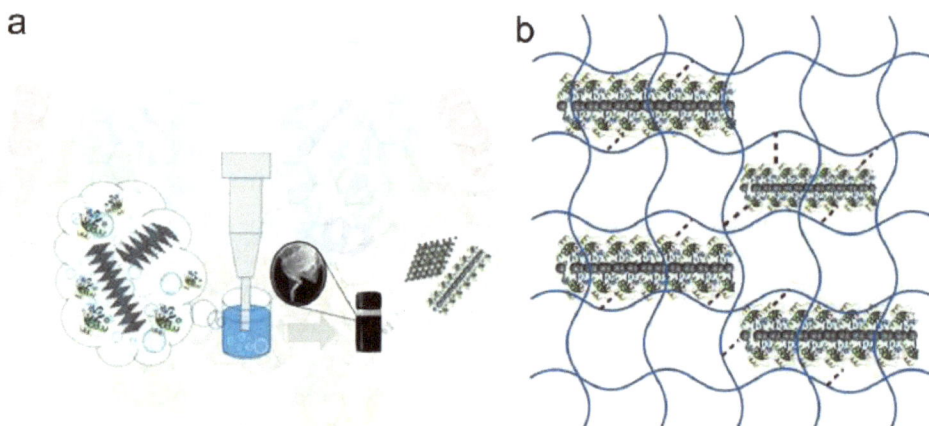

Fig. (2). a) Schematic of the synthesis of the amended graphene, protein-integrated graphene, **b)** Schematic illustration of the composite of gelatin-incorporated protein-integrated graphene (Askari *et al.*, 2021).

4.2. MICROSTRUCTURES

As mentioned before, the objective of fabricating a composite is to integrate the positive properties of each segment and cover the disadvantages of individual materials. The fraction of voids in to the total composite, processing circumstances, and the loaded fiber can highly impact the properties of carbon fiber-based polymeric nanocomposites. Polymers like epoxy, furfuryl, polyimide (PI), and polyetherimide (PEI) in the polymeric matrix have been used as thermoplastic in thermoset polymeric compounds. Usually, thermoset matrixes especially epoxies have been widely utilized with carbon fibers, because these polymers are reinforced under pressure and heat, due to the crosslink of polymers.

But thermoplastic polymers are utilized nowadays, due to their lower processing time, availability, durability in high temperature and ductility. In contrast, thermoset resins are treated gradually in a time-consuming manner. Therefore, thermoplastic-based composites are suitable for this reason. Particle size and pore structure are parameters which influence the release profile of drugs in mesoporous materials. Qu *et al.* demonstrated that the drug loading capacity in materials with mesoporous structure, depended on the pore architecture, surface area and pore volume. In other words, the pore size of these materials clarified the size of the loaded drug. Therefore, it is possible to control the drug release rate by managing the pore size (Das *et al.*, 2019, Gonzalez *et al.*, 2013).

Composites that have biocompatible elements are called biomedical composites or biocomposites. Biocomposites are anisotropic, structure-dependant and have adjustable properties such as cellular response (Kalantari *et al.*, 2019, Kalantari and Naghib, 2019). The structure of many tissues inside the body is similar to polymeric biocomposites. Although the microstructures inside the body are more complicated, including a combination of cells and organic or inorganic materials with significant properties. The morphology and structure of the elements in the microstructures control the performance of the organ. Factors such as geometry, shape, volume fraction and orientation of the secondary element, and properties of the matrix and the secondary element, affect the properties of the composite (Bogdan, 2015).

As mentioned before, modification is used to increase the dispersion and variation of carbon-based materials with different C/O ratio in the microstructure. The modification can adjust electrical conductivity, mechanical properties, functional groups and solubility of the microstructure. Ji *et al.* have reported that graphene-polymer nanocomposites are dispersed in polar solvents and form stable suspensions (Ji *et al.*, 2016).

Another important factor in the microstructure of nanocomposites, is the orientation of nanofillers. If the nanofillers are aligned with the strain direction, the reinforcement is higher. The alignment of nanofillers in graphene-based materials is easier due to the 2D structure of graphene. Fibers used in nanocomposites are categorized as continuous and discontinuous which are also referred to as long fiber and short fiber, respectively. The arrangement of the fibers in the composite matrix such as unidirectional fibers, random fibers, etc., highly depends on their application, (Papageorgiou *et al.*, 2020, Srivastava *et al.*, 2020).

Poly(ethylene glycol) (PEG) is a biodegradable polymer that isn't hydrolytically detached inside the body. PEG is processable and biocompatible due to its solubility in organic solvents and aqueous solutions. This polymer is hydrophilic, and has low toxicity and immunogenicity. PEG can form nanocomposites in combination with carbon-based nanofillers, and is tremendously utilized in drug delivery applications. PEG-g-SWNTs and PEG-g-MWNTs nanocomposites were loaded with paclitaxel (PTX), and used for cancer therapy. The loading capacity of PEG-g-SWNTs and PEG-g-MWNTs was 26% and 36% respectively. The high loading capacity of these nanocomposites was due to the hydrophobic interactions of carbon nanotubes and paclitaxel. The results demonstrated that these nanocomposites were able to kill cancer cells. The release ratio of the nanocomposite drug was higher than the conventional drug, which is related to the higher solubility of the nanocomposite drug in an aqueous medium. Toxicity analysis proved that PEG-g-SWNTs and PEG-g-MWNTs nanocomposites had low cytotoxicity and decreased the proliferation of cancer cells (Aram and Mehdipour-Ataei, 2020).

In another study, the dispersion of a polyurethane (PU) nanocomposite with different amounts of graphene in initial polymerization phase was studied for drug delivery purposes. In this study, the interactions between the graphene and PU were the result of T_m reduction and fusion heat of PU. The graphene was added with the aid of FTIR and the significant shifting of peak positions. The *in vitro* drug release activity of this nanocomposite was observed with a model drug (tetracycline hydrochloride), in T= 37˚C and in PBS medium utilizing UV-visible absorption technique. The results showed that by increasing the amount of graphene, sustained drug delivery was achieved, and the release rate was decreased due to the barrier impact of two-dimensional nanoparticles. Additionally, cell adhesion and MTT assays also confirmed the admissibility of this PU-based nanocomposite. Other groups of scientists developed a PVA/rGO hydrogel loaded with lidocaine hydrochloride as a DDS with an electrical-responsive carrier. The findings exhibited that higher graphene concentrations had higher amounts of loaded lidocaine hydrochloride. By increasing the rGO concentration in the nanocomposite, the negative charge increases, which develops electro-osmosis. The intermolecular interactions of the drug and rGO decreased the attachments and consequently led to more rapid drug release rate although, rGO acted as a physical barrier to reduce drug release in the matrix. Therefore stimuli-responsive drug release was enhanced using rGO nanosheets. By changing the composition of rGO or PVA, the drug release rate varied under the electrical field (Aram and Mehdipour-Ataei, 2020).

In a study, the release behavior of papaverine from poly(ε-caprolactone) was investigated. The results exhibited that the amorphous section of the polymer had an important role in drug diffusion. The samples prepared with higher polymer solution concentration had a slower drug release rate due to variations in the size of the particle, while in the samples with high MW, the microstructure had a coarse internal structure that resulted in a higher drug release rate. This outcome showed that the internal microstructure influenced the drug release performance. Furthermore, the crystalline microstructure of the polymer was easily controlled by using various thermal profiles without changing the total crystallinity. The model underwent annealing at higher temperatures demonstrated sustained drug release, showing the role of crystalline microstructure in drug release performance (Jeong *et al.*, 2003).

4.3. GLASS TRANSITION OF POLYMER MATRIX

Tg or glass transition temperature is one of the major properties of polymers, which highly affects the thermal stability of the polymer. In nanocomposites, Tg controls the higher temperature limit at which the material can be used. The variation of Tg in comparison with the Tg of primary polymer shows the interaction degree of nanofiller and matrices. In spite of many studies regarding the impact of the shape and size of nanoparticles on the Tg of polymeric matrix, it is hard to forecast how these changes may affect Tg. But generally, results achieved by many researchers show that some parameters influence the Tg of nanocomposites. The first parameter that can adjust chemical bonds and interactions of the nanoparticle and polymeric matrix is the chemical structure of the nanoparticle surface. The second parameter is the fabrication method. The third parameter is the stabilization technique of the nanoparticle in the bulk and if the surface modification is with high molecular or low molecular compounds. The last parameter is the thickness, size and aggregation of the nanoparticles. Experimentally, the Tg of the composite might be higher or lower than the Tg of the polymeric matrix, depending on the nanofiller size (Roldughin *et al.*, 2016, Ramanathan *et al.*, 2008).

In nanocomposites, nanofillers can stop the movement of polymeric chains caused by the interfacial interactions of nanofiller and matrices. This interaction controls the variation of Tg. Effectively interacted surfaces with polymer and even hydrogen bonds, have higher Tg compared to the bulk. Additionally, in graphene-based nanocomposites, graphene has a higher roughness, aspect ratio and suitable dispersion in the matrix, resulting in higher glass transition temperature. Researchers showed that, solvent blending with chemically modified graphene or GO or *in situ* polymerization method with unmodified graphene led to the increased glass transition temperature, which is a result of the covalent bondings between the polymer and graphene. On the contrary, solvent and melt blending techniques resulted in minor variation of glass transition temperature. The kind of polymer also influences the glass transition temperature. For instance, nanospherical silica incorporated with Poly(methyl methacrylate) (PMMA), polystyrene (PS) and Polyvinylpyrrolidone (PVP) demonstrated reduction, steady, and increase in Tg, respectively. The glass transition temperature of polymer/CNTs composites depends on the surface functionalization of CNTs (Bhattacharya, 2016, Rittigstein and Torkelson, 2006, Cheng *et al.*, 2016).

Polymers can be categorized based on the transition temperature. Semicrystallines are based on T_m, amorphous polymers are based on T_g, and thermoplastic and thermoset polymers are based on T_{trans}. Block copolymers are categorized as chemically and physically cross-linked amorphous polymers for $T_{trans}=T_g$, and chemically and physically cross-linked semicrystalline polymers for $T_{trans} = T_m$ (Melly *et al.*, 2020).

These changes in features can be related to the polymer properties near the nanoparticles, due to the interactions between the nanofiller and the polymer which is different from polymer-polymer interactions. Therefore, the results depend on the surface area to volume ratio of the nanofillers, and increase by reducing the filler size, especially when reaching nanoscale (Chen *et al.*, 2013).

In many graphene/polymer nanocomposites, there is a sharp increase in Tg, to impediment role of FGSs in the movement of polymeric chains with mechanical interlocking mechanism and also hydrogen bonding with oxygen functionalities at the surface of FGSs, in comparison with glass transition temperature of the polymer. For instance, in rGO/ PVA, there is a 20°C raise at 10% wt, in PS-grafted graphene oxide, there is a 15°C at 12% wt, and in (FGS)/PMMA (functionalized graphene sheet), there is a 30°C increase at 0.05%wt owing. Also, by adding 1%wt FGS to poly (acrylonitrile) (PAN), the glass transition temperature was raised by 46°C. In addition, elevated glass transition temperature of the mentioned nanocomposites over Polystyrene (PS) and Poly(vinyl alcohol) (PVA) is influenced by the decreased chain movement of rGO and graphene oxide owing to covalent bonds. Generally, the existence of graphene oxide in polymeric nanocomposites, increases glass transition temperature and decreases oxygen permeability. By adding constant amounts of carbon-based nanofillers such as carbon nanotubes, graphene and graphene oxide, to polymeric matrices, the increase in glass transition temperature is more obvious in graphene, owing to its 2 dimensional structure and higher surface-to-volume ratio to interact with the substrate (Lu *et al.*, 2019, Azizi-Lalabadi *et al.*, 2020, Liu *et al.*, 2019, Dhand *et al.*, 2013).

Glass transition temperature is highly dependent on the interaction of the polymer/substrate. When the interactions are weakened, Tg is reduced, and the movement of the polymeric chains is improved. On contrary, if more strong interactions occur, Tg rises. There is a repulsive interaction between nanoparticles and polymers. By increasing the volume fraction of nanoparticles, the glass transition temperature decreases due to the reduction of the interface area of the two segments. But for attractive forces between nanoparticles and polymer, the glass transition increases by increasing the volume fraction, which is due to the trapping movement of the polymers close to the interface. This data has been achieved by experimental techniques like nuclear magnetic resonance and calorimetry (Hagita and Morita, 2019, Khan *et al.*, 2016).

In some studies, the impact of carbon nanotubes on glass transition is ambiguous. Single wall carbon nanotubes will decrease Tg, owing to their bundling tendency. However, by using multi-wall carbon nanotubes, Tg remains constant or increases. Additionally, the usage of solvents may lower glass transition temperature because of the remaining effects even after evaporation (Allaoui and El Bounia, 2009, Lappe *et al.*, 2017).

In an investigation by Yoon *et al.*, the Tg of graphene oxide/PLGA (2%wt) nanocomposite increased to 66.7 ˚C, which was higher than Tg of graphene oxide/PLGA (1%wt) nanocomposite Tg=33 ˚C. This proves the presence of powerful chemical bonding and interfacial interactions between the sections of the (2%wt) nanocomposite. In another study by Wang the Tg of PVA/GO hybrids was reported 78 ˚C, while the glass transition of net PVA was 69˚ C. The increase in Tg of the hybrid was because of the hydrogen bonding of between the hydroxyl group of the polymer and graphene oxide (Ji *et al.*, 2016).

A group of researchers studied the variation of glass transition temperature of PS-grafted nanoparticles mixed with PS homopolymers nanocomposite under certain circumstances. However, the amount of the loaded nanoparticles were low with various Mw, and the Tg variations where matrix chains were longer than grafted chains were negative. Also, Tg was negative when the interfacial energy of the NPs-polymer was positive (Chen *et al.*, 2013, Desai *et al.*, 2005).

In another study, an injectable thermoresponsive hydrogel composed of GO/Pluronic block copolymer was prepared by a group of scientists, in which the Pluronic block copolymer acted as the physical crosslinker with no chemical modification of graphene oxide. The conversion of sol-gel happens near the body temperature with no chronic inflammatory reaction in mice. Also, the gel strength may be adjusted with the kind and concentrations of the pluronic. In this system, the photothermal property of graphene oxide was employed to obtain a light-sensitive material for rapid gelation of the system (Sahu *et al.*, 2012).

4.4. HYDROPHOBICITY AND HYDROPHILICITY OF COMPOSITES

A major challenge associated with many drug delivery systems is insolubility or low solubility of the loaded drug. Nanostructures may be used to overcome this issue, due to their delocalized electrons with surface π-conjugated feature and higher specific surface area, which help drugs with the mentioned features *via* π-π stacking and hydrophobic interactions. Bao and his coworkers developed a nanocarrier of chitosan in which the chains were grafted into the surface of GO through amide linkages and camptothecin. The nanocarrier was used as an insoluble drug for cancer therapy, which was loaded on the surface. Results demonstrated that the drug had a high loading capacity (20%) due to the π-π stacking and hydrophobic interactions. Additionally, the MTT analysis exhibited nontoxicity of the net nanocarrier and cytotoxicity of the chitosan-graphene oxide-camptothecin on cancerous cells, in comparison with the drug alone (Aram and Mehdipour-Ataei, 2020).

Interactions of the intestinal wall mucosal layer with hydrophobic materials and polymer chains, have been developed by the potent hydrogen bonding. These results extend residence time of the polymeric vesicles at the intestinal wall and enhance adsorption effectiveness (Gopi *et al.*, 2018).

In polymeric drug carriers, the drug release may be controlled by adjusting surface wettability. For instance, in polymeric carriers which include hydrophilic drug, the hydrophobicity of the surface highly influences drug release behavior, and usually higher hydrophobicity of the drug carrier surface will lead to slower drug release rates s(Xu *et al.*, 2013).

Surface functionalization may be used to enhance the dispersion of carbon nanotubes in polymeric solvents. The side walls in a CNT can be modified through the interaction of hydrophobic groups with long chains, which are used to break carbon nanotubes that aggregate. Consequently, the dispersion is enhanced and short hydrophilic groups are able to make hydrogen bonding with the host polymer. Generally, surface modification produces a balance between the entropic effects required for breaking carbon nanotube aggregates which enhances dispersion, and produces enthalpic effects required to improve interactions at the polymer/CNT interface. This method may be useful especially for thermoplastic polyurethane-(TPU) based nanocomposites, due to their distinguished phase-separated morphology. The hydrophobic hard parts and hydrophilic soft parts in TPU based nanocomposites supply readymade parts to interact with each other (Smart *et al.*, 2010).

A group of researchers, studied the impact of hydrophobicity and hydrophilicity of carbon nanotubes and also their surface chemistry on cell performance. In this study, the nanotubes were wrapped with different kinds of polysaccharides. The results demonstrated that the surface of CNTs which had been wrapped by amylase containing hydroxyl (OH) groups, were favorable to improve cell viability and adhesion properties. In another investigation, a multiwall carbon nanotube grafted polyethylene glycol (MWNT-g-PEG) was synthesized *via* a coupling reaction. Then inclusion complexes following selective threading of the polymer *via* the cavity of α-cyclodextrins units was performed. Due to the hydrophobic interaction and complexation of the polymer and cyclodextrin, a supramolecular injectable hydrogel with potent network, high thermal stability up to 100 °C and enhanced mechanical properties, was developed (Cirillo *et al.*, 2014).

Paclitaxel (PTX) delivery is an anticancer drug. Graphene-based nanomaterials/polymer nanocomposites have been widely utilized for PTX delivery. For example, GO/PEG nanocomposites loaded with PTX have demonstrated cytotoxicity against tumor cells. It is noteworthy that PEG polymers can develop biocompatibility and stability in physiological medium. The drug is attached to the nanocomposite *via* hydrophobic interactions and π-π stacking that improve loading capacity up to 11.2% wt. with the aid of inverted fluorescence microscopy. It was shown that A549 and MCF-7 cells received the cellular uptake of graphene oxide/polyethylene glycol loaded with PTX in 1 hour. In comparison with paclitaxel alone, this nanocomposite resulted in less cell viability, and also about 10% cell viability of MCF-7 and 30% A549 cell viability (Mohajeri *et al.*, 2019, Zhao *et al.*, 2017).

Poly(N-isopropylacrylamide) (PNIPAM) is a smart thermo-sensitive polymer used for tumor-targeted therapy with significant features (for example, lower critical solution temperature (LCST)). This polymer is usually hydrophobic in higher temperatures and hydrophilic under LCST. The improvement of LCST in this polymer, is due to the presence of hydrophilic monomers. Additionally, the hydrophilic state of this polymer turns into hydrophobic in hyperthermic tumor tissues media, which presents high effectiveness of cellular uptake and controlled drug delivery. In another case, a chitosan-modified graphene nanogel for noninvasive drug delivery, was studied. A near-infrared triggered DDS based on chitosan-modified RGO integrated with thermos-sensitive nanogel, was investigated. As a reaction to temperature variations, PNIPAM was turned from a hydrophilic to hydrophobic in water or from swelling to shrinking state which exhibits thermo-sensitivity of PNIPAM (Seo *et al.*, 2016, Zhang *et al.*, 2016).

A PNIPAM-graphene nanosheet-based composite which is composed of 50 percent polymer has suitable solubility in physiological medium. The nanocomposite shifted from hydrophilic state to hydrophobic state, at 33°C. This temperature is moderately less than that in PNIPAM homopolyemr owing to the interactions between polymer and PNIPAM. Most anticancer drugs are water-insoluble and, therefore can be loaded in nanocomposites, due to the hydrophobic interactions and π-π stacking between nanocomposites and the drug. For instance, this nanocomposite has a high loading capacity of 15.6 wt% for camptothecin (CPT) (Punetha *et al.*, 2017).

Wu and coworkers synthesized a novel biodegradable hybrid hydrogel from poly(ε-caprolactone) maleic acid (PGCL-Ma) and dextran derivatives of maleic acid (Dex-Ma) precursors with hydrophobic and hydrophilic characteristics, respectively, and different precursor feed ratio. A hydrophilic-hydrophobic hydrogel with controlled swelling behavior *via* diffusion relaxation or water diffusion methods. The diffusion method was highly dependent on the precursor feed ratio. Hydrogels with higher Dex-Ma component showed combined diffusion–relaxation method and those with higher hydrophobic PGCL-Ma preferred diffusion mechanism. Cocaine methiodide was utilized as a model drug to study the impact of precursor feed ratio on the release behavior and the possibility of drug release from the synthesized hydrogels. The results showed that the drug release behaviors highly depended on the precursor feed ratio. Due to the existence of PGCL-Ma in the PGCL-Ma/Dex-Ma hydrogel, there was a noteworthy reduction in drug burst release and sustained release behavior over a longer period was achieved (Wu and Chu, 2008).

4.5. MOLECULAR WEIGHT OF POLYMER MATRIX

A reasonable clarification in reducing the variation of drug release rate with rising molecular weight, is a dependency of the interfacial layer density on MW. In polymeric nanocomposites with less molecular weight, an extra densely packed interfacial layer results in a notable decrease in higher layer thickness and segmental dynamics. On the contrary, there is a contest between entropic and enthalpic impacts, frustrated chain packing and surface anchoring, respectively, affecting unpredicted dynamic variations in high molecular weight in polymeric nanocomposites (Cheng *et al.*, 2016). Molecular weight is a major property in polymers, which can highly influence physical, chemical and mechanical properties in polymers including Tg, solubility and diffusivity (Omelczuk and McGinity, 1992).

Also, MW in nanovectors significantly affects drug release. The size of nanovectors after systemic administration is less than 6 nanometers, and the MW is less than 50 KDa that can be cleared by the kidney. In contrast, for non-biodegradable polymers, size is important because the polymers are removed by the renal system. Nanovectors with high MW can aggregate in organs like kidney, liver and lung. Therefore, the standard MW of polymers depends on their applications. However, the MW of polymers is in the range of 30 to 100 KDa (Zhao *et al.*, 2017, Prakash *et al.*, 2011).

The functional groups of GO can interact with polymers during processing. For instance, carboxyl groups of GO can interact with hydroxyl groups of polymers *via* esterification. Also, GO can shape nanocomposites with various polymers like PVA. Researchers have investigated the impact of molecular weight on mechanical features of functionalized GO, and found that Young's modulus does not affect the MW of functional groups. Although with rising the level of functional groups, Young's modulus was reduced (Bhattacharya, 2016).

Oromucosal route is a drug delivery path; however, the induction of useful bioadhesion to the mucosal surface is a major limitation of this path. On the other hand, formulations of systemic or local drug delivery systems with low molecular weight materials, with a fast onset of pharmacological results, are effectively done that provide sustained DDSs. Chitosan composites have been widely utilized for wound healing purposes, due to their bioresorbablity, porosity, improved water absorbing capacity, gas permeation, interaction with drugs, cell proliferation, cell migration and cell adherence. This biomaterial is used for intense skin injuries and for immediate recovery through skin grafting. In a study, the delivery of chitosan in low and high MW as excipients to make a spray-dried microsphere for oromucosal drug delivery, has been investigated. According to the results, adding chitosan increased the drug release time and mucoadhesive interaction force of microspheres to the mucosal membrane, which could be an advantage for local therapy applications (Gopi *et al.*, 2018). In another study, the effect of MW on different kinds of PE/graphene nanocomposites, was studied. In this study, 3 kinds of PE with different MW, and comparable crystallinity were prepared (MW of PE1< PE2 < PE3), wherein crystallinity degree was reduced with rising MW. There was no obvious shift in diffraction peaks by adding graphene in polymers, but a graphene diffraction signal was detected in composites, representing the polymer intercalation in the filler interlayers. Morphology analysis of the nanocomposites demonstrated homogeneous dispersion of the fillers in low MW matrices and existence of numerous platelets as stacks, leading to diffraction signals in the X-ray diffractograms (Mittal *et al.*, 2016).

Vega *et al.* studied the impact of MW of polyethylene reinforced with carbon nanotubes on crystallization and rheology. Ethylene/1-hexene random copolymer, linear polyethylene, and ethylene/1-hexene random copolymers with different MWs were utilized. The results showed that matrices with low viscosity have a lower percolation threshold. Also, increasing the molecular weight of the matrices, enhanced the nucleation of nanotubes. As mentioned before, the dispersion of nanotubes is due to their functionalization through dipole-dipole interactions with the polymeric matrix. Khan *et al.* synthesized polystyrene/CNT which was functionalized with oleic acid. The attachment of functional groups on the CNT surface and aqueous dispersion was enhanced by the functionalization of nanotube with oleic acid. It was observed that the existence of carbon nanotube in the polymeric matrices reduced the polymer MW. The MW reduction was inversely related to the nanotube wt %. Employment of chain transfer agents together with carbon nanotubes improved MW with rising CNT wt %, but the overall MW was considerably less than that of the polymer itself (Al Sheheri *et al.*, 2019).

In a comparison study between pristine MWNT/PVDF and functionalized MWNT/PVDF, the functionalization of the composite with PVP *via* the noncovalent method in various MWs, was analyzed. The results demonstrated that the polymer MW could highly increase thermal conductivity. Also, in all polymer molecular weights, the dispersion degree of nanotubes in the polymeric matrix was increased. However, thermal conductivity had a better reaction with lower MW because short polymer chains could wrap the CNTs, developing the dispersion without compromising the connectivity in the nanotube network (Namasivayam *et al.*, 2019).

In a study, the impact of various processing factors on the properties of poly (butylene terephthalate)-based nanocomposites synthesized with ring-opening polymerization (ROP) of cyclic butylene terephthalate (CBT) with graphitic nano platelets, was studied. It was found that the average viscosimetric MW of pCBT in pCBT/GNP nanocomposites was highly influenced by nanoflakes, and MW was decreased in comparison with pure 40% pCBT. Inspite of restricted MW, an acceptable dispersion of graphite nanoparticles was detected (Colonna *et al.*, 2017).

(PLA–PEG)/ (NGO) nanocomposites were designed as DDSs for paclitaxel delivery in cancer therapy. The loading capacity of this nanocomposite was reported to be between 9% and 11%, and the entrapment effectiveness was between 15% and 17%. This system showed sustained *in vitro* drug delivery. The drug release rate was controllable by adjusting the copolymer MW. Additionally, this nanocomposite demonstrated cytotoxicity against A549 human lung cancer cells in culture, which increased with incubation time (Aram and Mehdipour-Ataei, 2020).

In a study, the release behavior of rifampicin (RFP) from Poly(DLlactide-*co*-glycolide) (PLGA) with an MW of 10,000- 20,000, was investigated *in vitro*. The results demonstrated that in lower MW, the impact of MW on drug release behavior was more than that of Tg. It was extensively recognized that MW highly influenced the drug release rate from nanoparticles. As the used temperature for tests, was lower than PLGA glass transition temperature and also the difference in Tg, was 4.8°C at the maximum, it was detected that the effect of Tg was negligible. In addition, the drug release profile of RFP from PLGA7510 and PLLGA7510, and their physical mixtures, were investigated and it was shown that the release profile of NPs can be manipulated *via* mixing PLGA7510 and PLLGA7510. Besides, it was confirmed that the impact of Tg on drug release profile, was more than that of crystallinity in similar MW conditions. In this research, the glass transition temperature of PLLGA7510 was 11.4°C higher than the ambient temperature. Consequently, the effect of Tg increased. This study revealed that not only MW and crystallinity of these copolymers were important, but also the difference between their *T*g and the surrounding temperature affected the release behavior of the drug from the nanoparticles (Takeuchi *et al.*, 2017, Park *et al.*, 2020).

In conclusion, MW plays an important role in the degradation of the polymeric matrix and, consequently, drug release. For the formation of reaction-erosion fronts, it is important to achieve a critical MW in which some oligomers must be soluble. In contrast, in some cases in which MW is low, almost 4000 g/mol, drug release happens in a few hours instead of several days, representing a rapid solution of the polymer. These findings demonstrate the non-linear effect of MW. In polymers, such as PGA, degradation and drug release rates can be altered by changing the MW of PGA. The small changes in the PGA MW resulted in considerable effects on the degradation rate of the polymer. In PGAs with high MW, drug release starts by obtaining critical MW. By reduction in initial MW, the degradation time is lowered, and the drug release initiates earlier. When high MW PGA is mixed with PGA, critical MW is significantly lowered, so the low MW polymer fraction is soluble, and drug release starts without delay. Additionally, models with high PGA with below critical MW show diffusion and dissolution mechanisms in drug release behavior rather than degradation mechanism (Braunecker *et al.*, 2004).

CONCLUSION

This chapter has summarized the attempts to develop LCDDSs based on carbon nanostructures/polymer nanocomposites. Carbon nanostructures like graphene and its derivatives have exceptional mechanical characteristics, versatile bio-functionalities and multipurpose functions for binding to different polymers and biopolymers. Commonly, the final performance and function can be remarkable and have already been depicted in several cases. The impacts of the most important properties and features of the nanocomposites such as composite microstructures, hydrophobicity and hydrophilicity of composites, glass transition and molecular weight of polymer matrix on LCDDS were described. Several factors like geometry, volume fraction and orientation of second element, features of matrix and shape influence the properties of the nanocomposites. Tg of composites regulates the higher limit of the temperature range that its variation in comparison with Tg of primary polymer depicts the interaction degree of nanofiller and matrix. Insolubility or low solubility of the loaded drug is a big challenge that could be addressed by nanostructures, because of their delocalized electrons with surface π-conjugated feature and higher specific surface area, which is able to help drugs with the mentioned features *via* π-π stacking and hydrophobic interactions. Standard Mw of polymers is subjected to their applications in LCDDSs. However, the polymer/composite Mw generally affect the degradation rate in the physiological medium and can alter the drug release rate.

REFERENCES

Al Sheheri, S.Z., Al-Amshany, Z.M., Al Sulami, Q.A., Tashkandi, N.Y., Hussein, M.A., El-Shishtawy, R.M. (2019). The preparation of carbon nanofillers and their role on the performance of variable polymer nanocomposites. *Des. Monomers Polym., 22*(1), 8-53.
[http://dx.doi.org/10.1080/15685551.2019.1565664] [PMID: 30833877]

Allaoui, A., El Bounia, N. (2009). How carbon nanotubes affect the cure kinetics and glass transition temperature of their epoxy composites? – A review. *Express Polym. Lett., 3*(9), 588-594.
[http://dx.doi.org/10.3144/expresspolymlett.2009.73]

Alubaidy, A., Venkatakrishnan, K., Tan, B. (2013). Nanofibers reinforced polymer composite microstructures. *Adv. Nanofiber, 7*, 165-184.

Aram, E., Mehdipour-Ataei, S. (2020). Carbon-based nanostructured composites for tissue engineering and drug delivery. *International Journal of Polymeric Materials and Polymeric Biomaterials,* 1-22.

Askari, E., Naghib, S.M., Zahedi, A., Seyfoori, A., Zare, Y., Rhee, K.Y. (2021). Local delivery of chemotherapeutic agent in tissue engineering based on gelatin/graphene hydrogel. *J. Mater. Res. Technol., 12*, 412-422.
[http://dx.doi.org/10.1016/j.jmrt.2021.02.084]

Azizi-Lalabadi, M., Hashemi, H., Feng, J., Jafari, S.M. (2020). Carbon nanomaterials against pathogens; the antimicrobial activity of carbon nanotubes, graphene/graphene oxide, fullerenes, and their nanocomposites. *Adv. Colloid Interface Sci., 284*, 102250.
[http://dx.doi.org/10.1016/j.cis.2020.102250] [PMID: 32966964]

Bhattacharya, M. (2016). Polymer nanocomposites—a comparison between carbon nanotubes, graphene, and clay as nanofillers. *Materials (Basel), 9*(4), 262.
[http://dx.doi.org/10.3390/ma9040262] [PMID: 28773388]

Bogdan, C. (2015). Simionescu Natural and Synthetic Polymers for Designing Composite Materials/C. Simionescu Bogdan, Ivanov Daniela.. Handbook of Bioceramics and Biocomposites.

Braunecker, J., Baba, M., Milroy, G.E., Cameron, R.E. (2004). The effects of molecular weight and porosity on the degradation and drug release from polyglycolide. *Int. J. Pharm., 282*(1-2), 19-34.
[http://dx.doi.org/10.1016/j.ijpharm.2003.08.020] [PMID: 15336379]

Chen, F., Clough, A., Reinhard, B.M., Grinstaff, M.W., Jiang, N., Koga, T., Tsui, O.K.C. (2013). Glass

transition temperature of polymer–nanoparticle composites: effect of polymer–particle interfacial energy. *Macromolecules, 46*(11), 4663-4669.
[http://dx.doi.org/10.1021/ma4000368]

Cheng, S., Holt, A.P., Wang, H., Fan, F., Bocharova, V., Martin, H., Etampawala, T., White, B.T., Saito, T., Kang, N.G., Dadmun, M.D., Mays, J.W., Sokolov, A.P. (2016). Unexpected molecular weight effect in polymer nanocomposites. *Phys. Rev. Lett., 116*(3), 038302.
[http://dx.doi.org/10.1103/PhysRevLett.116.038302] [PMID: 26849618]

Cirillo, G., Hampel, S., Spizzirri, U.G., Parisi, O.I., Picci, N., Iemma, F. (2014). Carbon nanotubes hybrid hydrogels in drug delivery: a perspective review. *BioMed Res. Int., 2014*, 1-17.
[http://dx.doi.org/10.1155/2014/825017] [PMID: 24587993]

Colonna, S., Bernal, M.M., Gavoci, G., Gomez, J., Novara, C., Saracco, G., Fina, A. (2017). Effect of processing conditions on the thermal and electrical conductivity of poly (butylene terephthalate) nanocomposites prepared *via* ring-opening polymerization. *Mater. Des., 119*, 124-132.
[http://dx.doi.org/10.1016/j.matdes.2017.01.067]

Das, T.K., Ghosh, P., Das, N.C. (2019). Preparation, development, outcomes, and application versatility of carbon fiber-based polymer composites: a review. *Adv. Compos. Hybrid Mater., 2*(2), 214-233.
[http://dx.doi.org/10.1007/s42114-018-0072-z]

Desai, T., Keblinski, P., Kumar, S.K. (2005). Molecular dynamics simulations of polymer transport in nanocomposites. *J. Chem. Phys., 122*(13), 134910.
[http://dx.doi.org/10.1063/1.1874852] [PMID: 15847505]

Dhand, V., Rhee, K.Y., Ju Kim, H., Ho Jung, D. (2013). A comprehensive review of graphene nanocomposites: research status and trends. *J. Nanomater., 2013*, 1-14.
[http://dx.doi.org/10.1155/2013/763953]

Díez-Pascual, A.M. (2020). *Carbon-based polymer nanocomposites for high-performance applications..* Multidisciplinary Digital Publishing Institute.

Fawaz, J., Mittal, V. (2015). Synthesis of polymer nanocomposites: review of various techniques. *Synthesis techniques for polymer Nanocomposites, *1-30.

Gonzalez, G., Sagarzazu, A., Zoltan, T. (2013). Infuence of microstructure in drug release behavior of silica nanocapsules. *J. Drug Deliv., 2013*, 1-8.
[http://dx.doi.org/10.1155/2013/803585] [PMID: 23986870]

Gooneh-Farahani, S., Naghib, S.M., Naimi-Jamal, M.R. (2020). A novel and inexpensive method based on modified ionic gelation for pH-responsive controlled drug release of homogeneously distributed chitosan nanoparticles with a high encapsulation efficiency. *Fibers Polym., 21*(9), 1917-1926.
[http://dx.doi.org/10.1007/s12221-020-1095-y]

Gooneh-Farahani, S., Naimi-Jamal, M.R., Naghib, S.M. (2019). Stimuli-responsive graphene-incorporated multifunctional chitosan for drug delivery applications: a review. *Expert Opin. Drug Deliv., 16*(1), 79-99.
[http://dx.doi.org/10.1080/17425247.2019.1556257] [PMID: 30514124]

Gopi, S., Amalraj, A., Sukumaran, N. P., Haponiuk, J. T., Thomas, S. (2018). Biopolymers and their composites for drug delivery: a brief review. *Macromolecular Symposia* Wiley Online Library.
[http://dx.doi.org/10.1002/masy.201800114]

Hagita, K., Morita, H. (2019). Effects of polymer/filler interactions on glass transition temperatures of filler-filled polymer nanocomposites. *Polymer (Guildf.), 178*, 121615.
[http://dx.doi.org/10.1016/j.polymer.2019.121615]

Jeong, J.C., Lee, J., Cho, K. (2003). Effects of crystalline microstructure on drug release behavior of poly(ε-caprolactone) microspheres. *J. Control. Release, 92*(3), 249-258.
[http://dx.doi.org/10.1016/S0168-3659(03)00367-5] [PMID: 14568406]

Ji, X., Xu, Y., Zhang, W., Cui, L., Liu, J. (2016). Review of functionalization, structure and properties of graphene/polymer composite fibers. *Compos., Part A Appl. Sci. Manuf., 87*, 29-45.

[http://dx.doi.org/10.1016/j.compositesa.2016.04.011]

Kalantari, E., Naghib, S.M. (2019). A comparative study on biological properties of novel nanostructured monticellite-based composites with hydroxyapatite bioceramic. *Mater. Sci. Eng. C, 98*, 1087-1096. [http://dx.doi.org/10.1016/j.msec.2018.12.140] [PMID: 30812992]

Kalantari, E., Naghib, S.M., Iravani, N.J., Esmaeili, R., Naimi-Jamal, M.R., Mozafari, M. (2019). Biocomposites based on hydroxyapatite matrix reinforced with nanostructured monticellite (CaMgSiO₄) for biomedical application: Synthesis, characterization, and biological studies. *Mater. Sci. Eng. C, 105*, 109912. [http://dx.doi.org/10.1016/j.msec.2019.109912] [PMID: 31546348]

Kazemi, F., Naghib, S.M. (2020). Smart controlled release of corrosion inhibitor from normal and stimuli-responsive micro/nanocarriers. *Corrosion Protection at the Nanoscale*. Elsevier.

Khan, W., Sharma, R., Saini, P. (2016). Carbon nanotube-based polymer composites: synthesis, properties and applications. *Carbon Nanotubes-Current Progress of their. Polym. Compos.*

Lappe, S., Mulac, D., Langer, K. (2017). Polymeric nanoparticles – Influence of the glass transition temperature on drug release. *Int. J. Pharm., 517*(1-2), 338-347. [http://dx.doi.org/10.1016/j.ijpharm.2016.12.025] [PMID: 27986475]

Liu, W., Ullah, B., Kuo, C.C., Cai, X. (2019). Two-dimensional nanomaterials-based polymer composites: fabrication and energy storage applications. *Adv. Polym. Technol., 2019*, 1-15. [http://dx.doi.org/10.1155/2019/4294306]

Liu, Y., Yin, P., Chen, J., Cui, B., Zhang, C., Wu, F. (2020). Conducting polymer-based composite materials for therapeutic implantations: from advanced drug delivery system to minimally invasive electronics. *Int. J. Polym. Sci., 2020*, 1-16. [http://dx.doi.org/10.1155/2020/5659682]

Lu, Q., Jang, H.S., Han, W.J., Lee, J.H., Choi, H.J. (2019). Stimuli-responsive graphene oxide-polymer nanocomposites. *Macromol. Res., 27*(11), 1061-1070. [http://dx.doi.org/10.1007/s13233-019-7176-3]

Melly, S.K., Liu, L., Liu, Y., Leng, J. (2020). Active composites based on shape memory polymers: overview, fabrication methods, applications, and future prospects. *J. Mater. Sci., 55*(25), 10975-11051. [http://dx.doi.org/10.1007/s10853-020-04761-w]

Mittal, V., Kim, S., Neuhofer, S., Paulik, C. (2016). Polyethylene/graphene nanocomposites: effect of molecular weight on mechanical, thermal, rheological and morphological properties. *Colloid Polym. Sci., 294*(4), 691-704. [http://dx.doi.org/10.1007/s00396-015-3827-x]

Mohajeri, M., Behnam, B., Sahebkar, A. (2019). Biomedical applications of carbon nanomaterials: Drug and gene delivery potentials. *J. Cell. Physiol., 234*(1), 298-319. [http://dx.doi.org/10.1002/jcp.26899] [PMID: 30078182]

Naghib, S.M., Kazemi, F. (2020). pH-responsive controlled release of corrosion inhibitor from nanocarriers/nanocapsules. *Corrosion Protection at the Nanoscale.*. Elsevier.

Namasivayam, M., Andersson, M.R., Shapter, J. (2019). Role of Molecular Weight in Polymer Wrapping and Dispersion of MWNT in a PVDF Matrix. *Polymers (Basel), 11*(1), 162. [http://dx.doi.org/10.3390/polym11010162] [PMID: 30960146]

Newcomb, B.A. (2016). Processing, structure, and properties of carbon fibers. *Compos., Part A Appl. Sci. Manuf., 91*, 262-282. [http://dx.doi.org/10.1016/j.compositesa.2016.10.018]

Omelczuk, M.O., McGinity, J.W. (1992). The influence of polymer glass transition temperature and molecular weight on drug release from tablets containing poly(DL-lactic acid). *Pharm. Res., 9*(1), 26-32. [http://dx.doi.org/10.1023/A:1018967424392] [PMID: 1589405]

Papageorgiou, D.G., Li, Z., Liu, M., Kinloch, I.A., Young, R.J. (2020). Mechanisms of mechanical reinforcement by graphene and carbon nanotubes in polymer nanocomposites. *Nanoscale, 12*(4), 2228-2267. [http://dx.doi.org/10.1039/C9NR06952F] [PMID: 31930259]

Park, K., Otte, A., Sharifi, F., Garner, J., Skidmore, S., Park, H., Jhon, Y.K., Qin, B., Wang, Y. (2020). Potential Roles of the Glass Transition Temperature o wf PLGA Microparticles in Drug Release Kinetics. *Mol. Pharm.*

Prakash, S., Malhotra, M., Shao, W., Tomaro-Duchesneau, C., Abbasi, S. (2011). Polymeric nanohybrids and functionalized carbon nanotubes as drug delivery carriers for cancer therapy. *Adv. Drug Deliv. Rev., 63*(14-15), 1340-1351. [http://dx.doi.org/10.1016/j.addr.2011.06.013] [PMID: 21756952]

Punetha, V.D., Rana, S., Yoo, H.J., Chaurasia, A., McLeskey, J.T., Jr, Ramasamy, M.S., Sahoo, N.G., Cho, J.W. (2017). Functionalization of carbon nanomaterials for advanced polymer nanocomposites: A comparison study between CNT and graphene. *Prog. Polym. Sci., 67*, 1-47. [http://dx.doi.org/10.1016/j.progpolymsci.2016.12.010]

Rahmanian, M., seyfoori, A., Dehghan, M.M., Eini, L., Naghib, S.M., Gholami, H., Farzad Mohajeri, S., Mamaghani, K.R., Majidzadeh-A, K. (2019). Multifunctional gelatin–tricalcium phosphate porous nanocomposite scaffolds for tissue engineering and local drug delivery: *In vitro* and *in vivo* studies. *J. Taiwan Inst. Chem. Eng., 101*, 214-220. [http://dx.doi.org/10.1016/j.jtice.2019.04.028]

Ramanathan, T., Abdala, A.A., Stankovich, S., Dikin, D.A., Herrera-Alonso, M., Piner, R.D., Adamson, D.H., Schniepp, H.C., Chen, X., Ruoff, R.S., Nguyen, S.T., Aksay, I.A., Prud'Homme, R.K., Brinson, L.C. (2008). Functionalized graphene sheets for polymer nanocomposites. *Nat. Nanotechnol., 3*(6), 327-331. [http://dx.doi.org/10.1038/nnano.2008.96] [PMID: 18654541]

Rittigstein, P., Torkelson, J.M. (2006). Polymer-nanoparticle interfacial interactions in polymer nanocomposites: Confinement effects on glass transition temperature and suppression of physical aging. *J. Polym. Sci., B, Polym. Phys., 44*(20), 2935-2943. [http://dx.doi.org/10.1002/polb.20925]

Roldughin, V.I., Serenko, O.A., Getmanova, E.V., Novozhilova, N.A., Nikifirova, G.G., Buzin, M.I., Chvalun, S.N., Ozerin, A.N., Muzafarov, A.M. (2016). Effect of hybrid nanoparticles on glass transition temperature of polymer nanocomposites. *Polym. Compos., 37*(7), 1978-1990. [http://dx.doi.org/10.1002/pc.23376]

Sahu, A., Choi, W.I., Tae, G. (2012). A stimuli-sensitive injectable graphene oxide composite hydrogel. *Chem. Commun. (Camb.), 48*(47), 5820-5822. [http://dx.doi.org/10.1039/c2cc31862h] [PMID: 22549512]

Said, R.A.M., Hasan, M.A., Abdelzaher, A.M., Abdel-Raoof, A.M. (2020). Review—Insights into the Developments of Nanocomposites for Its Processing and Application as Sensing Materials. *J. Electrochem. Soc., 167*(3), 037549. [http://dx.doi.org/10.1149/1945-7111/ab697b]

Seo, H.I., Cheon, Y.A., Chung, B.G. (2016). Graphene and thermo-responsive polymeric nanocomposites for therapeutic applications. *Biomed. Eng. Lett., 6*(1), 10-15. [http://dx.doi.org/10.1007/s13534-016-0214-6]

Smart, S., Fania, D., Milev, A., Kannangara, G.S.K., Lu, M., Martin, D. (2010). The effect of carbon nanotube hydrophobicity on the mechanical properties of carbon nanotube-reinforced thermoplastic polyurethane nanocomposites. *J. Appl. Polym. Sci., 117*, NA. [http://dx.doi.org/10.1002/app.31115]

Song, K., Zhang, Y., Meng, J., Green, E., Tajaddod, N., Li, H., Minus, M. (2013). Structural polymer-based carbon nanotube composite fibers: understanding the processing–structure–performance relationship. *Materials (Basel), 6*(6), 2543-2577. [http://dx.doi.org/10.3390/ma6062543] [PMID: 28809290]

Srivastava, V.K., Jain, P.K., Kumar, P., Pegoretti, A., Bowen, C.R. (2020). Smart Manufacturing Process of

Carbon-Based Low-Dimensional Structures and Fiber-Reinforced Polymer Composites for Engineering Applications. *J. Mater. Eng. Perform., 29*(7), 4162-4186.
[http://dx.doi.org/10.1007/s11665-020-04950-3]

Takeuchi, I., Yamaguchi, S., Goto, S., Makino, K. (2017). Drug release behavior of hydrophobic drug-loaded poly (lactide-co-glycolide) nanoparticles: Effects of glass transition temperature. *Colloids Surf. A Physicochem. Eng. Asp., 529*, 328-333.
[http://dx.doi.org/10.1016/j.colsurfa.2017.04.080]

Wu, D.Q., Chu, C.C. (2008). Biodegradable hydrophobic–hydrophilic hybrid hydrogels: swelling behavior and controlled drug release. *J. Biomater. Sci. Polym. Ed., 19*(4), 411-429.
[http://dx.doi.org/10.1163/156856208783719536] [PMID: 18318955]

Xiao, Y., Ye, X., He, L., Che, J. (2012). New carbon nanotube-conducting polymer composite electrodes for drug delivery applications. *Polym. Int., 61*(2), 190-196.
[http://dx.doi.org/10.1002/pi.3168]

Xu, H., Li, H., Chang, J. (2013). Controlled drug release from a polymer matrix by patterned electrospun nanofibers with controllable hydrophobicity. *J. Mater. Chem. B Mater. Biol. Med., 1*(33), 4182-4188.
[http://dx.doi.org/10.1039/c3tb20404a] [PMID: 32260972]

Zeinali Kalkhoran, A.H., Naghib, S.M., Vahidi, O., Rahmanian, M. (2018). Synthesis and characterization of graphene-grafted gelatin nanocomposite hydrogels as emerging drug delivery systems. *Biomed. Phys. Eng. Express, 4*(5), 055017.
[http://dx.doi.org/10.1088/2057-1976/aad745]

Zeinali Kalkhoran, A.H., Vahidi, O., Naghib, S.M. (2018). A new mathematical approach to predict the actual drug release from hydrogels. *Eur. J. Pharm. Sci., 111*, 303-310.
[http://dx.doi.org/10.1016/j.ejps.2017.09.038] [PMID: 28962856]

Zhang, B., Wang, Y., Zhai, G. (2016). Biomedical applications of the graphene-based materials. *Mater. Sci. Eng. C, 61*, 953-964.
[http://dx.doi.org/10.1016/j.msec.2015.12.073] [PMID: 26838925]

Zhao, H., Ding, R., Zhao, X., Li, Y., Qu, L., Pei, H., Yildirimer, L., Wu, Z., Zhang, W. (2017). Graphene-based nanomaterials for drug and/or gene delivery, bioimaging, and tissue engineering. *Drug Discov. Today, 22*(9), 1302-1317.
[http://dx.doi.org/10.1016/j.drudis.2017.04.002] [PMID: 28869820]

CHAPTER 5

Composites in Localized Controlled Drug Delivery Systems (LCDDSs)

Abstract: Localized controlled drug delivery systems (LCDDSs) have become the main topic in drug delivery, tissue engineering and pharmaceutical science by enhancing formulations and processes of controlled delivery. The side effects and problems of materials/biomaterials are critical and may lead to several issues, such as reducing the effective drug dose, delaying the treatment process, and not having a particular continuous treatment. Therefore, composites composed of hybrid materials/biomaterials with excellent release properties, biocompatibility, stability and biodegradability, with local adjusted release rates, are an alternate choice for protective drug delivery. Several approaches to fabricating composite-based LCDDSs include emulsification-solvent evaporation, spray drying, electrospraying, supercritical fluids processing, microfluidics, and nanoprecipitation/solvent displacement and emulsion. This chapter describes the advances in micro/nanoscaled composite-based LCDDSs and their fabrication methods.

Keywords: Drug delivery, Fabrication methods, Microfluidics, Microscaled composites, Nanoscaled composites, Release properties.

5.1. INTRODUCTION

Drug delivery systems are classified based on the intended action position and the administration route, which can both have systematic or localized methods (Ji and Kohane, 2019). Studies demonstrate that drug administration can be local with local or systemic impact or systemic with local effect (Askari *et al.*, 2021a, Gooneh-Farahani *et al.*, 2019). Pharmacological impacts of local drug action have been preferably limited to a specific part of the body, such as a particular nerve, or a specific organ, with benefits including enhanced efficacy, reduction in drug contact with off-target organs, and decreased toxicity. This method is able to supply the required dosage of the drug at the desired site with an acceptable therapeutic ratio, which results in a secure therapy. Local delivery is achieved *via* straight local administration, including inhalation, implantation or injection of DDSs at the target organ. Local administration can result in systemic effects throughout the water in the body. The drug dose in local administration is enough

Seyed Morteza Naghib, Samin Hoseinpour & Shadi Zarshad

to be distributed all over the body at therapeutic concentrations, and achieve a systemic effect. For local impact with local administration, such as free or encapsulated peripheral nerve blocks with local anesthetics, the dose of the drug is just enough for local impact. (Ji and Kohane, 2019).

The developed local drug delivery system has an advantage over systemic or conventional routes of drug administration. In oral, parenteral or inhalation delivery routes, high dosages of drugs are required to ensure sufficiency. Moreover, the pharmacological effectivity of novel drugs decreases due to their hydrophobicity and their disability to dissolve in water. The loss of blood circulation in the infected skeletal tissue results in inadequate drug distribution at the desired sites, which causes challenges in drug delivery. In contrast, efficient drug delivery to the desired site with minimum side effects and controlled drug release is achieved. Implants may cause infections due to the formation of well-defined bacterial networks on the implant surface. These bacterial networks are called biofilms and can highly resist antibiotics. However, the issue may be solved by local antibiotic delivery (Kumar *et al.*, 2019).

Intermittent oral drug delivery has been widely utilized for many diseases such as cancer. These techniques, introduce high dosages of the administered drug in the blood circulation, which may cause major side effects. Particularly in cancer therapy, where the drugs contain large amounts of toxic molecules, the high dosages may harm both normal and abnormal cells and consequently decrease the therapy efficacy. It has been observed that high concentrations of therapeutic molecules in the blood (more than 1%) may cause failure in organs such as the kidney. As a result, a local and controlled drug delivery system with minimum side effects, and high efficacy is required. Many polymer-based local drug delivery systems with various properties have been investigated in the art. These systems are responsive to environmental conditions, such as pH, enzymes, temperature, *etc.* Passive DDSs are based on the diffusion or slow release of a particular dose of drug over a period of time. Passive DDSs cannot be used for the administration of high drug doses and have a long drug release time. Another challenge of passive DDSs is controlling the drug release, such as the burst release of drugs with non-zero release kinetics in the first days of implantation (Mousavi *et al.*, 2018).

Carbon nanostructures are widely used in biomedical applications and specifically drug delivery due to their high specific surface area, low weight, ultra-high mechanical strength, release of heat in near-infrared radiation, stability at high temperatures and chemical properties. NIR may be used for local drug delivery and cancer treatment, due to its simple implementation. However, the use of NIR radiation may cause severe issues such as self-aggregation and toxicity, inside the body. However, surface functionalization with hydrophilic atoms may prevent the accumulation of carbon nanotubes. CNTs can be functionalized through covalent and non-covalent methods. They can interact with other molecules *via* π-π stacking on their inner and outer surface. Hydrogen bondings are also widely used in drug delivery to enhance the properties of the drug, which leads to bioavailability, biocompatibility, controlled drug delivery and also decreased drug toxicity. As a result, the functionalization of CNTs may enhance their performance as a drug carriers (Karimzadeh *et al.*, 2021, Jha *et al.*, 2020, Li *et al.*, 2020).

Most of the drugs used in cancer therapy are hydrophobic and insoluble in water. Consequently, the drug cannot be delivered to the specific site by hydrogels. Various methods have been used to develop drug solubility using hydrophilic polymer solutions. As an example, the anticancer drugs may be embedded inside micelles resulting in a hydrophilic combination. Graphene can interact with hydrophobic drugs due to its π structure. As a result, combining graphene-based materials with Pluronic F-127 hydrogels may be a suitable approach to enhance the properties of DDSs. In an investigation, DDSs based on injectable hydrogels have been used to deliver anti-cancer drugs. All hydrogel samples were produced *via* supramolecular self-assembly of α-CD and PEO blocks of Pluronic F-127. By increasing the graphene oxide and reduced-GO concentration, the hydrogel gelation time decreased. The dynamic viscoelastic performance of the samples revealed the elastomeric behavior of GO and rGO composite hydrogels. The hydrogel samples underwent erosion in Phosphate-buffered saline (PBS). The erosion rate of composite hydrogels was lower compared to native samples. CPT and DXR were used as model drugs, and had a higher drug release rate in Pluronic F- 127 solutions compared to functionalized GO or rGO solutions. Moreover, the drug release from composite hydrogel was controllable. The findings of this study demonstrated that graphene oxide and rGO composite hydrogels might be used as injectable carriers to deliver anti-cancer drugs (Hu *et al.*, 2014).

Substitutes used for bones are biodegradable, such as acrylic polymers and ceramics, with the ability to carry bone regeneration drugs. These implants must have properties such as bioactivity, efficient bone regeneration, and controlled drug release, which are difficult to obtain. But, implantable composites for bone substitute purposes can have the required properties. Several materials, such as stable polymers, glass, ceramics, etc., have been investigated for local delivery for bone regeneration purposes. Materials used for carrier formation must have specific characteristics, such as bioactivity, osteoconductivity, osteoinductivity, suitable release behavior, and mechanical and biological compatibility with the local bone tissue. Although every carrier material may have outstanding benefits over other carriers, limitations such as non-degradability, high cost, unfavorable tissue response of biodegradable polymer, and weak ductility may decrease the application of some materials. Decreasing adverse side effects, reducing hospitalization, low cost, sustained drug delivery, preventing parenteral administration, high drug concentration, and high drug stability for a long period of time are some advantages of local drug delivery (Soundrapandian *et al.*, 2009, Krisanapiboon *et al.*, 2006).

A nanocomposite hydrogel based on injectable carbohydrate bulk hydrogels, including entrapped, PNIPAAM- based microgel with soft structure, led to easier bupivacaine release in several weeks, was longer than the same time required for the hydrogel alone. Factors such as drug release time, drug release rate, and the drug burst are to be controlled by varying the phases in the nanocomposite. According to the art, both the nanocomposite hydrogel and gel precursors showed minimum toxicity even at higher concentrations. These materials might facilitate clinical requirements for long-time small molecule local drug delivery with the aid of injectable, in situ-gellable hydrogels (Sivakumaran *et al.*, 2011).

5.2. MICROSCALED COMPOSITES IN DDS

The concept of drug delivery is to deliver drugs to the targeted site inside the body. Challenges associated with DDSs are the production of drug carriers with sustainable and targeted drug release behavior, control of drug bioavailability after contact with the target tissue, enhancement of the specificity for target cells, and enhancement of macromolecule delivery into target cells. One method is the micro-encapsulation of drugs which provides controllable drug delivery and improves drug delivery accuracy with extended active drug effective time. In addition, drug encapsulation protects the protein from cells or enzymes in surrounding tissues, until it has been released (Liu *et al.*, 2020).

In an investigation, drugs with various hydrophobicities were encapsulated in Polylactic acid/ Polylactic-co-glycolic acid (PLA/PLGA) composites *via* ROP. PLA/PLGA composites had a lower weight distribution compared to industrialized composites, and the hydrophilicity was adjustable by manipulating the lactide content. Additionally, the stability and size of the composite were highly dependent on the solvents and stabilizers. Polymers with core-shell structures were achievable through coaxial electrospinning, wherein variations in voltage, and external and internal flows that affect fiber morphology, may remove the burst impact of coaxial electrospinning. The fibers demonstrated controllable fiber delivery with the existence of shells. The mouse preosteoblastic MC3T3-E1 proliferated and differentiated *via* the mixture of human bone morphogenetic protein-2 (BMP-2). PLA and Rifapentine were utilized as the drug carrier and sample drug, respectively, for sustained drug release. The microspheres were utilized as implants with HA/β-TCP or allogeneic bone, in osteoarticular tuberculosis therapy, which resulted in a drug loading efficacy of 78% and 36%, respectively. The results showed durable antibacterial properties and outstanding osteoinductive and osteoconductive features (Liu *et al.*, 2020).

5.3. NANOSCALED COMPOSITES IN DDS

Nanomaterials have been greatly used in biomedicines (Askari *et al.*, 2019, Askari *et al.*, 2021b, Kalkhoran *et al.*, 2018) and drug delivery (Ghorbanzade and Naghib, 2019, Ghorbanzade *et al.*, 2019, Gooneh-Farahani *et al.*, 2020, Rahmanian *et al.*, 2019, Seyfoori *et al.*, 2019, Zeinali Kalkhoran *et al.*, 2018). Localized drug delivery can decrease side effects and increase the drug delivery efficacy. In this regard, Weaver *et al.* investigated an electrically responsive graphene oxide/ conducting polymer nanocomposite loaded with dexamethasone. Drug release started as a reaction to voltage changes with a linear release behavior and significant toxicity. Also, the drug dosage was adjustable by varying the stimulation magnitude. Moreover, nano-delivery of graphene enhanced the antiproliferative impacts of gambogic acid (GA) on pancreatic and breast cancer cells without toxicity. Another group of scientists explored PLA/PEG copolymers to stabilize graphene oxide in an aqueous medium to be used as a paclitaxel carrier. The copolymer was able to stabilize graphene oxide for PTX delivery to A549 cancer cells. Graphene nanomaterials and their nanocomposites such as starch functionalized graphene, Pt(IV) conjugated nano-GO,96 PEGylated GO, GO stabilized in electrolyte solutions using hydroxyethyl cellulose, DNA–graphene hybrid nanoaggregates, and GO-wrapped mesoporous silica nanoparticles103 were used for various drug delivery systems (Singh, 2016).

Despite the improvements in cancer therapy, ineffective results due to low bioavailability and low delivery to the desired site are the main limitations. Graphene-based carriers may be used to solve the issues related to cancer therapy. Barahuie *et al.* showed that pH-responsive graphene oxide might be used as a chlorogenic acid (CA) carrier for controlled delivery. This platform exhibited maximum toxicity toward cancerous cells and minimum toxicity toward healthy cells. Studies show that the combination of folic acid with polyethyleneimine (PE1), functionalized GO, and carboxymethyl cellulose has no toxic impact on healthy cells meanwhile having controlled DOX release (Rajakumar *et al.*, 2020).

Additionally, GO-based hydrogels may be used to conjugate hydrophobic cancer therapy drugs and release the drug under control. Graphene/grapehenoxide-based hydrogels loaded with CPT and DOX can release anticancer drugs at a slower rate compared to Pluronic F-127 solution, resulting in a high binding interaction of hydrophobic drugs related to the G/GO content in the hydrogels. Another study stated that rGO/ AgNPs (Ag nanoparticles) stimulated the generation of free radicals (ROS) in A549 lung cancer cells, which may damage phospholipids and cause cell death *via* apoptosis (Rajakumar *et al.*, 2020).

In chemophotothermal synergistic treatment of colon cancerous cells, dual stimuli-sensitive polyelectrolyte NPs were fabricated *via* layer-by-layer assembly of carboxylated nanocellulose and aminated nanodextran on the graphene oxide surface. Studies on the HCT116 human colon cancer cell line showed that NPs led to the intracellular release of curcumin with NIR-sensitive and pH-sensitive behavior. Therefore, nanocellulose/graphene nanocomposites may be used as anticancer drug carriers with controlled release. Platforms such as nanocomposite carboxymethyl cellulose/GO hydrogel beads, and macroporous polyacrylamide hydrogels for DOX delivery were fabricated *via* the oil-in-water Pickering emulsion method, holding graphene oxide and hydroxyethyl cellulose with a quaternary ammonium group. Cellulose and carbon nanotubes-based nanocomposites can be utilized for drug delivery applications, as CNTs may be conjugated with many therapeutic agents and drugs. For instance, a system composed of multiwall CNT and cellulose acetate membrane was used for indomethacin delivery. The results showed that the system was able to eliminate cancer cells by nanocomposites even without a loaded drug (Bacakova *et al.*, 2020).

A smart thermo-responsive hydrogel drug carrier based on chitosan and dibasic sodium phosphate (DSP) was developed. *In vivo* and *in vitro* studies demonstrated the biodegradability and biocompatibility of hydrogel, making it an appropriate choice for local drug delivery. Camptothecin (CPT) nanocolloid with a diameter of 500nm was used as a sample drug. Camptothecin (CPT) nanocolloid was produced using sonication and microprecipitation method with trimethyl chitosan (TMC) stabilizer and polymeric surfactant. Then the drug was loaded in CS/DSP hydrogel. Lactone (Fig. **1**), which is the active mode of CPT, may be kept protected in the hydrogel for a minimum of one week, indicating the suitable microenvironment of the hydrogel. In the meantime, *in vitro* studies showed sustained release of lactone from the hydrogel for a long time with negligible toxicity in lower concentrations (Li *et al.*, 2011).

Researchers prepared CNT-reinforced PE nanocomposites with the functionalized surface *via* the chemical etching method. The interconnected micropores in the nanocomposite were filled with gentamicin-loaded CS. The nanocomposite exhibited sustained drug delivery for up to 21 days and effectively eliminated bacterial growth, consequently avoiding primary infection in the surgical area. Additionally, biocompatibility assays revealed the suitability of surface-modified

CNTs for clinical applications. The specific rate and the friction coefficient reduced up to 36% and 48%, respectively, compared to the net PE polymer, by adding 0.1 wt% of nanotubes to the polymer. Also, the hardness and elastic modulus of the CNT-reinforced UHMWPE improved up to 37% and 31%, respectively, due to the efficient load sharing. Implants loaded with a drug, have enhanced mechanical properties even after drug release, compared to unmodified polymer surfaces (Kumar *et al.*, 2019).

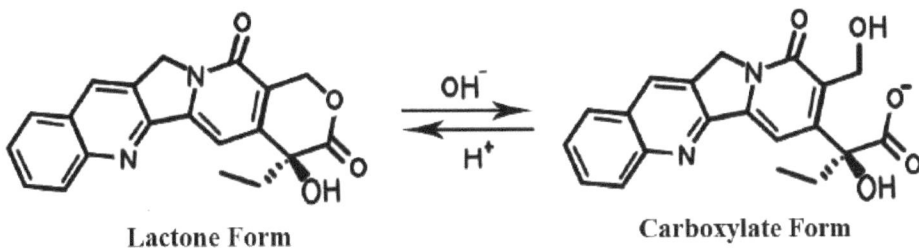

Lactone Form   **Carboxylate Form**

Fig. (1). Structure of camptothecin (lactone and carboxylate form).

PVA/GT/GO/TCH nanofiber scaffolds were used in transdermal drug delivery with lower cytotoxicity and biocompatibility (Gum Tragacanth (GT) and tetracycline hydrochloride (TCH)). In comparison with GO/ PVA/GT nanofibers, PVA/GT nanofibers had improved mechanical properties with smaller sizes and also a slower drug release due to the presence of GO. Antibacterial studies revealed no bacteria growth; therefore, the combination can be used as an appropriate system for controlled drug delivery (Abdoli *et al.*, 2020).

A dual stimuli-sensitive drug carrier to obtain pH and microwave-triggered drug release were designed with a flower-mesoporous sphere of 270 nm (Fig. **2**). Flower-like porous carbon (FPCS) containing a large specific surface area (101 m2/g) and plenty of channels were utilized for drug encapsulation. The surface of FPCS was modified with Fe_3O_4 NPs to obtain a magnetic targeting agent. DOX was loaded onto the carrier as a model drug. The outer layer of the carrier was functionalized with ZnO NPs as a sealing agent to inhibit premature drug leakage. ZnO dissolves in acidic circumstances, which may be used for pH-sensitive drug release. Simultaneously, the conductive loss of FPCS, the magnetic loss of Fe_3O_4 and the dielectric loss of ZnO result in a suitable microwave absorption carrier, thus providing microwave-triggered DOX delivery. The drug loading efficacy of the drug carrier was 99.1%. Drug release rate at 12 h was 8.2%, 19.0%, and 56.3% at pH of 7.4, 5.0 and 3.0 respectively. In addition, microwave radiation played an important role in drug delivery, since the drug release rate increased from 8.2% to 39.9% with microwave stimulation at pH of 7.4. Cytotoxicity assays showed the biocompatibility of the carrier (Yang *et al.*, 2020).

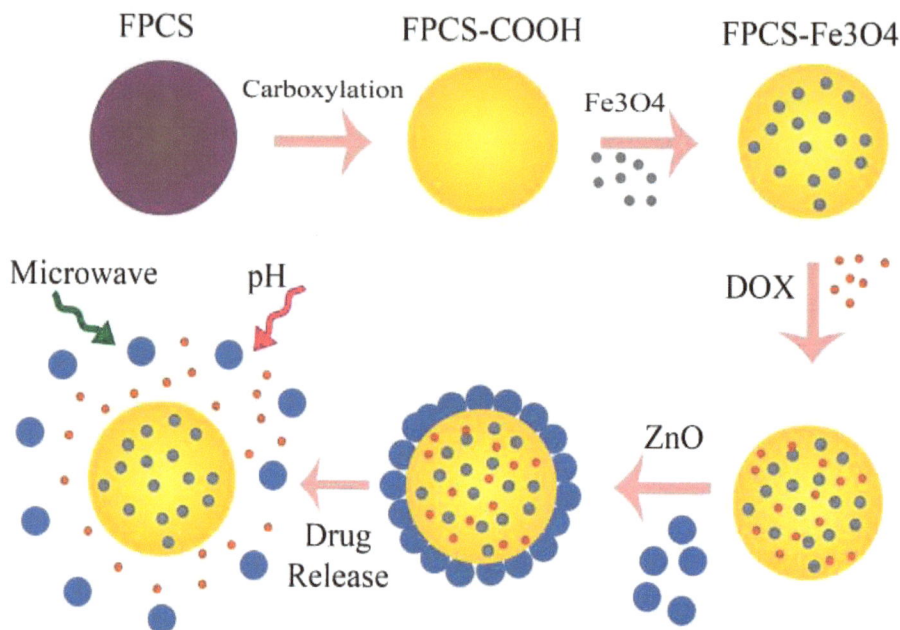

Fig. (2). Schematic of the synthesis, surface modification, DOX loading and bi-triggered release of the FPCS-Fe$_3$O$_4$-DOX-ZnO composite.

In another study, a NIR light-sensitive nanocomposite containing mesoporous silica (MS) shell coated with carbon nanotubes was designed. The combination was loaded with DOX and capped with plasma protein human serum albumin (HSA) as a biocompatible interface. The effect of parameters such as concentration and laser power on the photothermal features of this nanocomposite was explored. It was found that altering the power at 1 W/cm^2 is quite suitable for controlling temperature under the necrosis temperature (45°C). The CNT@MS@IBAM-DOX@HSA (isobutyramide(IBAM)) nanocomposite exhibited NIR release, with a primary burst release depending on the composite concentration. It was demonstrated that DOX delivery may be controllable using 1 W/cm^2 NIR (Li *et al.*, 2020).

5.4. THE EPR EFFECT

Passive targeting is defined as the natural reaction of the body to a molecule. The body directs the movement and accumulation of the drug at a specific site. Normally, this concept is based on drug delivery *via* the macrophage system or monocyte-phagocytic system of other cells relying on the properties and size of the drug. Therefore, drug carriers release the drug during circulation or entering the targeted tissue (Shukla *et al.*, 2019).

Tumor blood vessels are heterogeneous due to their specific structure, organization and functions. Tumor blood vessels have abnormal dynamics such as tortuosity, lack base membrane and are hyperpermeable in nature. So, there are basic differences between the vasculature system of a tumor tissue and normal tissue. The blood vessels in a tumor have different diameters, blind ends, irregular shape, and unusual bulges. When diffusion is restricted in blood vessels, new vasculatures are configured in order to absorb nutrition and oxygen and excrete waste, which is called angiogenesis. The deficiency of vasculature supportive tissues leads to the patterning of permeable vessels and the formation of pores through endothelial gaps with a diameter between 100 nm to 2 µm, influenced by the size and form of the tumor tissue. In addition, due to the weak lymphatic system of the tumor vasculature, the depletion of intratumoral components stops, which results in the accumulation of intratumoral components in the tumor tissue. This is referred to as the enhanced permeability and retention effect (EPR effect), which can be utilized in passive drug delivery to the tumor. Therefore, NPs with diameters smaller than the pore size can permeate into the tumor tissues through the permeable vasculature (Kalyane *et al.*, 2019, Hara *et al.*, 2010, Narayan, 2018, Shi *et al.*, 2020).

The main issue of anticancer chemotherapeutic drugs is low tumor selectivity. Defects of the tumor vasculature, *i.e.*, hypervascularization, abnormal vasculature structure, and lack of lymphatic drainage, are used to overcome this issue and deliver the drug to the tumor (Shukla *et al.*, 2019).

The endothelial lining of the blood vessel walls in specific conditions has a higher permeability compared to healthy and normal blood vessel walls. Consequently, large size molecules and particles with sizes ranging from 10 to 500 nm are able to abandon the vascular bed and aggregate inside the interstitial space, which can be seen in infracted areas and tumors. Therefore, large molecules or particles loaded with the drug are able to deliver the therapeutic agent to the required site due to the higher vascular permeability, and finally release the drug from the carrier. This passive targeting is called the EPR effect. Macromolecules and NPs can enter the tumor interstitial area due to the high permeability of the tumor vessels, and the compromised lymphatic filtration helps NPs remain in the tumor interstitial area. Unlike macromolecules, small drugs will not remain in tumors and may return to circulation *via* diffusion. Nowadays, EPR-mediated DDS is a method used to carry and release drugs and particularly macromolecular therapeutic agents, in tumors. The parameters and factors affecting EPR drug delivery must be studied to obtain optimum results. Many investigations have demonstrated data about EPR effect in different solid tumors, while parameters influencing its magnitude are still ambiguous. Studies have stated that the size and tumor type can highly influence EPR effect. Also, high vascular density, quick angiogenesis and vascular permeability may enhance EPR effect. As mentioned before, leaky and irregular vasculature systems in tumor tissues result in higher aggregation of NPs inside the tumor area. Also, NP-based systems improve the half-life of therapeutic agents owing to their ability to escape from renal clearance. Parameters including NPs accumulation and protein binding might influence EPR effect because of the increased size of NPs through complex formation. Also, observations stated that the reticuloendothelial system (RES) existing in the liver and spleen weakens EOR effect. Surface modification of carriers is a suitable method to enhance EPR effect and also solve the issue related to the adsorption of protein to nanoparticles and aggregation (Torchilin, 2011, Kalyane *et al.*, 2019, Rajora *et al.*, 2014, Shukla *et al.*, 2019).

Generally, both passive and active targeting methods can be utilized for cancer chemotherapy with nanoparticles. As mentioned before, intrinsic sized nanoparticles are used for passive targeting with the aid of exclusive anatomical and pathophysiological properties of tumor vasculature, such as EPR effect. Apparently, EPR effect connects developments in nanotechnology and progresses in knowledge about tumor vascular biology. Thus, it is called the gold standard in designing novel anti-cancer agents, which efficiently improve drug bioavailability and effectiveness. Maeda *et al.* were the first researchers who designed nano-anticancer drugs and exploited EPR effect to precisely deliver the drug to cancerous tissues. Defective vascular structure and extensive angiogenesis are the concepts of this phenomenon. Besides, many solid tumors have vascular permeability parameters, including oxide (NO), peroxynitrite (ONOO–) and bradykinin. The impact of various parameters on EPR-mediated uptake of NPs in solid tumors is not well established. The size and surface of the carrier greatly affect tumor drug uptake. It was observed that particles smaller than 200nm (<200nm) with a hydrophilic surface increase EPR effect, due to the longer existence of the carrier in the blood (Acharya and Sahoo, 2011).

Carbon nanotubes highly agglomerate in tumor tissues due to the deficiency of formed blood and lymphatic vessels, which provide fast tumor proliferation, and increase permeability and retention. Carbon nanotube DDSs have higher effectiveness, for example, folic acid may be combined with the drug-loaded CNT to help with active targeting capacity through receptor-mediated endocytosis or local accumulation activated by external stimuli. Current progresses in drug release *via* carbon nanotubes mostly focus on cancer pharmaceuticals. Additionally, carbon nanotubes may increase EPR effect and are functionalized easily. Therefore, single or multiple drugs can be attached to CNTs for cancer treatment. For instance, researchers functionalized single wall carbon nanotubes with an antibody, and loaded the SWCNTs with DOX. The manufactured carbon-nanotubes recognized leukemia cells (MDR K562) and precisely delivered the drug. Moreover, the manufactured carbon-nanotubes exhibited a more than two-fold increase in cytotoxicity in cells in comparison with free DOX, (A Stout, 2015).

CNT-based drug nanocarriers have been exploited for *in vivo* cancer therapy. In 2008, a group of scientists investigated *in vivo* cancer therapy by paclitaxel conjugated branched PEG-single wall CNT in 4T1 murine breast cancer. The drug embedded in SWCNT had a higher paclitaxel accumulation in tumor owing to the EPR effect compared to the ordinary drug, which led to higher treatment efficacy. CNTs conjugated with targeting ligands, demonstrate improved tumor uptake in comparison with non-targeted CNTs (Liu *et al.*, 2011).

In a study, the clinical results for PDCs, the magnitude of the EPR effect and the expression of enzymes (cathepsins) inside different tumor forms have been documented (Polymer-drug conjugates (PDCs)). Accordingly, lung, breast and ovarian cancer demonstrated a higher amount of clinical reactions to PDCs, which is related to the high amounts of cathepsins enzymes detected in these tumor forms, and the EPR effect (Rajora *et al.*, 2014).

5.5. FABRICATION METHODS OF MICRO/NANOSCALED COMPOSITES

5.5.1. Emulsification-solvent Evaporation

One of the most widespread methods for the production of polymeric micro and nano-sized particles is emulsification/solvent evaporation. This method is based on the preparation of oil in water emulsion of the polymer solution, which is in an aqueous solution including a surfactant. The polymer solvent is normally an unstable and organic which forms a stable emulsion after evaporation. The emulsion may be prepared using mechanical or magnetic stirring. The emulsification is done using ultrasonication. The surfactant is used to stabilize the emulsion, though the surfactant concentration affects the size of the droplets in the emulsion. The solvent is evaporated *via* long-time mild heating and under low pressure, leaving the polymeric micro and nanoparticles suspended in the aqueous phase. Poly(3-hydroxybutyrate-co-3-hydroxyvalerate) (PHBV) micro and nanoparticles can be synthesized using this technique. The size and morphology of the NPS may be manipulated by the process circumstances. The PHBV produced in this method has spherical porous particles with a huge size distribution. The porosity and size distribution of the particles may be controlled by manipulating the surfactant form, polymer concentration, surfactant concentration, and the emulsification method. Reducing the concentration of the polymer solution or increasing the surfactant concentration may result in the production of smaller microparticles. It is noteworthy that the surfactant concentration affects the size of the particles at higher polymer concentrations. Moreover, ultrasonication is critical to obtain nanosized particles (Farrag *et al.*, 2018). This technique is appropriate as a substitute to spray drying as a precursor to produce drug-loaded biopolymer particles for supercritical CO_2 foaming (Ong *et al.*, 2018).

The mini emulsion and solvent evaporation (MESE) technique is based on the homogenization of an organic solution of a polymer in an aqueous phase wherein the unstable organic solution is further evaporated. This method may be used to produce polymer nanoparticles. The shape and size of the NPs in MESE may be adjusted by controlling the synthesis factors such as the emulsifier and solvent kind, relative concentrations, viscosity, and homogenizer operating circumstances (temperature and time). Due to properties such as high stability against gravitational separation, and optical transparency of the nano-emulsions produced from this technique, they can be utilized as DDSs for lipophilic active components. Other applications for these products may include an application as drug delivery particles, multifunctional imaging agents, and optical sensors (Zhao *et al.*, 2014).

The process of emulsification followed by solvent evaporation, is one of the most commonly utilized methods for the fabrication of NPs with functional ingredients. For instance, a group of researchers investigated the features of β-carotene organized with different emulsifiers through this method. In another research, β-carotene was encapsulated by 3 water-insoluble proteins, including sodium caseinate, whey protein isolate and soybean protein isolate, through this technique to form 3 NPs with diameters of 78, 90 and 370 nm. Generally, this method is based on high-pressure emulsification with low toxicity solvents as functional ingredients carrier and water as the solvent. In an investigation, emulsification-solvent evaporation was used instead of anti-solvent precipitation method, in order to produce β-carotene loaded zein-PGA composite NPs, as β-carotene has weak solubility in aqueous ethanol solution. High-pressure emulsification treatment and the solvent-evaporation procedure can alter biopolymer microstructure. The biopolymers may interact with each other entirely, which may be used to decrease the size of NPs. Also, the impact of PGA polymer on this nanocomposite has been studied. The nanocomposite was produced with emulsification/solvent evaporation. Additionally, hydrogen bonding, electrostatic and hydrophobic interactions affected the formation of zein-PGA composite NPs.

Zein-PGA composite NPs prevent the degradation of β-carotene under light and heat (Wei *et al.*, 2018).

Vanderhoff *et al.* utilized solvent evaporation method to fabricate polymeric nanoparticles (PNPs) from a preformed polymer, which is the most widespread method to produce PNPs. In this technique, the preformed polymer is dissolved in an unstable organic solvent and then the oil-phase and aqueous-phase holding stabilizer/emulsifier are formed in water. The emulsion is formed by mixing the oil and aqueous phases in higher-speed homogenization. A suspension including the NPs is produced after the evaporation of the solvent, and then the NPs are collected *via* ultracentrifugation. There are 2 kinds of emulsions prepared in the solvent evaporation technique including 1) Single emulsion; o/w or w/o and 2) Double emulsion; w/o/w or o/w/o. In an emulsion, an oil droplet is suspended in water, while in a reverse emulsion, water is the suspended phase, and oil is the continuous phase. Depending on the solubility of the polymer in the aqueous or organic phase, both forms of emulsions may be utilized. In a single oil/water emulsion, small oil phase droplets are suspended in a continuous aqueous phase and are prepared by mixing the oil phase and aqueous phase using high-velocity homogenization. On the other hand, in water/oil/water, a main water/oil emulsion containing a suspended small aqueous phase in a continuous oil phase is combined with another aqueous phase using high-velocity homogenization. It has been observed that hydrophilic drugs are well-encapsulated in this emulsion (Saini *et al.*, 2018).

5.5.2. Spray Drying

Spray drying is a simple single-step technique to turn nanoparticles into powder and increase the physicochemical stability of nanoparticles. The properties of nanoparticles may be easily controlled in spray drying. In spray drying, the polymer is dissolved in an appropriate solvent and small droplets of the solution are sprayed into a high-temperature environment using an atomizer. When the droplets enter the high-temperature section, first the solvent is evaporated and then the nanoparticles precipitation in powder form (Saini *et al.*, 2018).

Powders obtained through this method have an amorphous structure and therefore have low physical stability. The nanoparticles produced using the spray drying method are hygroscopic, which is a threat to producing aerosols due to moisture uptake and agglomeration. One way to overcome this challenge, is fabricating dried powder NPs with a hydrophobic surface. The spray drying method includes three steps. 1) droplet formation, 2) drying, and 3) particle formation. Droplet formation starts from the bottom of the saturated solution, which is then dried at a constant rate until saturation. During the drying process, the component with lower water solubility undergoes precipitation, resulting in the formation of a solid shell. In the drying process, the droplet surface temperature is the same as the wet bulb, which is highly related to the inlet and outlet temperature. The solvent diffuses toward the surface due to the evaporation of the solvent from the droplet surface. Through solvent evaporation, the concentration of the solute will increase on the surface. The solute may precipitate on the surface or diffuse toward the droplet center due to the concentration gradient. The physiochemical characteristics of solvents and solutes such as MW have a major role in the segregation of the solute, in the spray-drying process. The particles are formed when the surface concentration reaches a specific level depending on the material solubility. The solute with low water solubility precipitates on the surface of the spray-dried particle. Accordingly, processing parameters have a considerable impact on the spray-drying process and the properties of the powder. Theoretically, when a compound is spray-dried, with a co-solvent system, wherein the second compound has a lower solubility in water and higher solubility in organic solvents, the second compound will precipitate on the surface of the composite particles when the organic solvents evaporate (Momin *et al.*, 2018).

One of the best techniques to increase drug solubility is to develop amorphous solid dispersions (ASD). For this reason, amphiphilic or biologically inert hydrophilic polymers, including PVP, have been widely utilized, wherein the formulation may lead to improved bioavailability, and quick dissolution rates. Generally, a solution of the drug and the polymer is prepared in a suitable solvent. Next, the solution is sprayed with a co-current flow of high-temperature gas inside a chamber. The quick evaporation of the solvent results in the production of amorphous particles. Spray drying factors affect the encapsulation effectiveness. For example, large size atomization droplets and high primary solid content may lead to higher encapsulation efficacy. Larger particles can be produced using an ultrasonic nozzle (Ruphuy *et al.*, 2020).

Spray drying is an extensively utilized method for mass production of powder granules in chemical and pharmaceutical industries. Although spray drying method has two main challenges. The first challenge is the stability of the feed solution having two or more various suspensions with diverse physicochemical properties. For instance, an aqueous solution of carbon nanotubes is not stable and the CNTs will agglomerate because of the Van der Waals attraction. Therefore, the aqueous solution of CNTs is not an appropriate choice for spray drying. The second challenge is the segregation of particles in spray drying because of different surface polarities and colloidal particle sizes. Current progresses in the spray drying method show that there has been an ongoing attempt to produce nanocomposite materials with this method. High drying rate, automation, scale-up ability, reproducibility, capability to create powders with various features, and continuous operation are some of the advantages of this method (Sarkar *et al.*, 2018, Mozaffar *et al.*, 2021).

5.5.3. Electrospraying

Electrospraying (Electrohydrodynamic spraying) is a method for the atomization of liquids using electrical forces. Electrospraying does not have a complicated process and does not require severe conditions. Therefore, it can be mentioned as an appropriate technique for the encapsulation of sensitive compounds. In this method, the liquid flows out of a nozzle, with high electric potential, and forms fine droplets due to the electric field. This one-step low-cost technique may be used for the fabrication of non-agglomerated NPs with a homogenous size distribution. ES may be used for pharmaceutical and biomedical applications due to the ability to use a wide range of materials with different setup configurations such as pressure and temperature. One of the main advantages of this method is the ability to produce droplets with sizes ranging from tens of nanometers to hundreds of micrometers. The size of the droplets may be controlled by the voltage of the capillary nozzle and the liquid flow rate. Electrospraying may be utilized for micro- and nano-encapsulation of drug compounds by optimizing parameters such as the polymer solution, the solvent, and process factors like applied flow rate, collector surface, and environment temperature (Tanhaei *et al.*, 2020, Jaworek and Sobczyk, 2008).

ES is the dispersion of highly charged droplets that are discharged into the gas phase *via* electrohydrodynamic (EHD) microjets. Thus, this method is also called electro-hydrodynamic atomization (EHDA) or electro-hydrodynamic spraying (EHDS). The droplet size in the ES method is in the micrometer scale or even less. The electrical field acts as the driving force in atomization. Therefore, there is no need for other energy sources like gas streams. As a result, this method has a low power consumption. Besides, this method is based on laminar (non-turbulent) microjet flows. Various liquids may be coaxially blended in the same jet to produce structured multi-phase droplets, which may be utilized for the fabrication of core-shell structures (Bodnár *et al.*, 2018).

The major parts of the ES system are a high voltage power supply, a syringe pump for delivering the polymer feed solution through a metal needle, and a grounded product collector, to collect the electrospun products. Different techniques such as solvent extraction/evaporation, spray drying, and sol–gel-based polymerization have been developed for the fabrication of nano and microparticles. Although each method may have disadvantages such as high-cost equipment, large particle size, wide size distribution, and high-temperature process, which will lead to product deterioration. ES is an easy, one-step and adaptable top-down method for the fabrication of micro and nanoparticles from polymers, from low amounts of solvent. This uses an electrical field to evaporate the solvent from a polymer solution. ES has high control over the size and final properties of the produced particles (Ozawa *et al.*, 2019, Liu *et al.*, 2018).

Electro spraying is an extensively utilized and effective method for the preparation of drug or protein-loaded NPs. ES has many benefits, such as low cost, monodisperse particle size, simple control over surface characteristics, and a fast preparation process. For instance, PTX-loaded PCL with sizes ranging from 7-11 mm in diameter have been produced for cancer treatment purposes. As another example, ampicillin-loaded chitosan NPs are utilized for sustained drug delivery. Electrospraying is an appropriate method for the preparation of biodegradable drug carriers, such as PLGA NPs,. In a study, electrosprayed antibodies resulted in the formation of biologically active spots with diameters ranging from 130 to 350 mm. A study revealed that the high voltage utilized for electrospraying a suspension of bovine serum albumin (BSA) molecules for the encapsulation of drugs does not degrade the molecules. Researchers in biotechnology and medicine utilize PLGA and PLG owing to immunogenicity, biocompatibility, low toxicity, solubility in many organic solvents, and controllable physical properties (Nguyen *et al.*, 2019, Jaworek and Sobczyk, 2008).

5.5.4. Supercritical Fluids Processing (SCF)

Supercritical fluids processing (SCF) is a practical method for most pharmaceutical applications. SCF is a substitute for usual material processing techniques. SCF may be used for the fabrication of 3D structures and injectable materials which are used in regenerative medicines. This method is based on the use of a dense phase with. a temperature and pressure above its critical point. A single phase in the critical point has mutual properties with liquids, such as density, and mutual properties with gases, such as viscosity and mass diffusion coefficient. The high density of the supercritical fluid facilitates solvation, meanwhile, lower viscosity results in higher diffusivity, which will facilitate the mass transfer. There are various implementations of this method. Therefore, the selection of an appropriate SCF highly depends on its physico-chemical characteristics (Duarte *et al.*, 2009).

Supercritical fluids comprise microscopically inhomogeneous and macroscopically homogenous areas (Fig. 3). Actually, supercritical fluids may change the reaction environment from liquid to gas and vice versa. The usual properties of the solvent are the same as the gas and liquid phases, meanwhile, properties such as polarity, surface tension, and density may be adjusted with temperature and pressure. Supercritical CO_2 (scCO_2) is the most known supercritical fluid in order to process graphene-based materials, owing to its environmental-friendly nature and simplicity in acquiring critical states. The properties of scCO_2 (31 °C, 7.38 MPa) as a solvent are like non-polar solvents such as hexane, and can dissolve non-polar or slightly polar compounds. The solubility limit of scCO_2 can increase with the aid of little amounts of co-solvent such as alcohol. Supercritical water (scH_2O) is not utilized for this reason because of its high critical pressure and temperature (374 °C, 22.1 MPa). Additionally, alcohols such as ethanol have more available critical conditions (240.9 °C, 6.1 MPa), and are extensively utilized in graphene process. The properties of SCFs may be simply manipulateds. SCFs may be used for the fabrication of graphene-based materials (Padmajan Sasikala *et al.*, 2016).

Critical factors of CO_2 and specifically its low critical temperature, have made it a desirable SCF for the process of thermoresponsive bioactive and pharmaceutical compounds. CO_2 has become the most known supercritical fluid. Other major advantages of scCO_2 are low-cost, environmentally friendly, corrosion resistance, non-flammability, safety, nontoxicity, and accessibility. The removal and recovery of scCO_2 is simpler in comparison with other processes (only *via* manipulation of pressure, a dry solid product is achievable), resulting in a method with a lower required energy. scCO_2 is also reusable and recoverable and thus, doesn't produce greenhouse gases. In compounds used for biomedical and pharmaceutical purposes, the existence of residual organic solvents is strictly controlled by international safety regulations. It is vital to guarantee the total clearance and absence of these substances, and no exposure of drugs to high temperatures, which would result in their degradation (Duarte *et al.*, 2009).

5.5.4.1. The Supercritical Anti-Solvent (SAS) Technique

This method is effective for the fabrication of graphene-polymer nanocomposites, which is another form of supercritical-based physical transformation technique. This method is based on controlling the solubility of components in a mixed solvent with at least one supercritical solvent. For example, a mixed solvent system containing scCO_2 and DMSO solution (Dimethyl Sulfoxide) is utilized for the fabrication of graphene-pyrene nanocomposites. Although, pyrene molecules are totally miscible in DMSO, they have a low affinity for CO_2. On the contrary, DMSO is totally miscible in scCO_2. Usually, a few layers of graphene are initially introduced to a solution where pyrene molecules are dissolved in Dimethyl Sulfoxide, then scCO_2 is introduced, which will result in a severe decrease in the solubility of pyrene molecules. Further, the system reaches supersaturated conditions, and the pyrene molecules precipitate from Dimethyl Sulfoxide into the graphene interlayer. Outstanding mass transfer and homogenous dispersion of polymers in carbon-based materials are some of the advantages of this method (Padmajan Sasikala *et al.*, 2016).

This is the most common supercritical anti-solvent precipitation method. The application of this method highly depends on the injection system. The injector is used to produce liquid jet break-up and form small droplets for a large mass transfer surface between the liquid and the gaseous phase. It is noteworthy that the findings achieved by SAS in the arrangement of composite microparticles are incomplete. Morphologies obtained from SAS precipitation include nano and microparticles and crystals. However, there are only outcomes about microparticles SAS precipitation produced *via* solvent removal from liquid droplets, but logically, polymer-drug composite particles can also be produced. Most studies have focused on the application of PLLA-drug microparticles. In addition, none of the studies have proposed a systematic investigation on drug encapsulation effectiveness and the impact of SAS factors on these results (Reverchon *et al.*, 2009).

5.5.4.2. Supercritical CO$_2$ Foaming (SF)

This method is utilized to produce polymer foams. As mentioned before, scCO$_2$ may be used as a foaming agent due to suitable properties such as nontoxicity and environmental friendliness. 3D graphene-based polymeric nanocomposite foams have been fabricated using this method. In general, during this process, graphene–polymer composites are placed in a high-pressure reactor filled with scCO$_2$, for a long period of time. Then the system pressure is decreased quickly, and the reactor is quenched in cold water. The CO$_2$ molecules move away from the composite when the pressure is decreased, which results in the antiplasticization of the polymer. Consequently, nucleation and growth of bubbles inside the polymer occurs. These nanocomposites have more nucleation sites compared to ordinary polymers, due to the higher surface area of graphene. The major challenge in graphene-based nanocomposites with desired properties is the aggregation of graphene sheets to obtain a homogeneous dispersion of graphene in the nanocomposite structure. The use of graphene oxide has been limited because of its insulating nature. In fact, graphene oxide has a higher dispersion in polymers compared to graphene due to the existence of inorganic NPs and oxygenated functional groups (Padmajan Sasikala *et al.*, 2016).

The properties of supercritical fluids are between gas and liquids and have high solubility. Supercritical CO$_2$ and H$_2$O are frequently utilized in the fabrication of various nanosized materials. NPs which are fabricated with this method are highly pure without any sign of solvents (Saini *et al.*, 2018).

5.5.5. Microfluidics

This method uses microfluidics to synthesize specialized NPs with considerable advantages, which has been a less investigated technique. This method utilizes microchannel technology to blend mixed phases under constant laminar flow, which is not able to be done with solvent emulsion. It was stated that this method can produce more uniform NPs in size and dispersity, which are highly reproducible and scalable, making it appropriate for drug delivery applications. This method was utilized to fabricate reproducible NPs with parameters that can be accurately controlled, compared to the regular emulsification method, which usually shows a large batch-to-batch variation (Essa *et al.*, 2020).

This is an effortless and potent technique to deliver various photocurable compounds to make composites with 3D microstructure. Also, it enables efficient washing and needs little value from reagents. A microstructure is prepared throughout every lithographic cycle, which can adhere to the channel surface and wash away the unpolymerized pre-polymer. In this method, the sample does not require elimination between lithographic cycles, and also time-consuming stages of alignment and re-registration are avoided. Three-dimensional structures of different materials can be produced with the help of microfluidics in multi-step lithography. This automated method does not require high-cost equipment (Cheung *et al.*, 2007).

5.5.6. ProLease Technique

During the 1970s and 1980s, most degradable drug-loaded microparticles were fabricated by phase separation or solvent evaporation methods. In the 1990s, a group of researchers discovered the Prolease® technique to prepare drug-loaded PLGA with the uniform-size property. This method utilized an ultrasonic sprayer, liquid nitrogen, and frozen ethanol bath to freeze the uniform-sized particles and eliminate the solvent. Prolease is a well-known method for fabricating novel drug-loaded, PLGA-based microparticle drug delivery systems (Fig. **3**) (Hoffman, 2008).

Despite solvent evaporation, spray drying and phase separation in microspheres preparation, prolease is a non-aqueous cryogenic technique. Prolease was investigated as a substitute process to prevent the instability of biological compounds such as protein at the oil/water interface. This method includes the preparation of lyophilized drug particles through micronization with stabilizing excipients and then the preparation of the drug-polymer suspension after sonication to decrease the drug particle size. The next step is the atomization of the suspension in liquid nitrogen with an ultrasonic spray nozzle, extraction using ethanol, and finally, filtration and vacuum drying. Low temperatures are maintained during the process. Prolease DDS has been used for protein/peptide encapsulation in the solid phase, which facilitates the encapsulation of protein/ peptides in microspheres made of polymers like PLGA. This method protects the protein integrity with required release kinetics. Also, this method is useful in high protein encapsulation efficiency owing to non-aqueous based entrapment since there is no oil/water interface (water is a reactant for the protein degradation process), and the interface is limited, which could lead to protein denaturation (Otte *et al.*, 2020, Tracy, 1998, Kumar Malik *et al.*, 2007).

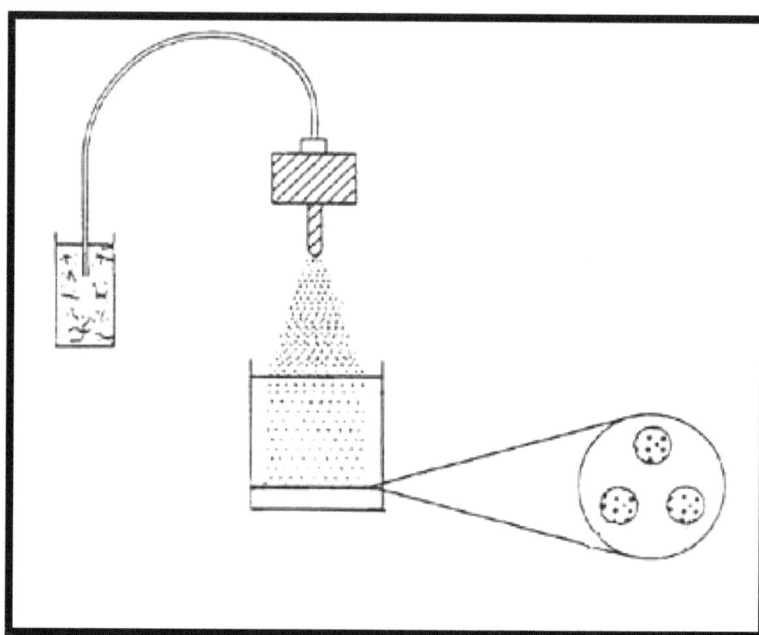

Fig. (3). Drug-loaded PLGA microparticles were prepared in "Prolease®" process (Hoffman, 2008).

5.5.7. Nanoprecipitation/Solvent Displacement

Nanoprecipitation or solvent displacement (SD) technique is a fast, single-step method for fabrication of nanoparticles owing to its low energy consumption, low cost and simplicity in implementation. Fessi *et al.* first investigated this technique in 1989 and stated that this method required an aqueous and organic phase, wherein the preformed polymer is dissolved in water-miscible organic solvents like ethanol, acetone, *etc.* with or without surfactant. In this method, first drugs and polymers in the organic solvent(s) are injected into the stabilizer, which is an aqueous solution, then they are mixed with a magnetic stirrer, and the nanoparticles are produced immediately through interfacial turbulence, which leads to quick, mutual diffusion during mixing. In most industrial processes, the mixing of ingredients or dispersion of one phase into the other is one of the most important sections. One of the advantages of this technique is that the polymeric nanoparticles are smaller compared to the emulsion-solvent evaporation method. Moreover, this technique permits the exploitation of non-halogenated organic solvents, which have lower toxicity compared to halogenated solvents regularly utilized in the emulsion-solvent evaporation technique. Also, the pouring and stirring rate highly influence the NPs size. Controlling the mixing conditions to obtain uniform size particles is one of the challenges of SD. This technique can be effectively used for the fabrication of nanosized capsules with oil-based central cavities in order to load lipophilic drugs. Nanosized capsules with oil-based central cavities may be prepared by adding a small amount of non-toxic oil in the organic phase. (García-Salazar *et al.*, 2018, Othmana *et al.*, 2016, Saini *et al.*, 2018).

Nanoprecipitation is the most extensively utilized technique for the fabrication of PLGA NPs. Acetone dissolved polymers are added in a drop-wised manner to the constantly stirring aqueous phase with or without an emulsifier/stabilizer. As a result, the organic phase is evaporated under reduced pressure. PCL (poly-ε-caprolactone) is one of the common polymers used in drug delivery applications. This polymer may be utilized in long-lasting implantable devices due to its slow degradation rate compared to polylactide. PCL NPs are mostly prepared using solvent displacement, solvent evaporation and nanoprecipitation methods (Kumari *et al.*, 2010).

5.5.8. Emulsion Techniques

In the emulsion freeze-drying technique, the polymer is dissolved in its solvent and water is added. Then the polymer-solvent solution and water are homogenized to form an emulsion. The emulsion is quickly cooled in order to lock in the liquid state structure, prior to the separation of 2 phases. At last, the water and solvent are eliminated using the freeze-drying method. The emulsion freeze-drying technique may be used to achieve high amounts of porosity (90%) and control the pore size through water phase percentage, solvent, freeze-drying factors, and polymer concentration. One of the benefits of this technique is the lack of a leaching step, although the use of organic solvents is an issue, particularly in tissue engineering applications. Hydroxyapatite/poly (hydroxybutyrate-co-valerate) composite scaffold has been fabricated *via* this method, and the impact of polymer solution concentration, solvent and water phase on the morphology of the composite scaffold has been studied. It was stated that at similar volume fractions of water, the scaffold porosity was reduced by increasing the polymer concentration. On the other hand, by increasing the volume fraction of water, the porosity increased. The scaffolds prepared *via* this technique were highly porous with an interconnected porous structure. It was observed that the pore size of these scaffolds was in the range of microns to 300 μm (Sampath *et al.*, 2016).

CONCLUSION

LCDDSs based on composites have attracted much attention in biomedicine, tissue engineering, pharmaceutical science and bioengineering due to their advantages in local delivery of therapeutic molecules from an implant/scaffold, amended loading and modified release of therapeutic agents, that are not achieved by the individual components alone. These composites can be utilized for releasing therapeutic molecules like drug, growth factors, gene and proteins from scaffolds in tissue engineering. This chapter surveys the various approaches to fabricate macro/micro/nanocomposite-based LCDDSs *via* simple, emerging and cost-effective techniques like emulsification-solvent evaporation, spray drying, electrospraying, supercritical fluids processing, microfluidics, prolease technique, nanoprecipitation/solvent displacement and emulsion techniques. These different synthesis methods are used to produce promising drug-loaded devices for loading various therapeutic agents, such as small biomolecules, biomacromolecules, genes, nucleic acid-based molecules like miRNA, polypeptides and proteins.

REFERENCES

Abdoli, M., Sadrjavadi, K., Arkan, E., Zangeneh, M.M., Moradi, S., Zangeneh, A., shahlaei, M., Khaledian, S. (2020). Polyvinyl alcohol/Gum tragacanth/graphene oxide composite nanofiber for antibiotic delivery. *J. Drug Deliv. Sci. Technol., 60*, 102044.
[http://dx.doi.org/10.1016/j.jddst.2020.102044]

Acharya, S., Sahoo, S.K. (2011). PLGA nanoparticles containing various anticancer agents and tumour delivery by EPR effect. *Adv. Drug Deliv. Rev., 63*(3), 170-183.
[http://dx.doi.org/10.1016/j.addr.2010.10.008] [PMID: 20965219]

Askari, E., Naghib, S.M., Seyfoori, A., Maleki, A., Rahmanian, M. (2019). Ultrasonic-assisted synthesis and *in vitro* biological assessments of a novel herceptin-stabilized graphene using three dimensional cell spheroid. *Ultrason. Sonochem., 58*, 104615.
[http://dx.doi.org/10.1016/j.ultsonch.2019.104615] [PMID: 31450294]

Askari, E., Naghib, S.M., Zahedi, A., Seyfoori, A., Zare, Y., Rhee, K.Y. (2021). Local delivery of chemotherapeutic agent in tissue engineering based on gelatin/graphene hydrogel. *J. Mater. Res. Technol., 12*, 412-422.
[http://dx.doi.org/10.1016/j.jmrt.2021.02.084]

Askari, E., Rasouli, M., Darghiasi, S.F., Naghib, S.M., Zare, Y., Rhee, K.Y. (2021). Reduced graphene oxide-grafted bovine serum albumin/bredigite nanocomposites with high mechanical properties and excellent osteogenic bioactivity for bone tissue engineering. *Biodes. Manuf., 4*(2), 243-257.
[http://dx.doi.org/10.1007/s42242-020-00113-4]

Bacakova, L., Pajorova, J., Tomkova, M., Matejka, R., Broz, A., Stepanovska, J., Prazak, S., Skogberg, A., Siljander, S., Kallio, P. (2020). Applications of nanocellulose/nanocarbon composites: Focus on biotechnology and medicine. *Nanomaterials (Basel),* *10*(2), 196.
[http://dx.doi.org/10.3390/nano10020196] [PMID: 31979245]

Bodnár, E., Grifoll, J., Rosell-Llompart, J. (2018). Polymer solution electrospraying: A tool for engineering particles and films with controlled morphology. *J. Aerosol Sci.,* *125*, 93-118.
[http://dx.doi.org/10.1016/j.jaerosci.2018.04.012]

Cheung, Y.K., Gillette, B.M., Zhong, M., Ramcharan, S., Sia, S.K. (2007). Direct patterning of composite biocompatible microstructures using microfluidics. *Lab Chip,* *7*(5), 574-579.
[http://dx.doi.org/10.1039/b700869d] [PMID: 17476375]

Duarte, A.R.C., Mano, J.F., Reis, R.L. (2009). Supercritical fluids in biomedical and tissue engineering applications: a review. *Int. Mater. Rev.,* *54*(4), 214-222.
[http://dx.doi.org/10.1179/174328009X411181]

Essa, D., Choonara, Y.E., Kondiah, P.P.D., Pillay, V. (2020). Comparative nanofabrication of PLGA-chitosan-PEG systems employing microfluidics and emulsification solvent evaporation techniques. *Polymers (Basel),* *12*(9), 1882.
[http://dx.doi.org/10.3390/polym12091882] [PMID: 32825546]

Farrag, Y., Montero, B., Rico, M., Barral, L., Bouza, R. (2018). Preparation and characterization of nano and micro particles of poly(3-hydroxybutyrate-co-3-hydroxyvalerate) (PHBV) *via* emulsification/solvent evaporation and nanoprecipitation techniques. *J. Nanopart. Res.,* *20*(3), 71.
[http://dx.doi.org/10.1007/s11051-018-4177-7]

García-Salazar, G., de la Luz Zambrano-Zaragoza, M., Quintanar-Guerrero, D. (2018). Preparation of nanodispersions by solvent displacement using the Venturi tube. *Int. J. Pharm.,* *545*(1-2), 254-260.
[http://dx.doi.org/10.1016/j.ijpharm.2018.05.005] [PMID: 29729406]

Ghorbanzade, S., Naghib, S.M. (2019). *Nanoscaled Materials for Drug Delivery into Cells/Stem Cells. Stem Cell Nanotechnology..* Springer.

Ghorbanzade, S., Naghib, S.M., Sadr, A., Fateminia, F.S., Ghaffarinejad, A., Majidzadeh, A.K., Sanati-nezhad, A. (2019). Multifunctional magnetic nanoparticles-labeled mesenchymal stem cells for hyperthermia and bioimaging applications.

Gooneh-Farahani, S., Naghib, S.M., Naimi-Jamal, M.R. (2020). A Novel and Inexpensive Method Based on Modified Ionic Gelation for pH-responsive Controlled Drug Release of Homogeneously Distributed Chitosan Nanoparticles with a High Encapsulation Efficiency. *Fibers Polym.,* *21*(9), 1917-1926.
[http://dx.doi.org/10.1007/s12221-020-1095-y]

Gooneh-Farahani, S., Naimi-Jamal, M.R., Naghib, S.M. (2019). Stimuli-responsive graphene-incorporated multifunctional chitosan for drug delivery applications: a review. *Expert Opin. Drug Deliv.,* *16*(1), 79-99.
[http://dx.doi.org/10.1080/17425247.2019.1556257] [PMID: 30514124]

Hoffman, A.S. (2008). The origins and evolution of "controlled" drug delivery systems. *J. Cont. Rel.,* *132*(3), 153-163.

Hara, T., Iriyama, S., Makino, K., Terada, H., Ohya, M. (2010). Mathematical description of drug movement into tumor with EPR effect and estimation of its configuration for DDS. *Colloids Surf. B Biointerfaces,* *75*(1), 42-46.
[http://dx.doi.org/10.1016/j.colsurfb.2009.08.013] [PMID: 19726170]

Hu, X., Li, D., Tan, H., Pan, C., Chen, X. (2014). Injectable graphene oxide/graphene composite supramolecular hydrogel for delivery of anti-cancer drugs. *Journal of Macromolecular Science. Part A,* *51*, 378-384.

Jaworek, A., Sobczyk, A.T. (2008). Electrospraying route to nanotechnology: An overview. *J. Electrost.,* *66*(3-4), 197-219.

[http://dx.doi.org/10.1016/j.elstat.2007.10.001]

Jha, R., Singh, A., Sharma, P.K., Fuloria, N.K. (2020). Smart carbon nanotubes for drug delivery system: A comprehensive study. *J. Drug Deliv. Sci. Technol., 58*, 101811.
[http://dx.doi.org/10.1016/j.jddst.2020.101811]

Ji, T., Kohane, D.S. (2019). Nanoscale systems for local drug delivery. *Nano Today, 28*, 100765.
[http://dx.doi.org/10.1016/j.nantod.2019.100765] [PMID: 32831899]

Kalyane, D., Raval, N., Maheshwari, R., Tambe, V., Kalia, K., Tekade, R.K. (2019). Employment of enhanced permeability and retention effect (EPR): Nanoparticle-based precision tools for targeting of therapeutic and diagnostic agent in cancer. *Mater. Sci. Eng. C, 98*, 1252-1276.
[http://dx.doi.org/10.1016/j.msec.2019.01.066] [PMID: 30813007]

Karimzadeh, S., Safaei, B., Jen, T.C. (2021). Theorical investigation of adsorption mechanism of doxorubicin anticancer drug on the pristine and functionalized single-walled carbon nanotube surface as a drug delivery vehicle: A DFT study. *J. Mol. Liq., 322*, 114890.
[http://dx.doi.org/10.1016/j.molliq.2020.114890]

Krisanapiboon, A., Buranapanitkit, B., Oungbho, K. (2006). Biocompatability of hydroxyapatite composite as a local drug delivery system. *J. Orthop. Surg. (Hong Kong), 14*(3), 315-318.
[http://dx.doi.org/10.1177/230949900601400315] [PMID: 17200535]

Kumar Malik, D., Baboota, S., Ahuja, A., Hasan, S., Ali, J. (2007). Recent advances in protein and peptide drug delivery systems. *Curr. Drug Deliv., 4*(2), 141-151.
[http://dx.doi.org/10.2174/156720107780362339] [PMID: 17456033]

Kumari, A., Yadav, S.K., Yadav, S.C. (2010). Biodegradable polymeric nanoparticles based drug delivery systems. *Colloids Surf. B Biointerfaces, 75*(1), 1-18.
[http://dx.doi.org/10.1016/j.colsurfb.2009.09.001] [PMID: 19782542]

Li, B., Harlepp, S., Gensbittel, V., Wells, C.J.R., Bringel, O., Goetz, J.G., Begin-Colin, S., Tasso, M., Begin, D., Mertz, D. (2020). Near infra-red light responsive carbon nanotubes@mesoporous silica for photothermia and drug delivery to cancer cells. *Mater. Today Chem., 17*, 100308.
[http://dx.doi.org/10.1016/j.mtchem.2020.100308]

Li, X., Kong, X., Zhang, J., Wang, Y., Wang, Y., Shi, S., Guo, G., Luo, F., Zhao, X., Wei, Y., Qian, Z. (2011). A novel composite hydrogel based on chitosan and inorganic phosphate for local drug delivery of camptothecin nanocolloids. *J. Pharm. Sci., 100*(1), 232-241.
[http://dx.doi.org/10.1002/jps.22256] [PMID: 20533555]

Liu, K., Li, H., Williams, G.R., Wu, J., Zhu, L.M. (2018). pH-responsive liposomes self-assembled from electrosprayed microparticles, and their drug release properties. *Colloids Surf. A Physicochem. Eng. Asp., 537*, 20-27.
[http://dx.doi.org/10.1016/j.colsurfa.2017.09.046]

Liu, S., Qin, S., He, M., Zhou, D., Qin, Q., Wang, H. (2020). Current applications of poly(lactic acid) composites in tissue engineering and drug delivery. *Compos., Part B Eng., 199*, 108238.
[http://dx.doi.org/10.1016/j.compositesb.2020.108238]

Liu, Z., Robinson, J.T., Tabakman, S.M., Yang, K., Dai, H. (2011). Carbon materials for drug delivery & cancer therapy. *Mater. Today, 14*(7-8), 316-323.
[http://dx.doi.org/10.1016/S1369-7021(11)70161-4]

Manoj Kumar, R., Rajesh, K., Haldar, S., Gupta, P., Murali, K., Roy, P., Lahiri, D. (2019). Surface modification of CNT reinforced UHMWPE composite for sustained drug delivery. *J. Drug Deliv. Sci. Technol., 52*, 748-759.
[http://dx.doi.org/10.1016/j.jddst.2019.05.044]

Momin, M.A.M., Tucker, I.G., Doyle, C.S., Denman, J.A., Das, S.C. (2018). Manipulation of spray-drying conditions to develop dry powder particles with surfaces enriched in hydrophobic material to achieve high aerosolization of a hygroscopic drug. *Int. J. Pharm., 543*(1-2), 318-327.

[http://dx.doi.org/10.1016/j.ijpharm.2018.04.003] [PMID: 29626509]

Mozaffar, S., Radi, M., Amiri, S., McClements, D.J. (2021). A new approach for drying of nanostructured lipid carriers (NLC) by spray-drying and using sodium chloride as the excipient. *J. Drug Deliv. Sci. Technol., 61*, 102212.
[http://dx.doi.org/10.1016/j.jddst.2020.102212]

Narayan, R. (2018). *Encyclopedia of biomedical engineering..* Elsevier.

Nguyen, D.T., Phan, V.H.G., Lee, D.S., Thambi, T., Huynh, D.P. (2019). Bioresorbable pH- and temperature-responsive injectable hydrogels-incorporating electrosprayed particles for the sustained release of insulin. *Polym. Degrad. Stabil., 162*, 36-46.
[http://dx.doi.org/10.1016/j.polymdegradstab.2019.02.013]

Ong, Y.X.J., Lee, L.Y., Davoodi, P., Wang, C.H. (2018). Production of drug-releasing biodegradable microporous scaffold using a two-step micro-encapsulation/supercritical foaming process. *J. Supercrit. Fluids, 133*, 263-269.
[http://dx.doi.org/10.1016/j.supflu.2017.10.018]

Othmana, R., Vladisavljevića, G. T., Thomasc, N. L., Nagya, Z. K. (2016). Fabrication of composite poly (D, L-lactide)/montmorillonite nanoparticles for controlled delivery of acetaminophen by solvent-displacement method using glass capillary microfluidics.

Otte, A., Sharifi, F., Park, K. (2020). Interfacial tension effects on the properties of PLGA microparticles. *Colloids Surf. B Biointerfaces, 196*, 111300.
[http://dx.doi.org/10.1016/j.colsurfb.2020.111300] [PMID: 32919245]

Padmajan Sasikala, S., Poulin, P., Aymonier, C. (2016). Prospects of Supercritical Fluids in Realizing Graphene-Based Functional Materials. *Adv. Mater., 28*(14), 2663-2691.
[http://dx.doi.org/10.1002/adma.201504436] [PMID: 26879938]

Rahmanian, M., seyfoori, A., Dehghan, M.M., Eini, L., Naghib, S.M., Gholami, H., Farzad Mohajeri, S., Mamaghani, K.R., Majidzadeh-A, K. (2019). Multifunctional gelatin–tricalcium phosphate porous nanocomposite scaffolds for tissue engineering and local drug delivery: *In vitro* and *in vivo* studies. *J. Taiwan Inst. Chem. Eng., 101*, 214-220.
[http://dx.doi.org/10.1016/j.jtice.2019.04.028]

Rajakumar, G., Zhang, X.H., Gomathi, T., Wang, S.F., Azam Ansari, M., Mydhili, G., Nirmala, G., Alzohairy, M.A., Chung, I.M. (2020). Current Use of Carbon-Based Materials for Biomedical Applications—A Prospective and Review. *Processes (Basel), 8*(3), 355.
[http://dx.doi.org/10.3390/pr8030355]

Rajora, A., Ravishankar, D., Osborn, H., Greco, F. (2014). Impact of the enhanced permeability and retention (EPR) effect and cathepsins levels on the activity of polymer-drug conjugates. *Polymers (Basel), 6*(8), 2186-2220.
[http://dx.doi.org/10.3390/polym6082186]

Reverchon, E., Adami, R., Cardea, S., Porta, G.D. (2009). Supercritical fluids processing of polymers for pharmaceutical and medical applications. *J. Supercrit. Fluids, 47*(3), 484-492.
[http://dx.doi.org/10.1016/j.supflu.2008.10.001]

Ruphuy, G., Saloň, I., Tomas, J., Šalamúnová, P., Hanuš, J., Štěpánek, F. (2020). Encapsulation of poorly soluble drugs in yeast glucan particles by spray drying improves dispersion and dissolution properties. *Int. J. Pharm., 576*, 118990.
[http://dx.doi.org/10.1016/j.ijpharm.2019.118990] [PMID: 31899318]

Saini, R.K., Bagri, L.P., Bajpai, A.K., Mishra, A. (2018). Government Autonomous Science College, Jabalpur, India, Graphic Era University, Dehradun, India. *Stimuli Responsive Polymeric Nanocarriers for Drug Delivery Applications, Types and triggers*

Sampath, U., Ching, Y., Chuah, C., Sabariah, J., Lin, P.C. (2016). Fabrication of porous materials from natural/synthetic biopolymers and their composites. *Materials (Basel), 9*(12), 991.

[http://dx.doi.org/10.3390/ma9120991] [PMID: 28774113]

Saneei Mousavi, M.S., Karami, A.H., Ghasemnejad, M., Kolahdouz, M., Manteghi, F., Ataei, F. (2018). Design of a remote-control drug delivery implantable chip for cancer local on demand therapy using ionic polymer metal composite actuator. *J. Mech. Behav. Biomed. Mater., 86,* 250-256.
[http://dx.doi.org/10.1016/j.jmbbm.2018.06.034] [PMID: 29986300]

Sarkar, D., Sen, D., Nayak, B.K., Bhatt, P., Deo, M.N., Dutta, B. (2018). Biopolymer assisted synthesis of silica-carbon composite by spray drying. *Colloids Surf. B Biointerfaces, 165,* 182-190.
[http://dx.doi.org/10.1016/j.colsurfb.2018.02.040] [PMID: 29482129]

Seyfoori, A., Ebrahimi, S.A.S., Omidian, S., Naghib, S.M. (2019). Multifunctional magnetic ZnFe2O4-hydroxyapatite nanocomposite particles for local anti-cancer drug delivery and bacterial infection inhibition: An *in vitro* study. *J. Taiwan Inst. Chem. Eng., 96,* 503-508.
[http://dx.doi.org/10.1016/j.jtice.2018.10.018]

Shi, Y., van der Meel, R., Chen, X., Lammers, T. (2020). The EPR effect and beyond: Strategies to improve tumor targeting and cancer nanomedicine treatment efficacy. *Theranostics, 10*(17), 7921-7924.
[http://dx.doi.org/10.7150/thno.49577] [PMID: 32685029]

Shukla, T., Upmanyu, N., Pandey, S.P., Sudheesh, M. (2019). *Site-specific drug delivery, targeting, and gene therapy. Nanoarchitectonics in Biomedicine..* Elsevier.

Singh, Z.S. (2016). Applications and toxicity of graphene family nanomaterials and their composites. *Nanotechnol. Sci. Appl., 9,* 15-28.
[http://dx.doi.org/10.2147/NSA.S101818] [PMID: 27051278]

Sivakumaran, D., Maitland, D., Hoare, T. (2011). Injectable microgel-hydrogel composites for prolonged small-molecule drug delivery. *Biomacromolecules, 12*(11), 4112-4120.
[http://dx.doi.org/10.1021/bm201170h] [PMID: 22007750]

Soundrapandian, C., Sa, B., Datta, S. (2009). Organic-inorganic composites for bone drug delivery. *AAPS PharmSciTech, 10*(4), 1158-1171.
[http://dx.doi.org/10.1208/s12249-009-9308-0] [PMID: 19842042]

Stout, D. (2015). Recent advancements in carbon nanofiber and carbon nanotube applications in drug delivery and tissue engineering. *Curr. Pharm. Des., 21*(15), 2037-2044.
[http://dx.doi.org/10.2174/1381612821666150302153406] [PMID: 25732658]

Tanhaei, A., Mohammadi, M., Hamishehkar, H., Hamblin, M.R. (2020). Electrospraying as a novel method of particle engineering for drug delivery vehicles. *J. Control. Release.*
[PMID: 33137365]

Torchilin, V. (2011). Tumor delivery of macromolecular drugs based on the EPR effect. *Adv. Drug Deliv. Rev., 63*(3), 131-135.
[http://dx.doi.org/10.1016/j.addr.2010.03.011] [PMID: 20304019]

Tracy, M.A. (1998). Development and scale-up of a microsphere protein delivery system. *Biotechnol. Prog., 14*(1), 108-115.
[http://dx.doi.org/10.1021/bp9701271] [PMID: 9496675]

Wahyudiono, Ozawa, H., Machmudah, S., Kanda, H., Goto, M. (2019). Electrospraying technique under pressurized carbon dioxide for hollow particle production. *React. Funct. Polym., 142,* 44-52.
[http://dx.doi.org/10.1016/j.reactfunctpolym.2019.05.016]

Wei, Y., Sun, C., Dai, L., Zhan, X., Gao, Y. (2018). Structure, physicochemical stability and *in vitro* simulated gastrointestinal digestion properties of β-carotene loaded zein-propylene glycol alginate composite nanoparticles fabricated by emulsification-evaporation method. *Food Hydrocoll., 81,* 149-158.
[http://dx.doi.org/10.1016/j.foodhyd.2018.02.042]

Yang, Z., Wang, L., Liu, Y., Liu, S., Tang, D., Meng, L., Cui, B. (2020). ZnO capped flower-like porous carbon-Fe_3O_4 composite as carrier for bi-triggered drug delivery. *Mater. Sci. Eng. C, 107,* 110256.

[http://dx.doi.org/10.1016/j.msec.2019.110256] [PMID: 31761234]

Zeinali Kalkhoran, A.H., Naghib, S.M., Vahidi, O., Rahmanian, M. (2018). Synthesis and characterization of graphene-grafted gelatin nanocomposite hydrogels as emerging drug delivery systems. *Biomed. Phys. Eng. Express, 4*(5), 055017.
[http://dx.doi.org/10.1088/2057-1976/aad745]

Zeinali Kalkhoran, A.H., Vahidi, O., Naghib, S.M. (2018). A new mathematical approach to predict the actual drug release from hydrogels. *Eur. J. Pharm. Sci., 111*, 303-310.
[http://dx.doi.org/10.1016/j.ejps.2017.09.038] [PMID: 28962856]

Zhao, X., Meng, Q., Liu, J., Li, Q. (2014). Hydrophobic dye/polymer composite colorants synthesized by miniemulsion solvent evaporation technique. *Dyes Pigments, 100*, 41-49.
[http://dx.doi.org/10.1016/j.dyepig.2013.07.028]

CHAPTER 6

Exogeneous-triggered Delivery in Localized Controlled Drug Delivery Systems (LCDDSs)

Abstract: Stimuli-sensitive materials and micro/nanostructures can be manipulated to release their therapeutic drugs in the target site. The release is based on a particular extracellular/cellular stimuli, triggered *via* physical, biochemical, and chemical changes. The trigger may change the carrier structure/chemistry to release the therapeutic drug at a specific site. When a therapeutic drug is encapsulated with a stimuli-triggered material/polymer, the release may start with changes in structures like charge switching, surface layers de-shedding and degradation of materials. Furthermore, the disruption of the bonds may result in the release of therapeutic agents that are covalently immobilized in the functional groups of materials. Exogenous stimuli are the activation of reactions/phenomena from outside the body, such as ultrasound, temperature and light. Herein, we will describe thermosensitive, light-sensitive, and ultrasound-sensitive controlled drug release of LCDDS, as the mentioned exogenous stimuli have been extensively used in LCDD applications.

Keywords: Exogenous stimuli, Light-responsive, Stimuli-responsive drug delivery system, Thermoresponsive, Ultrasound responsive.

6.1. INTRODUCTION

Most drugs are toxic to cells and often kill non-cancerous and healthy cells, which may cause several side effects (Campbell and Smeets, 2019, Gooneh-Farahani *et al.*, 2019b). As an example, conventional chemotherapy drugs are not tumor-specific and cause significant toxicity in healthy tissues (Rahmanian *et al.*, 2017, Seyfoori *et al.*, 2019, Palumbo *et al.*, 2013, Rahmanian *et al.*, 2019). Therefore, several DDSs were developed to enhance the therapeutic properties and increase the safety and effectiveness of drugs (Ghorbanzade and Naghib, 2019, Gooneh-Farahani *et al.*, 2020, Zeinali Kalkhoran *et al.*, 2018, Kalkhoran *et al.*, 2018). Localized drug delivery decreases systemic drug exposure, which results in an increase in efficacy, high levels of patient compliance and fewer side effects (Askari *et al.*, 2021). As a result, in recent years, smart drug delivery has gained increased attention and paved the way for more effective treatment of patients (De Souza *et al.*, 2010, Gooneh-Farahani *et al.*, 2019a).

Seyed Morteza Naghib, Samin Hoseinpour & Shadi Zarshad

Smart drug delivery systems (SDDSs) with stimuli-responsive characteristics are determined as a process in which the drug is not released until reaching the target site (Liu *et al.*, 2016a). This triggered release occurs due to the variations in the nano/microcarrier chemistry and structure, in response to endogenous and/ or exogenous stimulus, resulting in the release of the drugs at the exact site (Kamaly *et al.*, 2016).

Endogenous triggers such as pH, redox, enzyme concentration, and bio-molecules are related to the disease's pathological characteristics (Mura *et al.*, 2013). These triggers are described in detail in the next chapter. In exogeneous-triggered delivery, drug/gene release is controlled by an external stimulus. Light, magnetic field, temperature, electrical field, and ultrasound are some examples of exogenous triggers (Raza *et al.*, 2019b). Systems for localized drug delivery in response to temperature, light, and ultrasound are described in this chapter.

6.2. THERMO-RESPONSIVE DRUG RELEASE

Thermo-responsive drug delivery systems (TRDDSs) have a significant advantage over their counterparts. These systems have a high potential for designing high-performance delivery systems due to their tunable phase transition temperature, *in situ* phase transition in the body environment, and variety in design. Therefore, due to the unique properties of thermo-responsive materials, they can be used in smart delivery systems to overcome the challenges of normal delivery systems and reduce drug toxicity (Bikram and West, 2008). Thermo-responsive drug delivery systems (TRDDS) depend on temperature changes resulting in nonlinear sharp changes in the properties of the materials loaded with drugs. These systems are effective in cancer treatment as they can keep the drug at ~37 °C and release the drug into the tumor environment, which has a high temperature (~40–42 °C) (Mura *et al.*, 2013). Therefore, these systems have been extensively exploited in the gene, proteins and drug delivery (Gandhi *et al.*, 2015, Özdemir *et al.*, 2006, Li *et al.*, 2003, Talelli and Hennink, 2011).

In general, temperature-responsive polymers are divided into two categories: negative thermo-sensitive and positive thermo-sensitive polymers (Qiu and Park, 2001). Positively thermo-sensitive polymers have the upper critical solution temperature (UCST), so their water-solubility increases with increasing temperature and gelling occurs below their UCST (Taylor *et al.*, 2017). Interpenetrating polymer networks of P(AAm–co-BMA) or polyacrylamide (PAAm) and poly (acrylic acid) have positive thermosensitivity (Qiu and Park, 2001). Negative thermoresponsive polymers have a lower critical solution temperature (LCST) and show sol (solved coil)-gel (collapsed globule) transition by increasing the temperature. In fact, unlike positive thermo-sensitive polymers, the solubility of these polymers decreases by increasing the temperature, which leads to gel formation, shrinkage of a loaded structure and drug release. This phenomenon is based on the hydrogen bonding between the water molecules and the polymer hydrophilic groups at a low temperature. Therefore, the water molecules disperse between polymer chains and hydrate them. On the other hand, the hydrogen weakens above the LCST, and the hydrophobic interactions between the hydrophobic domains of the polymer chains are strengthened, causing coil-to-globule transition (Huang *et al.*, 2019, Miladinovic *et al.*, 2018, Calejo *et al.*, 2013). It should be mentioned that the phase transition of the mentioned polymers may be experimentally verified with techniques like differential scanning calorimetry (DSC) and spectroscopy (Klouda, 2015). In addition to the aforementioned thermosensitive polymers, there are also systems, that exhibit both LCST and UCST behavior, but these systems are not used for biomedical applications (Schmaljohann, 2006). Due to the unique properties of hydrogels, such as high drug loading capacity, they can be used for developing DDS. Therefore, many studies have focused on thermo-responsive hydrogels and nanogels (Askari *et al.*, 2020). Thermo-responsive hydrogels have a volume phase transition temperature (VPTT), wherein the hydrogel size and volume change. The VPTT is a key factor in thermosensitive hydrogels, which is used to develop SDDSs (Constantin *et al.*, 2011). Therefore, these hydrogels have a high capability for designing localized drug delivery systems. Since the temperature in most disease areas is slightly higher than normal body temperature, hydrogels, which have a VPTT slightly upper than 37°C, are suitable for SDDSs. Among the studied thermoresponsive hydrogels, poly(N-isopropyl acrylamide) (PNIPAM) is one of the most widely used hydrogels in SDDS owing to its good thermal reversibility and a VPTT close to the human body temperature (Wenceslau *et al.*, 2012).

Besides hydrogels, core-shell structures and micelles have also been used to develop temperature-responsive drug delivery systems (Karimi *et al.*, 2016). Negative thermo-sensitive polymers can be used as injectable systems in localized drug delivery. In fact, localized implantable drug delivery systems are not favorable due to their high price and implantation problems. Negative thermo-sensitive polymers were developed as injectable localized drug-delivery systems (Gou *et al.*, 2010). The sol-gel transition in these polymers enables a semi-solid DDS in the body environment with controlled drug release (Jiang *et al.*, 2014). To meet the requirement of designing an injectable hydrogel for LDD, the sol-gel transition must occur when the temperature changes. Generally, the sol-state of drug-loaded thermosensitive hydrogels can be injected into the target of the disease at a specific temperature T1, which is lower than the phase transition temperature. Then this drug-loaded sol is solidified at body temperature because of its LCST. The produced gel may be used for localized drug release in the target tissue (Li and Guan, 2011).

Therefore, (1) good and easy miscibility with the drug because of the low viscosity of the sol-state of a drug-loaded system before injection, (2) Creating a time-dependent and targeted drug delivery system and (3) developing a minimally invasive drug delivery system, are some of the advantages of an injectable thermosensitive drug delivery system (Deng *et al.*, 2019).

The aforementioned injectable thermosensitive systems have been employed for many DDS applications. As an example, Garie´py *et al.* synthesized an injectable thermosensitive system for localized delivery of paclitaxel to tumor resection sites. This system was made from a chitosan solution neutralized with β-glycerophosphate, which is a sol at room temperature but solidifies in the body environment. The *in vitro* drug release profiles of this SDDS demonstrated sustained delivery for over 1 month (Ruel-Gariépy *et al.*, 2004). Injectable thermo-sensitive systems can be used for wound dressing applications. For instance, Dong *et al.* designed a thermo-sensitive system of superoxide dismutase-loaded poly(γ-glutamic acid)/poly(N-isopropyl-acrylamide) (PP) for wound healing. This cytocompatible system has shown a controlled release of superoxide dismutase, which may be used for wound healing and tissue remodeling in diabetic models (Dong *et al.*, 2020).

One of the important points in designing smart thermoresponsive delivery systems in recent years is the use of thermoresponsive copolymers due to the regulation of LCS and thermoassociative properties (Liu *et al.*, 2009). As an example, the LCST of Poly(N-isopropyl acrylamide) (pNIPAAm), which is ~32°C, can be adjusted by grafting hydrophilic monomers (Soliman *et al.*, 2019).

As different tissues have diverse environmental temperatures, the sol-gel transition temperature is one of the properties of TRDDS, providing satisfactory results depending on the situation. For example, a TRDDS which is suitable for wound healing may not be appropriate for cancer therapy. Thus, proper tuning of sol-gel transition temperature is needed. Besides, the mechanism and gelation rates are influenced by the ratio of hydrophobic/hydrophilic monomers and the molecular weights of monomers, which may influence drug release kinetics (Hogan and Mikos, 2020). It should be noted that the sol-gel transition temperature is the temperature where the hydrophobic interaction in the polymer chain starts to exceed the water hydration energy. Therefore, increasing the hydrophobicity of the system reduces the gelation temperature, while increasing the hydrophilicity results in a higher gelation temperature (Li and Guan, 2011).

Therefore, the ratio of the repeating units and copolymerization can adjust the sol-gel transition temperature (Karimi *et al.*, 2016).

Particularly, block copolymers form gels easier in comparison with random copolymers. Besides, diblock copolymers are able to form stable gels compared to other ABA counterparts. By comparing different forms of triblock copolymers, it has been observed that the ABC triblock copolymers with a hydrophobic structure in B blocks demonstrated a better sol-gel transition with a more stable gel at high temperatures. On the other hand, when the hydrophobic and thermoresponsive monomers are the outer blocks, the polymers may form gels at all temperatures or have a very low Tgel (Constantinou and Georgiou, 2016). Mixing the hydrophilic polymer with temperature-sensitive hydrogels will also provide a beneficial way of mitigating the body reaction to the thermosensitive implantable system, which promotes the bioavailability of the drug (Sun *et al.*, 2012). Besides, the sol-gel transition temperature of the system could be tuned by this mixing method. For instance, biocompatible Poloxamer 407 (PX) is not an appropriate choice for designing injectable thermosensitive drug delivery systems. In fact, the sol-gel transition temperature of low concentration PX is close to the body temperature, but the gel is not stable. High concentrations of this polymer are more efficient in forming stronger gels, but in this case, the gelation temperature is lower than the desired temperature range (30–36°C). To prepare a novel PX-based system for *in situ* thermosensitive drug delivery, gelling near body temperature is needed. Therefore, the gelation temperature of PX was tuned by mixing poly(acrylic acid) (PAA) and PX, and the gelation temperature increased to the suitable temperature range of 30–36°C. This method developed an optimized PX and PAA combination for biocompatible localized drug delivery systems (Boonlai *et al.*, 2018).

In addition to chemical parameters, physical parameters, such as pressure affect the gelation temperature. For instance, by increasing the pressure (close to atmospheric pressure) on poly(N-vinyl isobutyramide), a slight increase in the LCST occurs. Nevertheless, in other findings by these authors, the reverse phenomenon was detected when the pressure was increased to higher than 150MPa. The same results have been reported for PNIPAM (Crespy and Rossi, 2007).

Thermo-responsive materials can be used in a wide range of DDS. For example, the regulation of drug release in a pulsatile pattern is a necessary key in designing a localized drug delivery system. According to Yang (Fig. **1**), a novel drug delivery device was made for the pulsatile on-demand release of rhodamine B. In this system, a Peltier electronic element is merged with a thermoresponsive film. Turning the current signal on and off provides the pulsatile release profile of the model drug, and the temperature controls drug release from the thermoresponsive film. In this case, the drug release rate will increase below the LCST, increasing the thermoresponsive size and resulting in a higher drug diffusion rate. On the other hand, increasing the temperature above the LCST reduces the drug release rate due to the collapse of the thermoresponsive polymer network (Yang *et al.*, 2013).

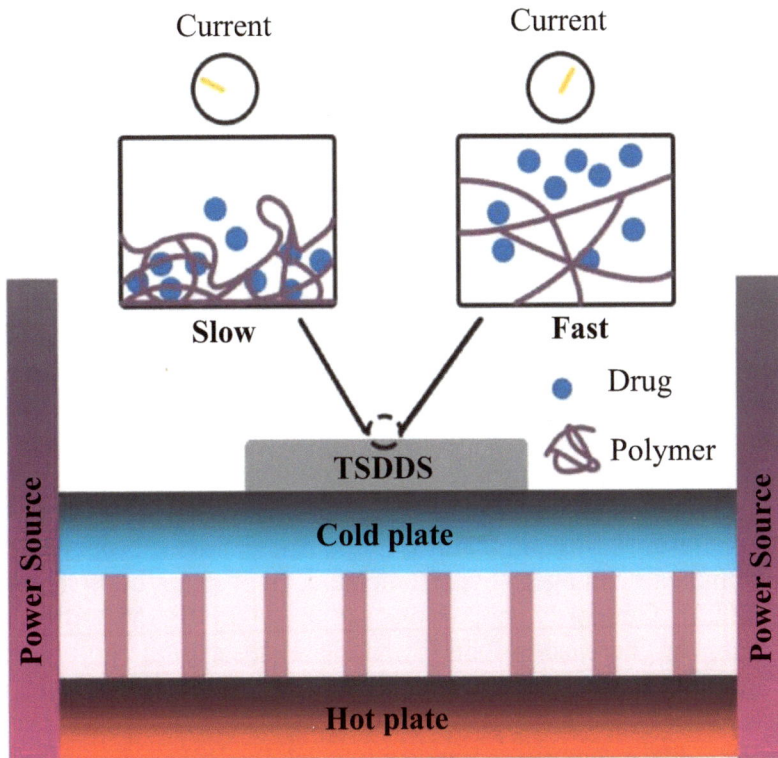

Fig. (1). Schematic of the thermosensitive Peltier drug delivery system.

6.2.1. Poly(N-isopropylacrylamide) *vs* poly(Nvinylcaprolactam)-based Composites

An increasing number of publications demonstrate that poly(N-isopropyl acrylamide) (PNIPAm) is one of the most important thermoresponsive polymers that has been studied extensively in tissue engineering scaffolds, SDDS, biosensors, and cell culture substrates (Subhash *et al.*, 2011). Thermo-reversible phase transition in aqueous solutions, solubility in water, and near body temperature gelation temperatures (32°C) are the most prominent properties of PNIPAm (Lanzalaco and Armelin, 2017). PNIPAm contains isopropylic as a hydrophobic moiety and amide as a hydrophilic moiety. The thermo-reversible rapid phase transition occurs by changing the temperature below or above the LCST as a result of hydration of the polymeric chains and dehydration in a hydrophilic globular state, respectively (Kokardekar *et al.*, 2012). The coil-to-globule transition causes a rapid reduction of the gel volume, which results in a fast drug release, followed by a linear and sustained release (Yoshida *et al.*, 1994).

LCSTs below the normal body temperature are not suitable for developing thermosensitive drug delivery systems. This issue is solved by applying changes to this polymer. The LCST of these polymers does not depend on the polymer MW and may be adjusted by integrating a hydrophobic or hydrophilic component which decreases and increases the LCST, respectively (Kamaly *et al.*, 2016). PNIPAM is simply available by radical polymerization with variable structures like different kinds of copolymers, gels, and grafted surfaces (Rao *et al.*, 2016). Several methods to enhance the properties of polymers based on PNIPAM systems, such as co-polymerization, should be highlighted. Co-polymerization is used to create copolymer systems and present other materials/nanostructures such as metallic nanoparticles, inorganic/ceramic nanoparticles, polymeric nanoparticles and carbon-based nanoparticles into the PNIPAM-derived polymers. Co-polymerization is used to produce interpenetrating polymer networks, which are two or more polymer chains with physical interactions or nanocomposite systems (Xu *et al.*, 2020). The properties of PNIPAM, such as transition temperature, biodegradability, and mechanical properties, may be adjusted with chitosan, collagen, hyaluronic acid, or other natural polymers (Chen and Cheng, 2006). Generally, copolymerization of PNIPAM with hydrophilic monomers causes an increase in LCST, making it closer to the body temperature. It is interesting to note that if the comonomer is an ionic polymer, such as *N*, *N*-dimethylaminoethyl methacrylate (DMAEMA), the final system is pH/temperature dual sensitive (Najafipour *et al.*, 2019). In a study, a thermoresponsive system comprised of hyaluronic acid/PNIPAM-containing chitosan-gacrylic acid coated with PLGA nano/micro-particles was prepared. The thermoresponsive injectable system had high bioactivity, improved mechanical characteristics and a suitable drug release rate. The C_C crosslinkers of PNIPAM established on the CH-g-AA shell of nanoparticles, improved the mechanical strength and controlled the melatonin release rate. This system may be injected into damaged parts and may fill irregular defects (Atoufi *et al.*, 2019).

PNIPAm has a great potential for designing medical systems. However, PNIPAM hydrogel is not a successful choice for designing clinical systems due to its hard degradation and incomplete drug release. Therefore, thermoresponsive and biodegradable hydrogels have been incorporated to design a biodegradable PNIPAM-based system for drug delivery and other biomedical purposes (Gan *et al.*, 2016). As an example, Li *et al.* fabricated a biodegradable thermosensitive poly(N-isopropylacrylamide-co-N,N-dimethylacrylamide-b-e-caprolactone) (PID 118-b-PCL60)/ poly(N-isopropylacrylamide-co-N,N-dimethylacrylamide-b-laci tde) (PID118-b-PLA59) block copolymer. As a result, the (VPTT) was set to the targeted tumor site temperature (39 °C) (Li *et al.*, 2011). In another study, Das *et al.* incorporated dextrin as a biodegradable polysaccharide, with PNIPAM hydrogel and created a biodegradable drug carrier for controlled ornidazole and ciprofloxacin delivery (Das *et al.*, 2015). Another disadvantage of these hydrogels is their poor mechanical properties which reduce their efficiency. IPN hydrogels may be used as a useful approach to improve the mechanical properties of the hydrogels based on PNIPAM. As an example, Kim *et al.* mixed hyaluronic acid with PNIPAM-derived hydrogels to create IPN-based hydrogels with improved mechanical properties (Xu *et al.*, 2020, Kim *et al.*, 2018). There are many studies on the application of PNIPAm-based composites in the biomedical field, which are summarized in Table **1**.

Table 1. PNIPAm-based composites used in SDDSs.

Polymer Composition	Drug Loaded	Type of System	References
PNIPAm-g-carboxymethyl chitosan	DOX	nanoparticle	(Antoniraj *et al.*, 2016)
PNIPAM–chitosan	curcumin	nanoparticles	(Yadavalli *et al.*, 2015)
mesoporous silica/PNIPAM-MAA/lanthanid--polyoxometalates	DOX	nanoparticles	(Wang *et al.*, 2020)
PMAA/PNIPAM	DOX	microgel	(Liu *et al.*, 2017)
poly(acrylic acid)-b-PNIPAm	DOX	micelle	(Li *et al.*, 2008)
chitosan-graft-PNIPAm/ carboxymethyl cellulose	5-fluorouracil	nanoparticle	(Zhang *et al.*, 2012)
ellulose nanofibril-PNIPAm hybrid	5-fluorouracil	microsphere	(Zhang *et al.*, 2016)

PVCL (Poly(N-vinylcaprolactam)) is another thermoresponsive polymer with similar features to a presented PNIPAM for biomedical application. This thermosensitive polymer has an LCST near body temperature (32C) (Vihola *et al.*, 2002, Vihola *et al.*, 2008). Similar to PNIPAm, Poly(N-Vinyl caprolactam) (PNVCL) can simply incorporate with biopolymers like chitosan and alginate to adjust LCST and biodegradability (Rejinold *et al.*, 2015). PNVCL consists of a hydrophilic amide group with a repeating unit, which contains a cyclic amide where the amide group nitrogen is directly attached to the hydrophobic polymer backbone. Therefore, unlike PNIPAm, it does not create small amide products upon hydrolysis [43]. Adjusting the polymerization molecular mass, and dispersity are some of the limitations of PNVCL. These limitations have been resolved by Cobalt and RAFT/MADIX-mediated polymerization techniques. Another problem is the change in the copolymerization capacity with the most common groups of monomers, including methacrylates, acrylates and styrenics (Cortez-Lemus and Licea-Claverie, 2016).

There are many biomedical systems based on poly(N-vinyl caprolactam), including hybrid nanostructures, self-assembly, and microgels. Along with the improvements of PNVCL-based systems, many studies have focused on the sol-gel transition behavior and mechanical strength under specific conditions of this polymer (Peng *et al.*, 2019). As an example, hydroxypropyl guar-graft-PNVCL had excellent thermoresponsive behavior and a reversible soluble-insoluble behavior at ~34 °C. This system may be used for the sustained release of injectable drugs. Besides, the HPG-g-PNVCL system acted as an excellent scaffold with high mechanical strength (Parameswaran-Thankam *et al.*, 2018). It should be noted that the LCST of PNVCL depends on the polymer concentration, chain length, and molecular weight (Ieong *et al.*, 2012). Water solubility, toxicity, and LCST represent the properties of PNVCL and PNIPAM. However, these two polymers are different in some features, such as the sol-gel transition thermodynamics and mechanisms. Moreover, the hydrolysis of PNIPAM under a concentrated acidic environment, produced toxic organic amine products, which were not favorable for biomedical applications, but the hydrolysis of PNVCL under a concentrated acidic environment, produced polymeric carboxylic acid rather than toxic amine products. (Mohammed *et al.*, 2018). There are many reported studies on PNVCL based composites that are used in the biomedical field which are summarized in Table **2**.

6.2.2. Oligoethylene Glycol-based Composites

Another group of thermosensitive polymers that can contend with or even surpass PNIPAm are oligo ethylene glycol-based polymers (Vancoillie *et al.*, 2014). Poly (oligo ethylene glycol acrylates) (OEG)-containing molecules have both the biocompatibility of (PEG) and controllable LCST performance. OEG polymers prepared by controlled radical polymerization methods from numerous monomers contain an asymmetrical OEG chain and a polymerizable group such as acrylamide, (meth)acrylate, or styrene (Vancoillie *et al.*, 2014). Thermosensitive polymers including oligo(ethylene glycol), are more useful in biomedical applications compared to PNIPAM-based polymers, due to their nonimmunogenic and nontoxic nature (Shao *et al.*, 2014). As an example, Soliman *et al.* demonstrated thermoresponsive star-shaped poly(oligoethylene glycol) copolymers *in situ* gels as nasal delivery carriers for risedronate and studied their *in vivo* efficacy for osteoporosis therapy in a rat model (Soliman *et al.*, 2018). In addition to the biocompatibility of OEG, LCST can be tuned by copolymerization, which means that LCST can be modulated without introducing comonomers of diverse chemical nature (París and Quijada-Garrido, 2009).

Table 2. PNVCL based composites used in SDDSs.

Polymer Composition	Drug Loaded	Type of System	References
chitosan-g PNVCL	5 fluorouracil	nanoparticle	(Rejinold *et al.*, 2011)
chitosan-graft-poly(Nvinylcaprolactam)	DOX	nanoparticle	(Fernández-Quiroz *et al.*, 2019)
poly(NVCL-co-AA)	ketoprofen	microparticle	(Medeiros *et al.*, 2017)
PNVCL-co-MAA	ketoprofen	nanofiber	(Liu *et al.*, 2016b)
PNIPA-co-NVC	Ciproflaxin	microsphere	(Mallikarjuna *et al.*, 2011)
fib-graft PNVCL	5-fluorouracil	nanogel	(Rejinold *et al.*, 2015)
poly (vinyl caprolactum-co-vinyl acetate)	5-fluorouracil	microsphere	(Yerriswamy *et al.*, 2014)
poly(NVCL-co-AGA)	5-fluorouracil	nanogel	(Rao *et al.*, 2013)

Polymers bearing a short (OEG) side chain can be used to produce dendrimers and fabricate thermosensitive scaffolds for biomedical purposes like drug delivery and tissue engineering.

The OEG groups of the dendrimers can develop particular hydrogen bonds with water molecules by virtue of the great compatibility between their geometrical structures. At high temperatures, when the thermal energy of the system exceeds the hydrogen bond energy, the interaction with water molecules is weakened, which results in thermosensitive performance (Wu *et al.*, 2014). Among all types of ethylene glycol-based macromonomers, OEG methacrylates (OEGMA) have been widely studied. In addition to biodegradability, injectability, and adjustable mechanical and chemical properties, poly(oligoethylene glycol methacrylate) (POEGMA) shows all of the essential protein and cell-repellent behaviors of conventional PEG hydrogels. According to the mentioned properties, OEGMA is a suitable choice for localized drug delivery, and injectable tissue engineering matrices (Smeets *et al.*, 2014). Lutz *et al.* verified the superior thermoresponsive behavior of OEGMA-based polymer (P(MEO2MA-co-OEGMA)) compared to polyNIPAAM (Lutz *et al.*, 2006).

6.2.3. Degradable Composites

In spite of the increasing number of publications on adjusting thermoresponsive properties, a small number of studies have focused on the post-delivery of polymer-based systems. This problem is of certain concern when TRDDS are derived from polymers prepared by methacrylamide and methacrylate monomers. Actually, in this case, after the hydrolysis of pendant groups, these polymers can leave behind hydrocarbon chains, which are not simply metabolized in the biological environment (Kamaly *et al.*, 2016). In fact, biodegradability is often necessary when using polymeric systems as biomaterials in the body environment. This factor allows materials to be metabolized and excreted from the body after treatment. Many studies have focused on thermosensitive poly(amino acid) and polyesters-derived materials, such as amphiphilic polyesters based on elastin-like polypeptide (ELP), poly(lactic acid) (PLA) and poly(ε-caprolactone) (PCL) (Komatsu *et al.*, 2017). As an example, Rainbolt *et al.* synthesized diblock copolymers, poly{γ -2-[2-(2-methoxyethoxy)ethoxy]ethoxy-ε-caprolactone}-b-poly{γ-(2-methoxyethoxy)-ε-caprolactone}, which exhibited biodegradable behavior and adjustable thermoresponsive performance (31–43 °C). The system had great potential for designing micellar TRDDS (Zhuo *et al.*, 2020) Besides, the mentioned polymers, aliphatic polycarbonates are biocompatible and degradable polymers which can be widely used in DDS. In spite of polyesters, which display bulk erosion degradation, polycarbonates are presented by surface erosion degradation, and do not create acidic byproducts (Kamaly *et al.*, 2016). It is worth to note that biodegradability is very important in localized drug delivery and injectable biodegradable hydrogels for biomedical applications, like drug/gene delivery and tissue engineering (Nguyen and Lee, 2010).

One of the important issues of poly(NIPAAm) in biomedical applications such as drug delivery systems is the non-degradable nature of NIPAAm, which limits its application in implantation and LDDS. The presence of non-degradable materials in the body environment may cause chronic inflammatory reactions. Therefore, improving the biodegradability of thermo-sensitive polymers, especially PNIPAm, is essential for designing smart and localized drug delivery systems (Cui *et al.*, 2007). For example, Niu *et al.* synthesized a thermosensitive and degradable PNIPAm-based hydrogel for delivering stem cells into infarcted heart and skeletal muscle tissues. The hydrogels were polymerized by (NIPAAm), 2-hydroxyethyl methacrylate (HEMA), 1-vinyl-2-pyrrolidinone (VP), and acrylateoligolactide (AOLA) and conjugated with hypericin (HYP). This degradable system was injected at 4 °C and quickly transformed to gel-state within 7s at normal body temperature. The degradable nature of this system allows the degradation of products by dissolving in body fluids and leaving the body through the urinary system (Niu *et al.*, 2019). In another study, Ziminska *et al.* synthesized a stable thermosensitive Cs-g-PNIPAAm hydrogel system. The storage modulus, swelling, degradation, and release rate from the hydrogel were adjusted by the chitosan ratio in the copolymer. This injectable system has a great potential for minimally invasive drug delivery and can be used as a sustained drug delivery system over a three-week period for localized and long-term delivery (Ziminska *et al.*, 2020).

6.3. LIGHT-RESPONSIVE DRUG DELIVERY

Light has many advantages in smart drug-delivery systems as an external stimulus. Some of these advantages are great spatial resolution, non-invasive nature, temporal control, and comfort of use. For these reasons, light has been broadly applied in a wide range of biomedical applications. The most common applications are drug delivery, image-guided surgery, degradation of tissue engineering scaffolds, and photodynamic therapy for cancer treatment. (Linsley and Wu, 2017). One of the most important light-based treatments is Photodynamic therapy (PDT). PDT is a clinical treatment, which uses photosensitizers (PS) to produce toxic reactive oxygen species (ROS) in the presence of light irradiation. Numerous fluorophores can be used as photosensitizers (PSs) that make toxic ROS along with fluorescence upon light irradiation. PDT can be used in combination with chemotherapy for the treatment of different types of cancers. PDT is an effective method for killing multi-drug-resistant cancer cells. In addition, the light radiation properties may be used to control the treatment (Son *et al.*, 2019). A photodynamic agent must have certain properties including: (1) strong absorption of near-infrared light, (2) biodegradability and biocompatibility, (3) great singlet oxygen quantum yield, (4) low or no dark toxicity, and (5) great photostability (Chen and Zhao, 2018).

Photocleavage-activated drug delivery systems enable the release of entrapped therapeutic drugs through the cleavage of photoscissible covalent bonds upon light irradiation. The most popular compounds used in photochemical-responsive drug delivery systems include nitrobenzyl, pyrene, and coumarin derivatives. The nitrobenzyl moiety can be irreversibly cleaved under UV irradiation to release free carboxylic acid and nitrosobenzaldehyde. The ester bonds in pyrene and coumarin can also be cleaved upon UV irradiation. These moieties can be employed as a photocage to prevent bioactivity of therapeutic drugs or as a cleavable linker in photo-controlled carriers for smart drug delivery purposes (Tao *et al.*, 2020).

Adjusting the hydrophilicity-hydrophobicity shift of amphiphilic polymers is another most common strategy to achieve photo-controlled disassembly of smart drug carriers. Drug carriers with photo-regulated hydrophobicity–hydrophilicity balance are designed to contain hydrophilic parts and another hydrophobic part supporting photochromic moieties on the backbone or side chains. The foundation and stability of photo-responsive drug carriers depend on the hydrophilic to hydrophobic balance. Under NIR irradiation, the photochemical reaction of the photochromic agents converts the hydrophobic part to hydrophilic, therefore causing the disassembly of carriers and drug release (Cho *et al.*, 2015).

Another strategy for achieving a light-triggered drug delivery system is photoisomerization which is a process that includes a conformational change about a bond that is restricted in rotation, typically a double bond. Organic molecules which have double bonds mostly contain isomerization from a trans orientation to a cis form followed by light irradiation. Azobenzenes, which have \N_N\ with phenyl rings on both sides, are the most popular used molecules for this aim. The key parameter which provides azobenzenes as an attractive choice for designing on-demand drug delivery systems is its reversible isomerization. It should be highlighted that the planar transform of azobenzenes is more hydrophobic than the nonplanar cis form (Fomina *et al.*, 2012).

As an example an azobenzene derivative (4-(3 triethoxysilyl propylureido) azobenzene; TSUA) was bound to MSNs. β- cyclodextrin (β-CD) was threaded onto the trans-TSUA stalks, to close the nanopores and prevent the release of drugs. Under UV irradiation (351 nm), the trans-cis transformation of TSUA resulted in the detachment of the β-CD rings from the stalks and the release of the drugs, followed by the opening of the nanopores (Barhoumi *et al.*, 2015).

Reversibly cross-linking/decrosslinking of a system is another effective strategy for designing photoinduced drug-loaded particles to deliver drugs at targeted sites. Coumarin, and cinnamoyl are the most used molecules to create crosslinked polymeric systems. These molecules may perform a cross-linking reaction *via* [2 + 2]-cycloaddition, under UV-light irradiation. The decrosslinking process happens unexpectedly when the system is exposed to radiation with photons with higher energy (shorter wavelength). As an example, Fluorouracil (5-Fu) was loaded into coumarin substitutes and cross-linked under365 nm UV light irradiation. The cross-linked assemblies were disrupted and exhibited an anticancer activity under UV light with a shorter wavelength (254 nm) (Zhao *et al.*, 2019).

The capability of NIR-absorbing plasmonic materials to transform photon energy into heat has been widely used to trigger the release of drugs from NIR-responsive devices. NIR-absorbing nanostructures such as carbon nanotubes, graphene oxide and gold nanoparticles may be used for designing light-responsive systems. In these cases, the NIR-absorbing nanostructures are incorporated in thermoresponsive carrier and convert NIR light into heat due to the photothermal effect, further the matrix is destroyed and the entrapped drugs are released (Ito, 2018).

It should be highlighted that based on the exposed light wavelengths, the most commonly used light for designing light-responsive delivery systems can be divided into three groups, including near-infrared (NIR) (700–1000 nm), visible light (Vis) (400–700 nm), and ultraviolet (UV) (200– 400 nm) (Chen and Zhao, 2018).

UV-responsive carriers are widely studied due to the adjustable wavelength and energy in a UV production setup and the low cost of the apparatus, which is simply set up in a laboratory. UV absorption happens through a one-photon process; though, ultraviolet and visible light can only diffuse shallow tissues (on the order of microns) due to the strong absorption and scattering by water and endogenous proteins such as hemoglobin in the body environment. Besides, UV light has harmful effects on tissues and cells, these disadvantages limit UV-responsive systems for biomedical purposes. Unlike UV light, absorption can occur through a two-photon process. Actually, two-photon absorption of NIR light makes similar energy to trigger the photoreactions of photochromic agents as one-photon absorption of UV light. Besides, NIR light can diffuse deeply into the tissues (on the order of several inches) because of the lower absorption and scattering by biomolecules and water. Moreover, NIR light has no noticeable harm to cells/tissues (Liu *et al.*, 2013a).

Therefore, light has a high potential for designing smart drug delivery systems. The combination of light with injectable localized systems makes an innovative, effective and minimally invasive drug delivery system with great physical properties and highly controlled drug release (Bisht *et al.*, 2016).

6.3.1. UV-light-responsive Drug Delivery

Reversible Photoisomerization of Azobenzenes from trans to cis form under UV light with a 300–380 nm wavelength and from cis to trans under visible light allows photo-controlled drug release (Mura *et al.*, 2013). Actually, These systems act differently due to the changes in hydrophobicity, polarity, conformation, and morphology (Yadav *et al.*, 2016). Mesoporous silica nanoparticles (MSNs) are the most common choices for developing photoisomerization-based drug delivery systems (Tao *et al.*, 2020). Mal *et al.* described the application of UV light in a reversible drug release system. The system used an MSNP wherein the pores were clogged with coumarin molecules which can suffer reversible dimerization in the presence of light irradiation. The same research group enhanced the treatment of the system using azobenzene molecules inside the pore networks. These molecules suffer cis-trans transformation followed by UV irradiation and they can act as nanoimpellers leading the drugs out of the channels (Fig. **2**) (Baeza *et al.*, 2015).

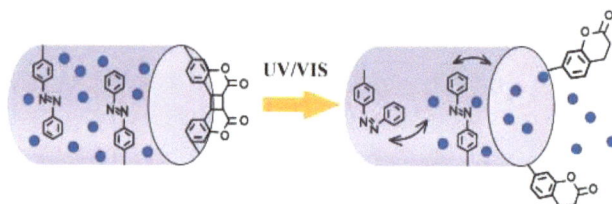

Fig. (2). Schematic of cis-trans isomerisation under UV irradiation of Coumarin-azobenzene-MSNPs.

In another study, a system was designed from surfactant, sodium dodecyl sulfate (SDS), and 4-cholesterocarbonyl-4′-(N, N, N-triethylamine butyloxyl bromide) azobenzene (CAB) in an aqueous solution. Reversible trans-to-cis photoisomerization of the CAB in vesicles upon UV light triggered the release of rhodamine B (RhB) and doxorubicin (DOX). Generally, the bent form of the cis structure of CAB molecules had more free space compared to the straight trans isomer, which caused the penetration of RhB through the micropore channels followed by UV irradiation. The carriers were treated with UV light 10 min every hour to avoid the cis-CAB from transforming back to the trans form in the absence of UV light, (Geng *et al.*, 2017). The hydrophobic–hydrophilic photo-transition can also be useful for designing smart carriers such as the hydrophobic trans- hydrophilic cis transformation of Azobenzene under UV radiation (340-380 nm). Similarly, the disassembly of micelle carriers due to the conversion of spiroypyran to its hydrophilic congener merocyanine results in the release of trapped drug molecules (Nair *et al.*, 2018). Another strategy is to investigate UV-cleavable systems. In this regard, a UV-cleavable star-like system that contains a 6-arm amphiphilic block copolymer and a UV-cleavable core with the photolabile o-nitrobenzyl group has been studied in Liu's work. Consequently, the detachment of unimolecular micelles and drug release can be controlled with UV irradiation and cleavage of the amphiphilic side chain from the inner core (Liu *et al.*, 2013c).

Sreejivungsa *et al.* studied a UV-controlled drug delivery system with noncovalently trapped drug molecules inside the monolayers of AuNPs. The structure of an alkanethiol monolayer contains hydrophobic pockets coupled with the aromatic character of dinitrobenzyl groups, which make more space to host hydrophobic drug molecules with controlled release, referred to Au-PC-COOH (Fig. **3**). Besides the anionic carboxylate groups in the exterior monolayer provide

EPR effect and reduce nonspecific binding to macromolecules. UV irradiation, and photocleavage of the monolayer of Au-PC-COOH results in the release of entrapped drug molecules, and the spatiotemporally controlled release of drug by UV irradiation, provides localized drug delivery and delivering drugs to the diseased tissue site (Sreejivungsa *et al.*, 2016).

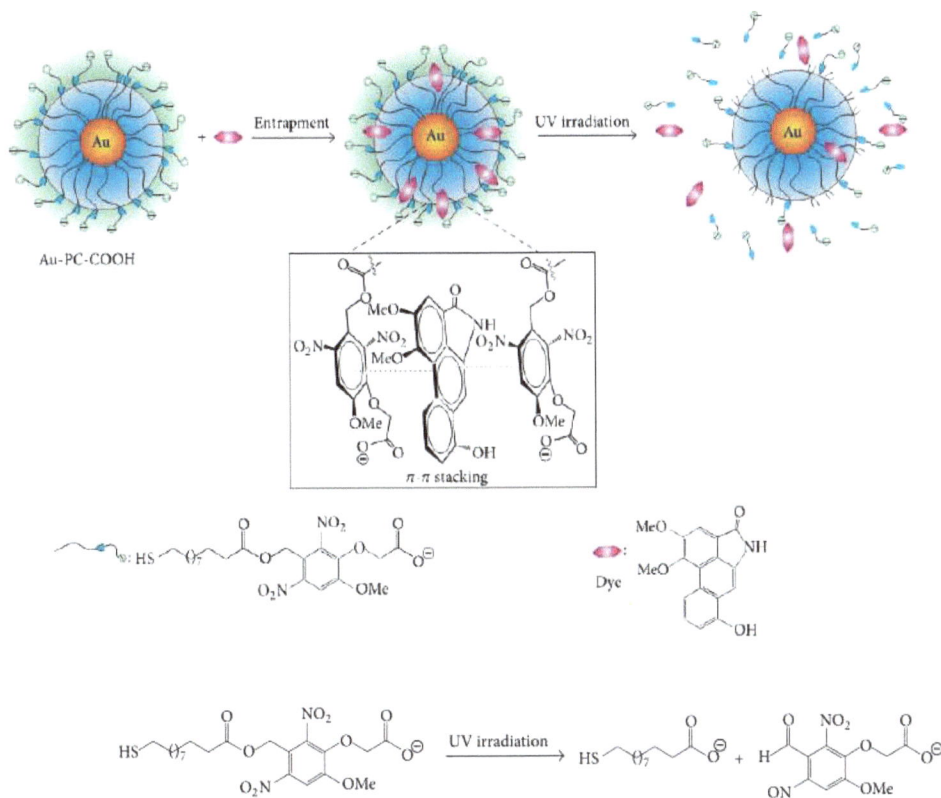

Fig. (3). A schematic of dye-loaded Au-PC-COOH, structure of dye, and release of entrapped molecules followed by UV irradiation, (b) photocleavage response of a PC ligand (Open access) (Sreejivungsa *et al.*, 2016).

6.3.2. NIR-light-responsive Drug Delivery

Near-infrared (NIR) light with a significant penetration feature is one of the most commonly used stimuli in designing smart drug delivery systems. Three strategies have been reported for drug release from NIR-light-responsive DDS: (a) Up-converting nanoparticles (UCNPs), (b) two-photonabsorption (TPA), and (c) photothermal effect (PTE) (Raza *et al.*, 2019a).

NIR-responsive DDS has been broadly considered, particularly those established by heating a thermoresponsive part *via* joining NIR-absorbing nanostructures. As an example, gold nanorods (GNRs) that can convert NIR light into heat were attached to liposomes (Lip-GNRs), enabling the NIR-induced phase transition of lipid bilayers with the subsequent release of drugs (Zhan *et al.*, 2016).

Since UV radiation has high energy with enough potential for the most relevant chemical changes, most light-responsive systems are activated only by UV, whilst NIR light has better tissue penetration but poor energy to initiate a chemical change. This problem has been solved with the development of TPA and UCNPs systems which absorb two photons of low-energy NIR light to make the same effects as with absorption of one photon of high-energy UV light (Olejniczak *et al.*, 2013). Using these two methods in the NIR region instead of high-energy lights has numerous advantages, including deeper penetration in body tissues, lower scattering losses, and three-dimensional spatial and temporal control of the drug release in a specific site(Croissant *et al.*, 2013). In the two-photon absorption strategy, simultaneous absorption of two photons excites a molecule from the lowest-energy state (ground state) to a higher energy level which then jumps back to the primary state by producing one photon which has higher energy than either of the absorbed photons (Zhu *et al.*, 2017). As an example, Ji *et al.* fabricated a unique nanocarrier by coating a light-responsive amphiphilic polymer onto modified HMSNs for controlled drug release in specific cancer cells. The multifunctional amphiphilic polymer was synthesized by RAFT polymerization of [7-(didodecylamino) coumarin-4-yl] methyl methacrylate (DDACMM) and hydroxyethylacrylate (HEA) and grafted with folic acid for selective cancer targeting. After modification of HMSNs with hydrophobic octadecyl chains (C18), core–shell nanocomposites (HMS@C18@HAMAFA-b-DDACMM) were obtained by coating the amphiphilic copolymers onto the core *via* a simple self-assembly strategy and DOX was entrapped in the mentioned system. The resulting nanocomposite could be disrupted by excitation with a femtosecond NIR light laser (800 nm) *via* a TPA process due to the high two-photon absorption cross-section of the coumarin moiety (Ji *et al.*, 2013).

The photoreaction triggered by TPA of NIR light has some disadvantages, including 1) low speed and ineffectiveness because of low two-photon-absorbing cross-sections of the chromophores. 2) the necessity of the use of a femtosecond pulse laser as the simultaneous absorption of two photons requires a laser with great power density in this case. Therefore, upconverting nanoparticles (UCNPs) were introduced recently. UCNPs absorb energy from two or more photons subsequently in the NIR range and convert it to photons with higher energy than each individual excitation photon in the UV, visible, and NIR regions. In contrast to TPA, the excitation of UCNPs by NIR light occurs *via* sequential, multiple absorptions with real energy levels. Therefore, a laser with a lower power density, such as a continuous-wave diode NIR laser may be used as the excitation source (Yan *et al.*, 2011). These UCNPs are usually made of lanthanide-based nanomaterials and can be used to activate photochemical changes for promoting drug release or to activate photosensitizers for photodynamic therapy (PDT) (Raza *et al.*, 2019a). The mechanisms for the development of UCNPs drug delivery systems can be divided into three groups: 1) NIR light-triggered redox reaction of photoactivated prodrug molecules, 2) NIR light-induced isomerization, 3) NIR light-induced photolysis of photoactivatable molecules (Zhao *et al.*, 2019).

To indicate the use of UCNPs, a study used poly(ethylene oxide)-block-poly(4-5-dimethoxy-2-nitrobenzyl methacrylate) as a UV-sensitive copolymer. The copolymer formed 100 nm micelles and UCNPs entrapped inside self-assemblies during their formation. Here, upon NIR irradiation (980 nm), simultaneous UV and visible emissions occurred from the UCNPs inside the micelles. As a result, o-nitrobenzyl groups were cleaved and the particles were destabilized, leading to drug release (Beauté *et al.*, 2019). Upconversion can also be used for photo-isomerization-triggered drug release. Liu *et al.* synthesized a NIR-triggered UCNPs coated with azobenzene-modified MSN (Liu *et al.*, 2013b). Here, Upon NIR irradiation, the UCNPs converted the light to higher-energy photons in visible and UV ranges, which were then absorbed by the photo-active azobenzene moiety in the MSN network, causing a reversible trans-cis isomerization. Finally, the sequential rotation inversion movements of azobenzene agents led to therapeutic drug release (Karimi *et al.*, 2017).

6.4. ULTRASOUND-RESPONSIVE DRUG DELIVERY

Using ultrasound-based methods is a safe method for designing drug/gene delivery and diagnosis systems due to its deep penetration into the tissue, and non-invasive nature. Ultrasound-responsive drug delivery systems have many advantages, including localized delivery and spatial drug release control. Microbubbles are the most recognized ultrasound-sensitive delivery systems.

Recently, nanoliposomes, micelles, droplets and nanobubbles have been studied widely as unique carriers (Cai *et al.*, 2020). Ultrasound permits the deposition of mechanical and thermal energies deep inside the body environment and can be focused with high intensity inside the desired tissue with a diameter of about 1 mm. It should be noted that the features of ultrasound can lead to local heating, cavitation, and radiation force, which can be useful for designing local drug delivery systems from nanocarriers with enhanced diffusivity of drugs (Deckers and Moonen, 2010). The efficiency of ultrasound-responsive drug delivery systems relies on the interaction between biocompatible materials as a carrier and an acoustic wave. Moreover, spatial drug release control is established by focusing the waves in the desired zone (Couture *et al.*, 2014).

The frequencies of the US used for biomedical applications are classified as high-frequency (5 MHz <frequency<10 MHz), medium (1 MHz <frequency<5 MHz) and low (frequency <1 MHz). US can noninvasively penetrate centimeters deep into the desired zone. Low-frequency US does not damage or excessively heat the tissues; however, it is hardly focused on a single point with high intensity and makes a larger focus point. Medium frequency US has a lower ability to penetrate into body tissues due to its higher scattering and attenuation. High-frequency US penetration into tissues is proportionally converted into heat, which can be harmful to tissues (Kamaly *et al.*, 2016).

US permits the deposition of mechanical or thermal energies deep inside the tissues. Thermal effects followed by the absorption of thermal energy by cells increase the temperature. In this case, hyperthermia causes the heating of carriers and drug release or may result in heating and damaging of the tumor tissues. In contrast, the mechanical effects occur because of oscillating bubbles, wave pressure, cavitation, and acoustic streaming (Elkhodiry *et al.*, 2016). It is worth noting that hyperthermia and thermal effect in US-responsive delivery systems can trigger release from thermo-responsive systems. Thermodox, is a well-known example of low-temperature-sensitive liposomes with encapsulated DOX (Boissenot *et al.*, 2016). The volumetric oscillations in compressible objects, such as microbubbles, when exposed to the acoustic waves, can facilitate designing SDDS with improved drug uptake and strong backscattered echoes that are useful for imaging purpose (Sirsi and Borden, 2014). Cavitation phenomena may be used as a mechanical effect to characterize the response of gas-filled bubbles under ultrasound exposure. This phenomenon is regarded as a key motivation to promote smart delivery systems and can be divided into stable and inertial cavitation based on the response of microbubbles (Yang *et al.*, 2019). Under stable cavitation, microbubbles oscillate periodically about their equilibrium radius without collapsing. The expansion of microbubbles occurs due to the rarefaction phase of an ultrasound wave, while their contract occurs due to the compression phase. This non-Inertial phenomenon leads to microstreaming, which enhances the micropump of drugs to the surrounding liquid due to the momentum transfer. The inertial cavitation and microbubble expansion start when the pressure increases, resulting in unstable bubble growth. Due to this transient phenomenon, microbubbles collapse rapidly to a small division of their primary volume. Inertial cavitation has a tendency to produce heat, shock waves, free radicals, shear forces, and microstreams. So this effect will play a key role in Ultrasound-responsive DDS for delivering drugs deep into solid tumors (Mo *et al.*, 2012).

US-responsive drug delivery systems contain microbubbles (Ahmadi *et al.*, 2020), nanobubbles (Suzuki *et al.*, 2005), liposomes (Schroeder *et al.*, 2007, Schroeder *et al.*, 2009), and micelles (Rapoport, 2004, Husseini *et al.*, 2000). Since the 1990s, many research groups have tried to develop microbubbles that can carry therapeutic drugs. Microbubbles are attractive choices for US-responsive drug delivery systems due to (a) the visualization of drug-loaded microbubbles with low acoustic pressures and potential for 'image-guided drug delivery'; (b) several drugs, specific biopharmaceuticals such as nucleic acids and proteins must be protected from degradation upon administration, which can be done by formulation associated with microbubbles; (c) the drugs entrapped into microbubbles can also stop their uptake in undesirable tissue and thus decrease side-effects; (d) both localized drug delivery and cell membrane permeabilization can happen upon exposure to ultrasound (Geers *et al.*, 2012).

Microbubbles, as appropriate ultrasound contrast agents are micro-sized (1–10 μm) gas bubbles with a shell composed of phospholipids, polymers, or proteins. Many approaches may be used to create drug-loaded microbubbles, which involve the association of drugs with the shell, covalent linkage with the building blocks, and drugs entrapped in an oil reservoir within the microbubble core. Another approach includes trapping the drugs into nanoparticles, which are attached to the microbubble surface at a subsequent time (Zhao *et al.*, 2013). However, because of the size of microparticles (1-10 μm), MB-based drug delivery systems suffer from confinement to the vasculature and poorly penetration into tumor tissues, so their applications for *in vivo* tumor treatment are limited (Wang *et al.*, 2010). Nanobubbles (NBs) have developed as favorable choices for US-triggered drug delivery, with great penetration into the desired site because of their small size and extravasation from blood vessels into surrounding tissues (Batchelor *et al.*, 2020).

Nanobubbles as a further generation of US responsive carriers, have high efficiency for designing drug delivery systems for *in vivo* studies. Nanobubbles can be loaded with gases, hydrophilic or lipophilic and small or macromolecules.

Several approaches have been suggested for loading drugs and genes on nanobubbles: a) incorporation of drugs within the core, b) encapsulation of drugs at the interface with the gas core, c) incorporation of drugs within the bubble shell d) dissolution of cargoes in an inner oil layer added to the shell; (e) electrostatic interaction between drugs and the bubble shell and (f) trapping the drugs into nanoparticles then linking to the bubble surface (Cavalli *et al.*, 2016).

In addition to microbubbles and nanobubbles, numerous studies have focused on the application of US as a stimulus for drug delivery from liposomes. Liposomes include an aqueous core enclosed by single or concentric bilayers. The liposome membrane usually includes phospholipids with polar hydrophilic heads and nonpolar lipophilic tails. Hydrophilic drugs are entrapped in the aqueous core, whereas lipophilic drugs are dissolved in the hydrophilic membrane (Ahmadi *et al.*, 2020). The common liposome-based drugs described in the literature are temperature-sensitive liposomes (TSL). TSLs release entrapped drugs close to the melting phase transition temperature (Tm) of the lipid bilayer, at which the lipid membrane structure converts from a gel to a liquid crystalline phase (Ninomiya *et al.*, 2014). Inspired by the concept of TSL, Dormi *et al.* proposed pulsed-high intensity focused ultrasound (HIFU) as a source of hyperthermia with TSL to noninvasively produce improved and localized DOX delivery in tumor (Dromi *et al.*, 2007, Wang and Kohane, 2017)

Polymeric micelles (PMs) have shown a great potential for designing drug delivery systems upon exposure to US by physical/chemical disruption of the micelles (Zhou *et al.*, 2018). A micelle is composed of an amphiphilic molecule as a hydrophobic core and a hydrophilic shell. The hydrophobic/hydrophilic interactions of the molecules control the structure of the micelle. The commonly studied micelles for US-triggered drug delivery are based on Pluronic block copolymers that are composed of triblock copolymers of poly (propylene oxide) (PPO) and poly(ethylene oxide) (Husseini and Pitt, 2008). The PMs are disrupted or disassembled upon exposure to US due to the ultrasonic cavitation and the drugs are released from the micelles. For this approach, the micelle disassembly is temporary and the drug release is reversible. Actually, as the US ceases, the micelle can be reassembled again, and the payload can be re-entrapped. As an example, Xia and Zhao developed a new US- triggered drug release system based on the usage of amphiphilic block copolymers of designed US-susceptible molecular structures. When the micelle solution was subjected to ultrasound perturbation, the US-responsive copolymer was degraded and the amphiphilic copolymer structure was broken. The hydrophobic/ hydrophilic balance was shifted, and therefore the micelle was disrupted and the entrapped drugs were irreversibly released (Xia *et al.*, 2016).

CONCLUSION

Based on the developments in drug delivery, biology and materials chemistry, a stimuli-sensitive strategy to release a therapeutic molecule in dosage-controlled, temporal-controlled and spatial-controlled frames has been widely used. The application of these carriers requires the utilization of bio/cyto-compatible biomaterials that are sensitive to a precise physico-chemical stimulus or a supramolecular conformational variation. Exogeneous-triggered delivery in LCDDS, is the promising approach for spatiotemporal regulation upon the drug release. In this chapter, we discussed important advances and progress in the design and fabrication of stimuli-sensitive LCDDS that are capable of regulating the distribution of therapeutic molecules (drugs) in response to a specific exogenous stimulus (changes in light, ultrasound and temperature).

REFERENCES

Ahmadi, A., Hosseini-Nami, S., Abed, Z., Beik, J., Aranda-Lara, L., Samadian, H., Morales-Avila, E., Jaymand, M., Shakeri-Zadeh, A. (2020). Recent advances in ultrasound-triggered drug delivery through lipid-based nanomaterials. *Drug Discov. Today, 25*(12), 2182-2200.
[http://dx.doi.org/10.1016/j.drudis.2020.09.026] [PMID: 33010479]

Antoniraj, M.G., Kumar, C.S., Kandasamy, R. (2016). Synthesis and characterization of poly (N-isopropylacrylamide)-g-carboxymethyl chitosan copolymer-based doxorubicin-loaded polymeric nanoparticles for thermoresponsive drug release. *Colloid Polym. Sci., 294*(3), 527-535.
[http://dx.doi.org/10.1007/s00396-015-3804-4]

Askari, E., Naghib, S.M., Zahedi, A., Seyfoori, A., Zare, Y., Rhee, K.Y. (2021). Local delivery of chemotherapeutic agent in tissue engineering based on gelatin/graphene hydrogel. *J. Mater. Res. Technol., 12*, 412-422.
[http://dx.doi.org/10.1016/j.jmrt.2021.02.084]

Askari, E., Seyfoori, A., Amereh, M., Gharaie, S.S., Ghazali, H.S., Ghazali, Z.S., Khunjush, B., Akbari, M. (2020). Stimuli-responsive hydrogels for local post-surgical drug delivery. *Gels, 6*(2), 14.
[http://dx.doi.org/10.3390/gels6020014] [PMID: 32397180]

Atoufi, Z., Kamrava, S.K., Davachi, S.M., Hassanabadi, M., Saeedi Garakani, S., Alizadeh, R., Farhadi, M., Tavakol, S., Bagher, Z., Hashemi Motlagh, G. (2019). Injectable PNIPAM/Hyaluronic acid hydrogels containing multipurpose modified particles for cartilage tissue engineering: Synthesis, characterization, drug release and cell culture study. *Int. J. Biol. Macromol., 139*, 1168-1181.
[http://dx.doi.org/10.1016/j.ijbiomac.2019.08.101] [PMID: 31419553]

Baeza, A., Colilla, M., Vallet-Regí, M. (2015). Advances in mesoporous silica nanoparticles for targeted stimuli-responsive drug delivery. *Expert Opin. Drug Deliv., 12*(2), 319-337.
[http://dx.doi.org/10.1517/17425247.2014.953051] [PMID: 25421898]

Barhoumi, A., Liu, Q., Kohane, D.S. (2015). Ultraviolet light-mediated drug delivery: Principles, applications, and challenges. *J. Control. Release, 219*, 31-42.
[http://dx.doi.org/10.1016/j.jconrel.2015.07.018] [PMID: 26208426]

Batchelor, D.V.B., Abou-Saleh, R.H., Coletta, P.L., McLaughlan, J.R., Peyman, S.A., Evans, S.D. (2020). Nested nanobubbles for ultrasound-triggered drug release. *ACS Appl. Mater. Interfaces, 12*(26), 29085-29093.
[PMID: 32501014]

Beauté, L., McClenaghan, N., Lecommandoux, S. (2019). Photo-triggered polymer nanomedicines: From molecular mechanisms to therapeutic applications. *Adv. Drug Deliv. Rev., 138*, 148-166.
[http://dx.doi.org/10.1016/j.addr.2018.12.010] [PMID: 30553952]

Bikram, M., West, J.L. (2008). Thermo-responsive systems for controlled drug delivery. *Expert Opin. Drug Deliv., 5*(10), 1077-1091.
[http://dx.doi.org/10.1517/17425247.5.10.1077] [PMID: 18817514]

Bisht, R., Jaiswal, J.K., Chen, Y.S., Jin, J., Rupenthal, I.D. (2016). Light-responsive *in situ* forming injectable implants for effective drug delivery to the posterior segment of the eye. *Expert Opin. Drug Deliv., 13*(7), 953-962.
[http://dx.doi.org/10.1517/17425247.2016.1163334] [PMID: 26967153]

Boissenot, T., Bordat, A., Fattal, E., Tsapis, N. (2016). Ultrasound-triggered drug delivery for cancer treatment using drug delivery systems: From theoretical considerations to practical applications. *J. Control. Release, 241*, 144-163.
[http://dx.doi.org/10.1016/j.jconrel.2016.09.026] [PMID: 27667179]

Boonlai, W., Tantishaiyakul, V., Hirun, N., Sangfai, T., Suknuntha, K. (2018). Thermosensitive poloxamer 407/poly (acrylic acid) hydrogels with potential application as injectable drug delivery system. *AAPS PharmSciTech, 19*(5), 2103-2117.
[http://dx.doi.org/10.1208/s12249-018-1010-7] [PMID: 29696613]

Cai, X., Jiang, Y., Lin, M., Zhang, J., Guo, H., Yang, F., Leung, W., Xu, C. (2020). Ultrasound-Responsive Materials for Drug/Gene Delivery. *Front. Pharmacol., 10*, 1650.
[http://dx.doi.org/10.3389/fphar.2019.01650] [PMID: 32082157]

Calejo, M.T., Sande, S.A., Nyström, B. (2013). Thermoresponsive polymers as gene and drug delivery vectors: architecture and mechanism of action. *Expert Opin. Drug Deliv., 10*(12), 1669-1686.
[http://dx.doi.org/10.1517/17425247.2013.846906] [PMID: 24125490]

Campbell, S., Smeets, N. (2019). *Drug delivery: localized and systemic therapeutic strategies with polymer systems. Functional polymers. Polymers and polymeric composites: a reference series.*. Cham: Springer.

Cavalli, R., Soster, M., Argenziano, M. (2016). Nanobubbles: a promising efficienft tool for therapeutic delivery. *Ther. Deliv., 7*(2), 117-138.
[http://dx.doi.org/10.4155/tde.15.92] [PMID: 26769397]

Chen, H., Zhao, Y. (2018). Applications of light-responsive systems for cancer theranostics. *ACS Appl. Mater. Interfaces, 10*(25), 21021-21034.
[http://dx.doi.org/10.1021/acsami.8b01114] [PMID: 29648777]

Chen, J.P., Cheng, T.H. (2006). Thermo-responsive chitosan-graft-poly(N-isopropylacrylamide) injectable hydrogel for cultivation of chondrocytes and meniscus cells. *Macromol. Biosci., 6*(12), 1026-1039.
[http://dx.doi.org/10.1002/mabi.200600142] [PMID: 17128421]

Cho, H.J., Chung, M., Shim, M.S. (2015). Engineered photo-responsive materials for near-infrared-triggered drug delivery. *J. Ind. Eng. Chem., 31*, 15-25.
[http://dx.doi.org/10.1016/j.jiec.2015.07.016]

Constantin, M., Cristea, M., Ascenzi, P., Fundueanu, G. (2011). Lower critical solution temperature versus volume phase transition temperature in thermoresponsive drug delivery systems. *Express Polym. Lett., 5*(10), 839-848.
[http://dx.doi.org/10.3144/expresspolymlett.2011.83]

Constantinou, A.P., Georgiou, T.K. (2016). Tuning the gelation of thermoresponsive gels. *Eur. Polym. J., 78*, 366-375.
[http://dx.doi.org/10.1016/j.eurpolymj.2016.02.014]

Cortez-Lemus, N.A., Licea-Claverie, A. (2016). Poly(N-vinylcaprolactam), a comprehensive review on a thermoresponsive polymer becoming popular. *Prog. Polym. Sci., 53*, 1-51.

[http://dx.doi.org/10.1016/j.progpolymsci.2015.08.001]

Couture, O., Foley, J., Kassell, N.F., Larrat, B., Aubry, J-F. (2014). Review of ultrasound mediated drug delivery for cancer treatment: updates from pre-clinical studies. *Transl. Cancer Res., 3*, 494-511.

Crespy, D., Rossi, R.M. (2007). Temperature-responsive polymers with LCST in the physiological range and their applications in textiles. *Polym. Int., 56*(12), 1461-1468.
[http://dx.doi.org/10.1002/pi.2277]

Croissant, J., Maynadier, M., Gallud, A., Peindy N'Dongo, H., Nyalosaso, J.L., Derrien, G., Charnay, C., Durand, J.O., Raehm, L., Serein-Spirau, F., Cheminet, N., Jarrosson, T., Mongin, O., Blanchard-Desce, M., Gary-Bobo, M., Garcia, M., Lu, J., Tamanoi, F., Tarn, D., Guardado-Alvarez, T.M., Zink, J.I. (2013). Two-photon-triggered drug delivery in cancer cells using nanoimpellers. *Angew. Chem. Int. Ed., 52*(51), 13813-13817.
[http://dx.doi.org/10.1002/anie.201308647] [PMID: 24214916]

Cui, Z., Lee, B.H., Vernon, B.L. (2007). New hydrolysis-dependent thermosensitive polymer for an injectable degradable system. *Biomacromolecules, 8*(4), 1280-1286.
[http://dx.doi.org/10.1021/bm061045g] [PMID: 17371066]

Das, D., Ghosh, P., Ghosh, A., Haldar, C., Dhara, S., Panda, A.B., Pal, S. (2015). Stimulus-responsive, biodegradable, biocompatible, covalently cross-linked hydrogel based on dextrin and poly (N-isopropylacrylamide) for *in vitro/in vivo* controlled drug release. *ACS Appl. Mater. Interfaces, 7*(26), 14338-14351.
[http://dx.doi.org/10.1021/acsami.5b02975] [PMID: 26069986]

De Souza, R., Zahedi, P., Allen, C.J., Piquette-Miller, M. (2010). Polymeric drug delivery systems for localized cancer chemotherapy. *Drug Deliv., 17*(6), 365-375.
[http://dx.doi.org/10.3109/10717541003762854] [PMID: 20429844]

Deckers, R., Moonen, C.T.W. (2010). Ultrasound triggered, image guided, local drug delivery. *J. Control. Release, 148*(1), 25-33.
[http://dx.doi.org/10.1016/j.jconrel.2010.07.117] [PMID: 20709123]

Deng, H., Dong, A., Song, J., Chen, X. (2019). Injectable thermosensitive hydrogel systems based on functional PEG/PCL block polymer for local drug delivery. *J. Control. Release, 297*, 60-70.
[http://dx.doi.org/10.1016/j.jconrel.2019.01.026] [PMID: 30684513]

Dong, Y., Zhuang, H., Hao, Y., Zhang, L., Yang, Q., Liu, Y., Qi, C., Wang, S. (2020). Poly (N-Isopropy-Acrylamide)/Poly (γ-Glutamic Acid) thermo-sensitive hydrogels loaded with superoxide dismutase for wound dressing application. *Int. J. Nanomedicine, 15*, 1939-1950.
[http://dx.doi.org/10.2147/IJN.S235609] [PMID: 32256070]

Dromi, S., Frenkel, V., Luk, A., Traughber, B., Angstadt, M., Bur, M., Poff, J., Xie, J., Libutti, S.K., Li, K.C.P., Wood, B.J. (2007). Pulsed-high intensity focused ultrasound and low temperature-sensitive liposomes for enhanced targeted drug delivery and antitumor effect. *Clin. Cancer Res., 13*(9), 2722-2727.
[http://dx.doi.org/10.1158/1078-0432.CCR-06-2443] [PMID: 17473205]

Elkhodiry, M.A., Momah, C.C., Suwaidi, S.R., Gadalla, D., Martins, A.M., Vitor, R.F., Husseini, G.A. (2016). Synergistic nanomedicine: passive, active, and ultrasound-triggered drug delivery in cancer treatment. *J. Nanosci. Nanotechnol., 16*(1), 1-18.
[http://dx.doi.org/10.1166/jnn.2016.11124] [PMID: 27398430]

Fernández-Quiroz, D., Loya-Duarte, J., Silva-Campa, E., Argüelles-Monal, W., Sarabia-Sainz, A., Lucero-Acuña, A., del Castillo-Castro, T., San Román, J., Lizardi-Mendoza, J., Burgara-Estrella, A.J., Castaneda, B., Soto-Puebla, D., Pedroza-Montero, M. (2019). Temperature stimuli-responsive nanoparticles from chitosan-*graft* -poly(*N* -vinylcaprolactam) as a drug delivery system. *J. Appl. Polym. Sci., 136*(32), 47831.
[http://dx.doi.org/10.1002/app.47831]

Fomina, N., Sankaranarayanan, J., Almutairi, A. (2012). Photochemical mechanisms of light-triggered release from nanocarriers. *Adv. Drug Deliv. Rev., 64*(11), 1005-1020.

[http://dx.doi.org/10.1016/j.addr.2012.02.006] [PMID: 22386560]

Gan, J., Guan, X., Zheng, J., Guo, H., Wu, K., Liang, L., Lu, M. (2016). Biodegradable, thermoresponsive PNIPAM-based hydrogel scaffolds for the sustained release of levofloxacin. *RSC Advances, 6*(39), 32967-32978.
[http://dx.doi.org/10.1039/C6RA03045A]

Gandhi, A., Paul, A., Sen, S. O., Sen, K. K. (2015). Studies on thermoresponsive polymers: Phase behaviour, drug delivery and biomedical applications. *Asian J Pharmaceutical Sciences, 10*, 99-107.

Geers, B., Dewitte, H., De Smedt, S.C., Lentacker, I. (2012). Crucial factors and emerging concepts in ultrasound-triggered drug delivery. *J. Control. Release, 164*(3), 248-255.
[http://dx.doi.org/10.1016/j.jconrel.2012.08.014] [PMID: 23320295]

Geng, S., Wang, Y., Wang, L., Kouyama, T., Gotoh, T., Wada, S., Wang, J.Y. (2017). A light-responsive self-assembly formed by a cationic azobenzene derivative and SDS as a drug delivery system. *Sci. Rep., 7*(1), 39202.
[http://dx.doi.org/10.1038/srep39202] [PMID: 28051069]

Ghorbanzade, S., Naghib, S.M. (2019). Nanoscaled materials for drug delivery into cells/stem cells. *Stem Cell Nanotechnology.*. Springer.

Gooneh-Farahani, S., Naghib, S.M., Naimi-Jamal, M.R. (2019). A critical comparison study on the pH-sensitive nanocomposites based on graphene-grafted chitosan for cancer theragnosis. *Multidisciplinary Cancer Investigation, 3*(1), 05-16. a
[http://dx.doi.org/10.30699/acadpub.mci.3.1.5]

Gooneh-Farahani, S., Naghib, S.M., Naimi-Jamal, M.R. (2020). A novel and inexpensive method based on modified ionic gelation for pH-responsive controlled drug release of homogeneously distributed chitosan nanoparticles with a high encapsulation efficiency. *Fibers Polym., 21*(9), 1917-1926.
[http://dx.doi.org/10.1007/s12221-020-1095-y]

Gooneh-Farahani, S., Naimi-Jamal, M.R., Naghib, S.M. (2019). Stimuli-responsive graphene-incorporated multifunctional chitosan for drug delivery applications: a review. *Expert Opin. Drug Deliv., 16*(1), 79-99. b
[http://dx.doi.org/10.1080/17425247.2019.1556257] [PMID: 30514124]

Gou, M., Gong, C., Zhang, J., Wang, X., Wang, X., Gu, Y., Guo, G., Chen, L., Luo, F., Zhao, X., Wei, Y., Qian, Z. (2010). Polymeric matrix for drug delivery: honokiol-loaded PCL-PEG-PCL nanoparticles in PEG-PCL-PEG thermosensitive hydrogel. *J. Biomed. Mater. Res. A, 93*(1), 219-226.
[PMID: 19557789]

Hogan, K.J., Mikos, A.G. (2020). Biodegradable thermoresponsive polymers: Applications in drug delivery and tissue engineering. *Polymer (Guildf.), 211*, 123063.
[http://dx.doi.org/10.1016/j.polymer.2020.123063]

Huang, H., Qi, X., Chen, Y., Wu, Z. (2019). Thermo-sensitive hydrogels for delivering biotherapeutic molecules: A review. *Saudi Pharm. J., 27*(7), 990-999.
[http://dx.doi.org/10.1016/j.jsps.2019.08.001] [PMID: 31997906]

Husseini, G.A., Myrup, G.D., Pitt, W.G., Christensen, D.A., Rapoport, N.Y. (2000). Factors affecting acoustically triggered release of drugs from polymeric micelles. *J. Control. Release, 69*(1), 43-52.
[http://dx.doi.org/10.1016/S0168-3659(00)00278-9] [PMID: 11018545]

Husseini, G.A., Pitt, W.G. (2008). The use of ultrasound and micelles in cancer treatment. *J. Nanosci. Nanotechnol., 8*(5), 2205-2215.
[http://dx.doi.org/10.1166/jnn.2008.225] [PMID: 18572632]

Ieong, N.S., Hasan, M., Phillips, D.J., Saaka, Y., O'Reilly, R.K., Gibson, M.I. (2012). Polymers with molecular weight dependent LCSTs are essential for cooperative behaviour. *Polym. Chem., 3*(3), 794-799.
[http://dx.doi.org/10.1039/c2py00604a]

Ito, Y. (2018). Drug delivery systems. *Photochemistry for Biomedical Applications.*. Springer.

Ji, W., Li, N., Chen, D., Qi, X., Sha, W., Jiao, Y., Xu, Q., Lu, J. (2013). Coumarin-containing photo-responsive nanocomposites for NIR light-triggered controlled drug release *via* a two-photon process. *J. Mater. Chem. B Mater. Biol. Med., 1*(43), 5942-5949.
[http://dx.doi.org/10.1039/c3tb21206h] [PMID: 32261061]

Jiang, G., Sun, J., Ding, F. (2014). PEG-g-chitosan thermosensitive hydrogel for implant drug delivery: cytotoxicity, *in vivo* degradation and drug release. *J. Biomater. Sci. Polym. Ed., 25*(3), 241-256.
[http://dx.doi.org/10.1080/09205063.2013.851542] [PMID: 24160458]

Kalkhoran, Z., Naghib, S.M., Vahidi, O., Rahmanian, M. (2018). Synthesis and characterization of graphene-grafted gelatin nanocomposite hydrogels as emerging drug delivery systems. *Biomed. Phys. Eng. Express, 4*(5), 055017.
[http://dx.doi.org/10.1088/2057-1976/aad745]

Kamaly, N., Yameen, B., Wu, J., Farokhzad, O.C. (2016). Degradable controlled-release polymers and polymeric nanoparticles: mechanisms of controlling drug release. *Chem. Rev., 116*(4), 2602-2663.
[http://dx.doi.org/10.1021/acs.chemrev.5b00346] [PMID: 26854975]

Karimi, M., Sahandi Zangabad, P., Baghaee-Ravari, S., Ghazadeh, M., Mirshekari, H., Hamblin, M.R. (2017). Smart nanostructures for cargo delivery: uncaging and activating by light. *J. Am. Chem. Soc., 139*(13), 4584-4610.
[http://dx.doi.org/10.1021/jacs.6b08313] [PMID: 28192672]

Karimi, M., Sahandi Zangabad, P., Ghasemi, A., Amiri, M., Bahrami, M., Malekzad, H., Ghahramanzadeh Asl, H., Mahdieh, Z., Bozorgomid, M., Ghasemi, A., Rahmani Taji Boyuk, M.R., Hamblin, M.R. (2016). Temperature-responsive smart nanocarriers for delivery of therapeutic agents: applications and recent advances. *ACS Appl. Mater. Interfaces, 8*(33), 21107-21133.
[http://dx.doi.org/10.1021/acsami.6b00371] [PMID: 27349465]

Kim, A.R., Lee, S.L., Park, S.N. (2018). Properties and *in vitro* drug release of pH- and temperature-sensitive double cross-linked interpenetrating polymer network hydrogels based on hyaluronic acid/poly (N-isopropylacrylamide) for transdermal delivery of luteolin. *Int. J. Biol. Macromol., 118*(Pt A), 731-740.
[http://dx.doi.org/10.1016/j.ijbiomac.2018.06.061] [PMID: 29940230]

Klouda, L. (2015). Thermoresponsive hydrogels in biomedical applications. *Eur. J. Pharm. Biopharm., 97*(Pt B), 338-349.
[http://dx.doi.org/10.1016/j.ejpb.2015.05.017] [PMID: 26614556]

Kokardekar, R.R., Shah, V.K., Mody, H.R. (2012). PNIPAM Poly (N-isopropylacrylamide): A thermoresponsive "smart" polymer in novel drug delivery systems. *Internet Journal of Medical Update-E Journal, 7.*

Komatsu, S., Asoh, T.A., Ishihara, R., Kikuchi, A. (2017). Facile preparation of degradable thermoresponsive polymers as biomaterials: Thermoresponsive polymers prepared by radical polymerization degrade to water-soluble oligomers. *Polymer (Guildf.), 130*, 68-73.
[http://dx.doi.org/10.1016/j.polymer.2017.09.073]

Lanzalaco, S., Armelin, E. (2017). Poly (n-isopropylacrylamide) and copolymers: A review on recent progresses in biomedical applications. *Gels, 3*(4), 36.
[http://dx.doi.org/10.3390/gels3040036] [PMID: 30920531]

Li, G., Song, S., Guo, L., Ma, S. (2008). Self-assembly of thermo- and pH-responsive poly(acrylic acid)- *b* -poly(*N* -isopropylacrylamide) micelles for drug delivery. *J. Polym. Sci. A Polym. Chem., 46*(15), 5028-5035.
[http://dx.doi.org/10.1002/pola.22831]

Li, W., Li, J., Gao, J., Li, B., Xia, Y., Meng, Y., Yu, Y., Chen, H., Dai, J., Wang, H., Guo, Y. (2011). The fine-tuning of thermosensitive and degradable polymer micelles for enhancing intracellular uptake and drug release in tumors. *Biomaterials, 32*(15), 3832-3844.
[http://dx.doi.org/10.1016/j.biomaterials.2011.01.075] [PMID: 21377724]

Li, Z., Guan, J. (2011). Thermosensitive hydrogels for drug delivery. *Expert Opin. Drug Deliv., 8*(8), 991-

1007.
[http://dx.doi.org/10.1517/17425247.2011.581656] [PMID: 21564003]

Li, Z., Ning, W., Wang, J., Choi, A., Lee, P-Y., Tyagi, P., Huang, L. (2003). Controlled gene delivery system based on thermosensitive biodegradable hydrogel. *Pharm. Res., 20*(6), 884-888.
[http://dx.doi.org/10.1023/A:1023887203111] [PMID: 12817892]

Linsley, C.S., Wu, B.M. (2017). Recent advances in light-responsive on-demand drug-delivery systems. *Ther. Deliv., 8*(2), 89-107.
[http://dx.doi.org/10.4155/tde-2016-0060] [PMID: 28088880]

Liu, D., Yang, F., Xiong, F., Gu, N. (2016). The smart drug delivery system and its clinical potential. *Theranostics, 6*(9), 1306-1323. a
[http://dx.doi.org/10.7150/thno.14858] [PMID: 27375781]

Liu, G., Liu, W., Dong, C.M. (2013). UV- and NIR-responsive polymeric nanomedicines for on-demand drug delivery. *Polym. Chem., 4*(12), 3431-3443. a
[http://dx.doi.org/10.1039/c3py21121e]

Liu, J., Bu, W., Pan, L., Shi, J. (2013). NIR-triggered anticancer drug delivery by upconverting nanoparticles with integrated azobenzene-modified mesoporous silica. *Angew. Chem. Int. Ed., 52*(16), 4375-4379. b
[http://dx.doi.org/10.1002/anie.201300183] [PMID: 23495013]

Liu, L., Bai, S., Yang, H., Li, S., Quan, J., Zhu, L., Nie, H. (2016). Controlled release from thermo-sensitive PNVCL- co -MAA electrospun nanofibers: The effects of hydrophilicity/hydrophobicity of a drug. *Mater. Sci. Eng. C, 67*, 581-589. b
[http://dx.doi.org/10.1016/j.msec.2016.05.083] [PMID: 27287157]

Liu, L., Zeng, J., Zhao, X., Tian, K., Liu, P. (2017). Independent temperature and pH dual-responsive PMAA/PNIPAM microgels as drug delivery system: Effect of swelling behavior of the core and shell materials in fabrication process. *Colloids Surf. A Physicochem. Eng. Asp., 526*, 48-55.
[http://dx.doi.org/10.1016/j.colsurfa.2016.11.007]

Liu, R., Fraylich, M., Saunders, B.R. (2009). Thermoresponsive copolymers: from fundamental studies to applications. *Colloid Polym. Sci., 287*(6), 627-643.
[http://dx.doi.org/10.1007/s00396-009-2028-x]

Liu, X., Tian, Z., Chen, C., Allcock, H.R. (2013). UV-cleavable unimolecular micelles: synthesis and characterization toward photocontrolled drug release carriers. *Polym. Chem., 4*(4), 1115-1125. c
[http://dx.doi.org/10.1039/C2PY20825C]

Lutz, J.F., Akdemir, Ö., Hoth, A. (2006). Point by point comparison of two thermosensitive polymers exhibiting a similar LCST: is the age of poly(NIPAM) over? *J. Am. Chem. Soc., 128*(40), 13046-13047.
[http://dx.doi.org/10.1021/ja065324n] [PMID: 17017772]

Mallikarjuna, B., Rao, K.M.S., Prasad, C., Rao, K., Rao, K.K., Subha, M. (2011). Synthesis, characterization and use of Poly (N-isopropylacrylamide-co-N-vinylcaprolactam) crosslinked thermoresponsive microspheres for control release of Ciproflaxin hydrochloride drug. *J. Appl. Pharm. Sci., 1*, 171.

Medeiros, S.F., Lopes, M.V., Rossi-Bergmann, B., Ré, M.I., Santos, A.M. (2017). Synthesis and characterization of poly(*N* -vinylcaprolactam)-based spray-dried microparticles exhibiting temperature and pH-sensitive properties for controlled release of ketoprofen. *Drug Dev. Ind. Pharm., 43*(9), 1519-1529.
[http://dx.doi.org/10.1080/03639045.2017.1321660] [PMID: 28436310]

Mo, S., Coussios, C.C., Seymour, L., Carlisle, R. (2012). Ultrasound-enhanced drug delivery for cancer. *Expert Opin. Drug Deliv., 9*(12), 1525-1538.
[http://dx.doi.org/10.1517/17425247.2012.739603] [PMID: 23121385]

Mohammed, M.N., Yusoh, K.B., Shariffuddin, J.H.B.H. (2018). Poly(N-vinyl caprolactam) thermoresponsive polymer in novel drug delivery systems: A review. *Mater. Express, 8*(1), 21-34.
[http://dx.doi.org/10.1166/mex.2018.1406]

Mura, S., Nicolas, J., Couvreur, P. (2013). Stimuli-responsive nanocarriers for drug delivery. *Nat. Mater.,*

12(11), 991-1003.
[http://dx.doi.org/10.1038/nmat3776] [PMID: 24150417]

Nair, H.A., Rajawat, G.S., Nagarsenker, M.S. (2018). *Stimuli-responsive micelles: A nanoplatform for therapeutic and diagnostic applications. Drug Targeting and Stimuli Sensitive Drug Delivery Systems.*. Elsevier.
[http://dx.doi.org/10.1016/B978-0-12-813689-8.00008-2]

Najafipour, A., Mahdavian, A.R., Aliabadi, H.S., Fassihi, A. (2019). Dual thermo-and pH-responsive poly (N-isopropylacrylamide-co-(2-dimethylamino) ethyl methacrylate)-g-PEG nanoparticle system and its potential in controlled drug release. *Polym. Bull.,* •••, 1-14.

Nguyen, M.K., Lee, D.S. (2010). Injectable biodegradable hydrogels. *Macromol. Biosci., 10*(6), 563-579.
[http://dx.doi.org/10.1002/mabi.200900402] [PMID: 20196065]

Ninomiya, K., Kawabata, S., Tashita, H., Shimizu, N. (2014). Ultrasound-mediated drug delivery using liposomes modified with a thermosensitive polymer. *Ultrason. Sonochem., 21*(1), 310-316.
[http://dx.doi.org/10.1016/j.ultsonch.2013.07.014] [PMID: 23948493]

Niu, H., Li, X., Li, H., Fan, Z., Ma, J., Guan, J. (2019). Thermosensitive, fast gelling, photoluminescent, highly flexible, and degradable hydrogels for stem cell delivery. *Acta Biomater., 83*, 96-108.
[http://dx.doi.org/10.1016/j.actbio.2018.10.038] [PMID: 30541703]

Olejniczak, J., Sankaranarayanan, J., Viger, M.L., Almutairi, A. (2013). Highest efficiency two-photon degradable copolymer for remote controlled release. *ACS Macro Lett., 2*(8), 683-687.
[http://dx.doi.org/10.1021/mz400256x] [PMID: 24044102]

Özdemir, N., Tuncel, A., Kang, M., Denkbş, E.B. (2006). Preparation and characterization of thermosensitive submicron particles for gene delivery. *J. Nanosci. Nanotechnol., 6*(9), 2804-2810.
[http://dx.doi.org/10.1166/jnn.2006.463] [PMID: 17048486]

Palumbo, M.O., Kavan, P., Miller, W.H., Jr, Panasci, L., Assouline, S., Johnson, N., Cohen, V., Patenaude, F., Pollak, M., Jagoe, R.T., Batist, G. (2013). Systemic cancer therapy: achievements and challenges that lie ahead. *Front. Pharmacol., 4*, 57.
[http://dx.doi.org/10.3389/fphar.2013.00057] [PMID: 23675348]

Parameswaran-Thankam, A., Parnell, C.M., Watanabe, F., RanguMagar, A.B., Chhetri, B.P., Szwedo, P.K., Biris, A.S., Ghosh, A. (2018). Guar-based injectable thermoresponsive hydrogel as a scaffold for bone cell growth and controlled drug delivery. *ACS Omega, 3*(11), 15158-15167.
[http://dx.doi.org/10.1021/acsomega.8b01765] [PMID: 30555998]

París, R., Quijada-Garrido, I. (2009). Swelling behaviour of thermo-sensitive hydrogels based on oligo(ethylene glycol) methacrylates. *Eur. Polym. J., 45*(12), 3418-3425.
[http://dx.doi.org/10.1016/j.eurpolymj.2009.09.012]

Peng, J., Tang, D., Lv, H., Wang, N., Yang, X., Sun, Z., Yu, Z. (2019). Thermal phase transition of poly(N-vinyl caprolactam)-based copolymers: the distribution of hydrophilic units within polymeric chains. *Colloid Polym. Sci., 297*(10), 1255-1264.
[http://dx.doi.org/10.1007/s00396-019-04537-y]

Qiu, Y., Park, K. (2001). Environment-sensitive hydrogels for drug delivery. *Adv. Drug Deliv. Rev., 53*(3), 321-339.
[http://dx.doi.org/10.1016/S0169-409X(01)00203-4] [PMID: 11744175]

Rahmanian, M., seyfoori, A., Dehghan, M.M., Eini, L., Naghib, S.M., Gholami, H., Farzad Mohajeri, S., Mamaghani, K.R., Majidzadeh-A, K. (2019). Multifunctional gelatin–tricalcium phosphate porous nanocomposite scaffolds for tissue engineering and local drug delivery: *In vitro* and *in vivo* studies. *J. Taiwan Inst. Chem. Eng., 101*, 214-220.
[http://dx.doi.org/10.1016/j.jtice.2019.04.028]

Rahmanian, M., Naghib, S., Seyfoori, A., Zare, A. (2017). Tricalcium phosphate nanostructures loaded with bisphosphonate as potential anticancer agents. *J Ceram Sci Technol, 8*, 505-512.

Madhusudana Rao, K., Mallikarjuna, B., Krishna Rao, K.S.V., Siraj, S., Chowdoji Rao, K., Subha, M.C.S. (2013). Novel thermo/pH sensitive nanogels composed from poly(N-vinylcaprolactam) for controlled release of an anticancer drug. *Colloids Surf. B Biointerfaces, 102*, 891-897.
[http://dx.doi.org/10.1016/j.colsurfb.2012.09.009] [PMID: 23107966]

Rao, K., Rao, K., Ha, C.S. (2016). Stimuli responsive poly (vinyl caprolactam) gels for biomedical applications. *Gels, 2*(1), 6.
[http://dx.doi.org/10.3390/gels2010006] [PMID: 30674138]

Rapoport, N. (2004). Combined cancer therapy by micellar-encapsulated drug and ultrasound. *Int. J. Pharm., 277*(1-2), 155-162.
[http://dx.doi.org/10.1016/j.ijpharm.2003.09.048] [PMID: 15158978]

Raza, A., Hayat, U., Rasheed, T., Bilal, M., Iqbal, H.M.N. (2019). "Smart" materials-based near-infrared light-responsive drug delivery systems for cancer treatment: A review. *J. Mater. Res. Technol., 8*(1), 1497-1509. a
[http://dx.doi.org/10.1016/j.jmrt.2018.03.007]

Raza, A., Rasheed, T., Nabeel, F., Hayat, U., Bilal, M., Iqbal, H. (2019). Endogenous and exogenous stimuli-responsive drug delivery systems for programmed site-specific release. *Molecules, 24*(6), 1117. b
[http://dx.doi.org/10.3390/molecules24061117] [PMID: 30901827]

Rejinold, N.S., Baby, T., Chennazhi, K.P., Jayakumar, R. (2015). Multi drug loaded thermo-responsive fibrinogen-graft-poly (N-vinyl caprolactam) nanogels for breast cancer drug delivery. *J. Biomed. Nanotechnol., 11*(3), 392-402.
[http://dx.doi.org/10.1166/jbn.2015.1911] [PMID: 26307823]

Rejinold, N.S., Chennazhi, K.P., Nair, S.V., Tamura, H., Jayakumar, R. (2011). Biodegradable and thermo-sensitive chitosan-g-poly(N-vinylcaprolactam) nanoparticles as a 5-fluorouracil carrier. *Carbohydr. Polym., 83*(2), 776-786.
[http://dx.doi.org/10.1016/j.carbpol.2010.08.052]

Rogic Miladinovic, Z., Micic, M., Mrakovic, A., Suljovrujic, E. (2018). Smart hydrogels with ethylene glycol propylene glycol pendant chains. *J. Polym. Res., 25*(1), 1.
[http://dx.doi.org/10.1007/s10965-017-1408-z]

Ruel-Gariépy, E., Shive, M., Bichara, A., Berrada, M., Le Garrec, D., Chenite, A., Leroux, J.C. (2004). A thermosensitive chitosan-based hydrogel for the local delivery of paclitaxel. *Eur. J. Pharm. Biopharm., 57*(1), 53-63.
[http://dx.doi.org/10.1016/S0939-6411(03)00095-X] [PMID: 14729080]

Schmaljohann, D. (2006). Thermo- and pH-responsive polymers in drug delivery. *Adv. Drug Deliv. Rev., 58*(15), 1655-1670.
[http://dx.doi.org/10.1016/j.addr.2006.09.020] [PMID: 17125884]

Schroeder, A., Avnir, Y., Weisman, S., Najajreh, Y., Gabizon, A., Talmon, Y., Kost, J., Barenholz, Y. (2007). Controlling liposomal drug release with low frequency ultrasound: mechanism and feasibility. *Langmuir, 23*(7), 4019-4025.
[http://dx.doi.org/10.1021/la0631668] [PMID: 17319706]

Schroeder, A., Honen, R., Turjeman, K., Gabizon, A., Kost, J., Barenholz, Y. (2009). Ultrasound triggered release of cisplatin from liposomes in murine tumors. *J. Control. Release, 137*(1), 63-68.
[http://dx.doi.org/10.1016/j.jconrel.2009.03.007] [PMID: 19303426]

Seyfoori, A., Ebrahimi, S.A.S., Omidian, S., Naghib, S.M. (2019). Multifunctional magnetic ZnFe2O4-hydroxyapatite nanocomposite particles for local anti-cancer drug delivery and bacterial infection inhibition: An *in vitro* study. *J. Taiwan Inst. Chem. Eng., 96*, 503-508.
[http://dx.doi.org/10.1016/j.jtice.2018.10.018]

Shao, Y., Jia, Y.G., Shi, C., Luo, J., Zhu, X.X. (2014). Block and random copolymers bearing cholic acid and oligo(ethylene glycol) pendant groups: aggregation, thermosensitivity, and drug loading. *Biomacromolecules,*

15(5), 1837-1844.
[http://dx.doi.org/10.1021/bm5002262] [PMID: 24725005]

Sirsi, S.R., Borden, M.A. (2014). State-of-the-art materials for ultrasound-triggered drug delivery. *Adv. Drug Deliv. Rev., 72*, 3-14.
[http://dx.doi.org/10.1016/j.addr.2013.12.010] [PMID: 24389162]

Smeets, N.M.B., Bakaic, E., Patenaude, M., Hoare, T. (2014). Injectable and tunable poly(ethylene glycol) analogue hydrogels based on poly(oligoethylene glycol methacrylate). *Chem. Commun. (Camb.), 50*(25), 3306-3309.
[http://dx.doi.org/10.1039/c3cc48514e] [PMID: 24531402]

Soliman, K.A., Ullah, K., Shah, A., Jones, D.S., Singh, T.R.R. (2019). Poloxamer-based *in situ* gelling thermoresponsive systems for ocular drug delivery applications. *Drug Discov. Today, 24*(8), 1575-1586.
[http://dx.doi.org/10.1016/j.drudis.2019.05.036] [PMID: 31175956]

Soliman, M.E., Elmowafy, E., Casettari, L., Alexander, C. (2018). Star-shaped poly(oligoethylene glycol) copolymer-based gels: Thermo-responsive behaviour and bioapplicability for risedronate intranasal delivery. *Int. J. Pharm., 543*(1-2), 224-233.
[http://dx.doi.org/10.1016/j.ijpharm.2018.03.053] [PMID: 29604369]

Son, J., Yi, G., Yoo, J., Park, C., Koo, H., Choi, H.S. (2019). Light-responsive nanomedicine for biophotonic imaging and targeted therapy. *Adv. Drug Deliv. Rev., 138*, 133-147.
[http://dx.doi.org/10.1016/j.addr.2018.10.002] [PMID: 30321619]

Sreejivungsa, K., Suchaichit, N., Moosophon, P., Chompoosor, A. (2016). Light-regulated release of entrapped drugs from photoresponsive gold nanoparticles. *J. Nanomater., 2016*, 1-7.
[http://dx.doi.org/10.1155/2016/4964693]

Subhash, D., Mody, H., Banerjee, R., Bahadur, D., Srivastava, R. (2011). Poly (N-isopropylacrylamide) based polymer nanogels for drug delivery applications. *11th IEEE International Conference on Nanotechnology.,* IEEE.1741-1744.

Sun, J., Jiang, G., Wang, Y., Ding, F. (2012). Thermosensitive chitosan hydrogel for implantable drug delivery: Blending PVA to mitigate body response and promote bioavailability. *J. Appl. Polym. Sci., 125*(3), 2092-2101.
[http://dx.doi.org/10.1002/app.36297]

Suzuki, M., Koshiyama, K., Shinohara, F., Mori, S., Ono, M., Tomita, Y., Yano, T., Fujikawa, S., Vassaux, G., Kodama, T. (2005). Nanobubbles enhanced drug susceptibility of cancer cells using ultrasound. *International Congress Series.* Elsevier.

Talelli, M., Hennink, W.E. (2011). Thermosensitive polymeric micelles for targeted drug delivery. *Nanomedicine (Lond.), 6*(7), 1245-1255.
[http://dx.doi.org/10.2217/nnm.11.91] [PMID: 21929459]

Tao, Y., Chan, H.F., Shi, B., Li, M., Leong, K.W. (2020). Light: A magical tool for controlled drug delivery. *Adv. Funct. Mater., 30*(49), 2005029.
[http://dx.doi.org/10.1002/adfm.202005029] [PMID: 34483808]

Taylor, M., Tomlins, P., Sahota, T. (2017). Thermoresponsive Gels. *Gels, 3*(1), 4.
[http://dx.doi.org/10.3390/gels3010004] [PMID: 30920501]

Vancoillie, G., Frank, D., Hoogenboom, R. (2014). Thermoresponsive poly(oligo ethylene glycol acrylates). *Prog. Polym. Sci., 39*(6), 1074-1095.
[http://dx.doi.org/10.1016/j.progpolymsci.2014.02.005]

Vihola, H., Laukkanen, A., Hirvonen, J., Tenhu, H. (2002). Binding and release of drugs into and from thermosensitive poly(N-vinyl caprolactam) nanoparticles. *Eur. J. Pharm. Sci., 16*(1-2), 69-74.
[http://dx.doi.org/10.1016/S0928-0987(02)00076-3] [PMID: 12113893]

Vihola, H., Laukkanen, A., Tenhu, H., Hirvonen, J. (2008). Drug release characteristics of physically cross-linked thermosensitive poly(N-vinylcaprolactam) hydrogel particles. *J. Pharm. Sci., 97*(11), 4783-4793.

[http://dx.doi.org/10.1002/jps.21348] [PMID: 18306245]

Wang, J., Huang, N., Peng, Q., Cheng, X., Li, W. (2020). Temperature/pH dual-responsive and luminescent drug carrier based on PNIPAM-MAA/lanthanide-polyoxometalates for controlled drug delivery and imaging in HeLa cells. *Mater. Chem. Phys., 239*, 121994.
[http://dx.doi.org/10.1016/j.matchemphys.2019.121994]

Wang, Y., Kohane, D.S. (2017). External triggering and triggered targeting strategies for drug delivery. *Nat. Rev. Mater., 2*(6), 17020.
[http://dx.doi.org/10.1038/natrevmats.2017.20]

Wang, Y., Li, X., Zhou, Y., Huang, P., Xu, Y. (2010). Preparation of nanobubbles for ultrasound imaging and intracelluar drug delivery. *Int. J. Pharm., 384*(1-2), 148-153.
[http://dx.doi.org/10.1016/j.ijpharm.2009.09.027] [PMID: 19781609]

Wenceslau, A.C., dos Santos, F.G., Ramos, É.R.F., Nakamura, C.V., Rubira, A.F., Muniz, E.C. (2012). Thermo- and pH-sensitive IPN hydrogels based on PNIPAAm and PVA-Ma networks with LCST tailored close to human body temperature. *Mater. Sci. Eng. C, 32*(5), 1259-1265.
[http://dx.doi.org/10.1016/j.msec.2012.04.001]

Wu, W., Driessen, W., Jiang, X. (2014). Oligo(ethylene glycol)-based thermosensitive dendrimers and their tumor accumulation and penetration. *J. Am. Chem. Soc., 136*(8), 3145-3155.
[http://dx.doi.org/10.1021/ja411457r] [PMID: 24506735]

Xia, H., Zhao, Y., Tong, R. (2016). *Ultrasound-mediated polymeric micelle drug delivery. Therapeutic Ultrasound.*. Springer.

Xu, X., Liu, Y., Fu, W., Yao, M., Ding, Z., Xuan, J., Li, D., Wang, S., Xia, Y., Cao, M. (2020). Poly (N-isopropylacrylamide)-based thermoresponsive composite hydrogels for biomedical applications. *Polymers (Basel), 12*(3), 580.
[http://dx.doi.org/10.3390/polym12030580] [PMID: 32150904]

Yadav, S., Deka, S.R., Verma, G., Sharma, A.K., Kumar, P. (2016). Photoresponsive amphiphilic azobenzene–PEG self-assembles to form supramolecular nanostructures for drug delivery applications. *RSC Advances, 6*(10), 8103-8117.
[http://dx.doi.org/10.1039/C5RA26658K]

Yadavalli, T., Ramasamy, S., Chandrasekaran, G., Michael, I., Therese, H.A., Chennakesavulu, R. (2015). Dual responsive PNIPAM–chitosan targeted magnetic nanopolymers for targeted drug delivery. *J. Magn. Magn. Mater., 380*, 315-320.
[http://dx.doi.org/10.1016/j.jmmm.2014.09.035]

Yan, B., Boyer, J.C., Branda, N.R., Zhao, Y. (2011). Near-infrared light-triggered dissociation of block copolymer micelles using upconverting nanoparticles. *J. Am. Chem. Soc., 133*(49), 19714-19717.
[http://dx.doi.org/10.1021/ja209793b] [PMID: 22082025]

Yang, C., Li, Y., Du, M., Chen, Z. (2019). Recent advances in ultrasound-triggered therapy. *J. Drug Target., 27*(1), 33-50.
[http://dx.doi.org/10.1080/1061186X.2018.1464012] [PMID: 29659307]

Yang, R., Gorelov, A.V., Aldabbagh, F., Carroll, W.M., Rochev, Y. (2013). An implantable thermoresponsive drug delivery system based on Peltier device. *Int. J. Pharm., 447*(1-2), 109-114.
[http://dx.doi.org/10.1016/j.ijpharm.2013.02.051] [PMID: 23467083]

Yerriswamy, B., Reddy, C. L. N., Prasad, C. V., Subha, M., Rao, K. C., Venkatareddy, G. (2014). Controlled release studies of 5-Fluorouracil through poly (vinyl caprolactum-co-vinyl acetate) microspheres. *Asian Journal of Pharmaceutics (AJP): Free full text articles from Asian J Pharm, 4*.

Yoshida, R., Kaneko, Y., Sakai, K., Okano, T., Sakurai, Y., Bae, Y.H., Kim, S.W. (1994). Positive thermosensitive pulsatile drug release using negative thermosensitive hydrogels. *J. Control. Release, 32*(1), 97-102.
[http://dx.doi.org/10.1016/0168-3659(94)90229-1]

Zeinali Kalkhoran, A.H., Vahidi, O., Naghib, S.M. (2018). A new mathematical approach to predict the actual drug release from hydrogels. *Eur. J. Pharm. Sci., 111*, 303-310.
[http://dx.doi.org/10.1016/j.ejps.2017.09.038] [PMID: 28962856]

Zhan, C., Wang, W., McAlvin, J.B., Guo, S., Timko, B.P., Santamaria, C., Kohane, D.S. (2016). Phototriggered local anesthesia. *Nano Lett., 16*(1), 177-181.
[http://dx.doi.org/10.1021/acs.nanolett.5b03440] [PMID: 26654461]

Zhang, F., Wu, W., Zhang, X., Meng, X., Tong, G., Deng, Y. (2016). Temperature-sensitive poly-NIPAm modified cellulose nanofibril cryogel microspheres for controlled drug release. *Cellulose, 23*(1), 415-425.
[http://dx.doi.org/10.1007/s10570-015-0799-4]

Zhang, T., Li, G., Guo, L., Chen, H. (2012). Synthesis of thermo-sensitive CS-g-PNIPAM/CMC complex nanoparticles for controlled release of 5-FU. *Int. J. Biol. Macromol., 51*(5), 1109-1115.
[http://dx.doi.org/10.1016/j.ijbiomac.2012.08.033] [PMID: 22981819]

Zhao, W., Zhao, Y., Wang, Q., Liu, T., Sun, J., Zhang, R. (2019). Remote Light-Responsive Nanocarriers for Controlled Drug Delivery: Advances and Perspectives. *Small, 15*(45), 1903060.
[http://dx.doi.org/10.1002/smll.201903060] [PMID: 31599125]

Zhao, Y-Z., Du, L-N., Lu, C-T., Jin, Y-G., Ge, S-P. (2013). Potential and problems in ultrasound-responsive drug delivery systems. *Int. J. Nanomedicine, 8*, 1621-1633.
[PMID: 23637531]

Zhou, Q., Zhang, L., Yang, T., Wu, H. (2018). Stimuli-responsive polymeric micelles for drug delivery and cancer therapy. *Int. J. Nanomedicine, 13*, 2921-2942.
[http://dx.doi.org/10.2147/IJN.S158696] [PMID: 29849457]

Zhu, X., Su, Q., Feng, W., Li, F. (2017). Anti-Stokes shift luminescent materials for bio-applications. *Chem. Soc. Rev., 46*(4), 1025-1039.
[http://dx.doi.org/10.1039/C6CS00415F] [PMID: 27966684]

Zhuo, S., Zhang, F., Yu, J., Zhang, X., Yang, G., Liu, X. (2020). pH-Sensitive Biomaterials for Drug Delivery. *Molecules, 25*(23), 5649.
[http://dx.doi.org/10.3390/molecules25235649] [PMID: 33266162]

Ziminska, M., Wilson, J.J., McErlean, E., Dunne, N., McCarthy, H.O. (2020). Synthesis and Evaluation of a Thermoresponsive Degradable Chitosan-Grafted PNIPAAm Hydrogel as a "Smart" Gene Delivery System. *Materials (Basel), 13*(11), 2530.
[http://dx.doi.org/10.3390/ma13112530] [PMID: 32498464]

CHAPTER 7

Endogenous-triggered Delivery in Localized Controlled Drug Delivery Systems (LCDDSs)

Abstract: Responsive and smart materials/biomaterials are responsive/sensitive to signals originating from physiological systems, or to abnormalities originating from pathological defects that can interact with or be triggered by the biological environments. Responsive and smart materials/biomaterials are interesting in drug delivery platforms/devices for developing next-generation accurate medicines. For a deeper consideration of the different endogenous-responsive mechanisms of materials and biomaterials, many researches have been established for the development of micro/nano-fabrication, pharmaceutical science, biomedical engineering and materials chemistry to improve endogenous-responsive biomaterials for various drug delivery applications, such as medical bio-devices, drug delivery, localized controlled drug delivery systems (LCDDS), tissue engineering and theranostics. This chapter reports and discusses significant developments and progresses in the design and fabrication of endogenous-responsive LCDDS that have the ability to control or regulate the distribution of therapeutic agents (drugs) in response to a specific endogenous stimulus (changes in redox, pH, enzyme and oxidation).

Keywords: Endogenous stimuli, Enzyme-sensitive materials, Oxidation-sensitive materials, pH-sensitive materials, Redox-sensitive drug delivery, Stimuli-responsive biomaterials.

7.1. INTRODUCTION

In recent years, smart drug delivery systems have gained increased attention and paved the way for more effective treatment of patients (Askari *et al.*, 2021, Kalkhoran *et al.*, 2018a, Kalkhoran *et al.*, 2018b, Rahmanian *et al.*, 2019). In these systems with stimuli-responsive characteristics, the drugs are not released before reaching the target site (Gooneh-Farahani *et al.*, 2020, Gooneh-Farahani *et al.*, 2019, Kazemi and Naghib, 2020, Naghib *et al.*, 2020). This triggered release occurs due to the changes in the system structure or chemistry in response to endogenous and/ or exogenous stimuli that result in the local effect and release of the drugs at the disease site. The endogenous triggers such as pH, redox, enzyme concentration, and bio-molecules are related to the disease's pathological characteristics (Torchilin, 2018). This chapter will focus on endogenous stimuli-

Seyed Morteza Naghib, Samin Hoseinpour & Shadi Zarshad

sensitive LCDDSs for programmed/on-demand site-specific release in recently published studies.

The pathological characteristics of the disease are key parameters as physiological triggers for designing programmed delivery devices that may be used for the non-invasive and effective treatment of a wide range of pathological conditions, such as cancer, infections, diabetes, cardiovascular diseases, autoimmune disorders, stroke and chronic wounds, and degenerative diseases. In general, these physiological triggers exist at the organ, tissue, and cell levels (Lu *et al.*, 2016). For instance, different sites of the body (like blood vessels, vagina, gastrointestinal tract, tumor environment and *etc.*) represent their own pH (Gupta *et al.*, 2002) that may be utilized for triggering the selective release of therapeutic agents in the target site. So, endogenously triggered drug release is the same as exogenously triggered drug release, and can lead to enhanced release of therapeutic molecules at the target place in its therapeutic concentration, reducing local toxicity and side effects, thereby reducing the need for repeated administrations, and increasing patient compliance.

However, these systems have their own limitations and challenges. One of the most important challenges is related to their degradability or insufficient biocompatibility with most smart delivery system materials (Alsehli, 2020). Another challenge is related to the application of 2D *in vitro* models or *in vivo* animal studies to evaluate the performance of these systems, and there is a poor relationship between such results and human clinical trials. Thus, these incompatibilities can lead to the failure of numerous smart systems in clinical studies (Abdo *et al.*, 2020).

7.2. REDOX-SENSITIVE DRUG DELIVERY

One of the main challenges in DDSs is site-specific delivery and improved release of therapeutic molecules at the target site. Redox-sensitive DDSs are capable of overcoming these limitations. The gradient of redox potential between the intracellular/extracellular environment of abnormal cells/tissues can be used as an internal stimulus for controlled-release drug delivery (Kamaly *et al.*, 2016). As an example, Glutathione (a tripeptide containing cysteine, GSH)-mediated release systems represent a way in which therapeutic drugs can be released in a controlled manner. These systems are designed based on the gradient of GSH concentrations between intracellular and extracellular fluids, which is in the range of (2–10 mM) and (2-20 µM), respectively (Duncan *et al.*, 2010, Kamaly *et al.*, 2016, Wu *et al.*, 2004). Based on the in-vivo research, in tumor cells, this GSH difference is four times higher than their counterparts in normal cells. Therefore, polymer-based DDSs with redox-sensitive components can take advantage of this approach for the local release of therapeutic agents (Askari *et al.*, 2020). Disulfide bond (–S–S–) is one of the most widely used reduction-responsive linkages in many types of research and may be simply broken down by reduction of glutathione into thiols, whilst it is stable in blood circulation. Therefore, this phenomenon can lead to the degradation of DDSs with disulfide bonds and rapid release of the loaded cargoes in a reductive environment (Wen *et al.*, 2015).

There is a wide range of redox-sensitive delivery systems, including hydrogels (Gong *et al.*, 2017), mesoporous silica nanoparticles (Chen *et al.*, 2016b), gold nanoparticles (Guo *et al.*, 2021), polymeric vesicles (Chang *et al.*, 2014), polymeric micelles (Zhang *et al.*, 2016b), nanogels (Kumar *et al.*, 2019), *etc.* As an example, to overcome the poor site-specific release of therapeutic molecules in cancer therapy, Chang *et al.* developed a redox-sensitive release platform comprised of polyethylene glycol-poly(b-benzyl-L-aspartate)-SS-paclitaxel (PPSP) with disulfide linkages. Under high GSH concentration in the tumor environment, disulfide bonds in PPSP molecules break easily, and the size of the system increases, leading to the site-specific delivery of PTX in cancer cells (Chang *et al.*, 2019). In general, as shown in Fig. (**1**), in redox-mediated delivery systems, reduction-responsive linkages may be present in the backbone, side chain, on the surface of a nanoparticle, or as a linker between two agents. Moreover, the disulfide linkage core/shell cross-linked polymeric micelles were developed recently (Guo *et al.*, 2018).

Reduction-responsive linkages, such as disulfide bonds, may be located in the polymer backbone with two distinct approaches, including directly utilizing monomers containing disulfide bonds or installing thiol functionality followed by oxidation to establish the S–S-links. For example, Wu *et al.* prepared L-cystein--based poly(disulfide amide) *via* polycondensation of L-cystine and fatty acids for creating redox-sensitive delivery nanocarriers (Monteiro *et al.*, 2021). However, the poor stability of redox-sensitive DDSs with reduction-responsive linkages in the backbone makes them less attractive than other redox-mediated delivery counterparts, as presented in Fig. (**1**) (Guo *et al.*, 2018).

In another approach, reduction-responsive linkages may be used in the side chain to modify the main chain and provide a redox-sensitive delivery system. For instance, PEG chains are grafted onto the polyaspartamide backbone through disulfide linkages, preparing a sheddable shell for the preparation of redox-sensitive DOX-loaded polymeric micelles (Gong *et al.*, 2016). In another study, DOX was attached to the HA backbone *via* disulfide and hydrazine linkages for designing redox/pH dual-sensitive delivery micelles. This system exhibited a site-specific DOX release in response to acidic pH and/or high concentration levels of GSH that is presented in A549 human lung cancer cells (Yin *et al.*, 2018).

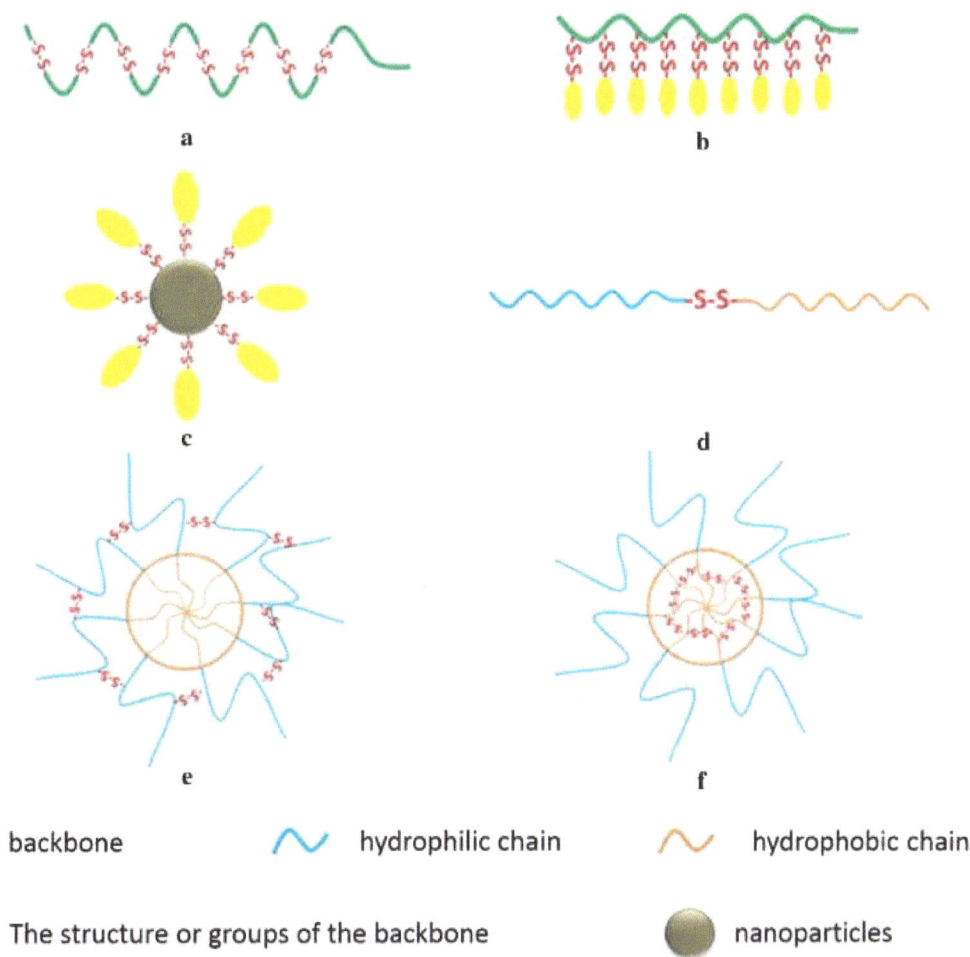

Fig. (1). Schematic representation of redox-mediated delivery systems with disulfide linkages. A) Disulfide linkages are present in the backbone. B) Disulfide linkages are present in side chains. C) Disulfide bonds attached to the surface of nanoparticles. D) Disulfide bond as a linker between two agents. E) Shell cross-linked micelles. f) Core cross-linked micelles (open access) (Guo *et al.*, 2018).

Using nanotechnology for developing redox-responsive systems is greatly increasing. Nanoparticles such as MSNPs, gold nanoparticles, liposomes, nanogels, *etc.*, may be used to produce redox-sensitive systems. In this regard, reduction-responsive bonds can be used for linking modified structures to the surface of nanostructures (Lin *et al.*, 2017). For example, Zhang *et al.* used disulfide bonds for linking HA onto the surface of mesoporous silica nanoparticles (MSNs) to create an MSNs/SS/HA@DOX system. This nanoscale delivery system exhibited a great redox-sensitive drug release in response to the high concentration of GSH existing in tumor cells (Zhang *et al.*, 2016a). In another study, Zhao *et al.* used disulfide bonds to link siRNAs to the surface of MSNs to develop an MSNs-SS-siRNA@Dox nanocarrier with redox-controlled co-delivery of gene and therapeutic agents for cancer treatment (Zhao *et al.*, 2017b).

In another approach, redox-mediated delivery micelles composed of reduction-responsive bonds as a linker between hydrophilic and hydrophobic polymers were destabilized to release therapeutic agents under reduction environment (Pham *et al.*, 2020). For instance, Zhao *et al.* designed a GSH-responsive delivery micelle composed of triple-disulfide bonds which were introduced into an amphiphilic copolymer to create a triblock copolymer of PEG-SS-PCL-SSPCL- SS-PEG. This system demonstrated great structural stability under physiological circumstances, outside the cancerous area, while it would disassemble easily under high GSH concentration in the tumor environment due to the cleaving of the triple disulfide bonds (Zhao *et al.*, 2017a).

In the last approach, reduction-responsive bonds can exist as cross-linkers in core-shell structures (such as core cross-linked/shell cross-linked micelles). As an instance, the redox-sensitive core cross-linked polymeric micelles of amphiphilic (PEO-b-PFMA) block co-polymers were prepared effectively in le's work. This delivery system was composed of a DOX-loaded core with PFMA cross-linked *via* disulfide cross-linking agents and the PEO corona. This system demonstrated great stability during blood circulation, while disassociated through the cleaving of disulfide linkages in the presence of 1,4-dithiothreitol (DTT) (Le *et al.*, 2016). In another study, Sun *et al.* designed a diblock terpolymer PDPA-b-P(NMS-co-OEG), which was further cross-linked with redox-sensitive cystamine, which reacted with the NMS ester groups to prepare a shell-cross-linked polymeric micelle with great pH/redox-dual responsive release characteristic. This smart delivery system was composed of a pH-sensitive PDPA core and redox-sensitive cystamine-containing shell for camptothecin (CPT) delivery (Sun *et al.*, 2019).

Selenide- or diselenide-containing systems could also respond to redox potential with lower bond energy (172 kJ/mol) than disulfide bonds (268 kJ/mol) (Mi, 2020, Monteiro *et al.*, 2021). Moreover, selenium-containing systems are much more sensitive to H_2O_2 than sulphide-based systems. Diselenide-based systems can be used as carriers for the combination of drug delivery with radiotherapy or photodynamic therapy. Besides, these smart delivery systems can be used for more than one medication carrier for combination therapy (Mollazadeh *et al.*, 2020). As an example, diselenide-rich amphiphilic diblock copolymers were synthesized successfully in Zhai's work for combination therapy and loading two anticancer drugs, CPT and DOX. Then the visible-light-induced dynamic exchange of diselenide bonds in the hydrophobic core was amended to form the core cross-linked micelles, CPT/DOX-CCM. This delivery system showed a great tunable combined delivery of DOX and CPT, under a cancer-related reductive environment (Zhai *et al.*, 2017).

Besides disulfide and diselenide linkages, numerous redox-sensitive linkages are less explored. For example, succinimide-thioether can be used as a reduction-responsive linkage that can be cleaved in response to GSH, leading to the disassembly of the succinimide-thioether-containing system and efficient intracellular release of drugs. Drug delivery systems with "trimethyl-locked" benzoquinone (TMBQ) were used for designing redox-sensitive delivery systems (Guo *et al.*, 2018, Huo *et al.*, 2014). For instance, a paclitaxel-loaded delivery system has been developed in Cho's work using TMBQ as a redox-sensitive group. As a result, in response to the reduction of sodium dithionite, shedding of the TMBQ from the polymer backbone, led to the release of therapeutic cargos (Cho *et al.*, 2012).

In addition to the aforementioned systems, Mn^{2+} ions released from MnO_2 nanosheets in response to the intracellular GSH, were used for GSH-responsive delivery of anticancer agents (Cho *et al.*, 2017). In this context, MnO_2 nanosheets can be applied as gatekeepers for developing gated MSNPs as a redox-sensitive delivery system. For instance, Meng *et al.* utilized this method to design a multifunctional nanosystem for contrast-enhanced bimodal cellular imaging and controlled drug delivery in cancer therapy. As a result, under high concentration levels of GSH observed in tumor cells, MnO_2 nanosheets were reduced to Mn^{2+} ions, leading to the delivery of cargos to the target site and contrast-enhanced two-photon fluorescence (Fig. **2**) (Chen *et al.*, 2016a).

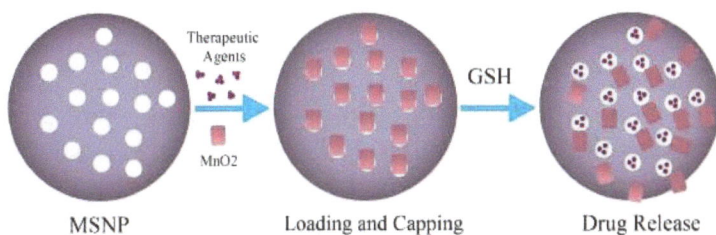

MSNP   Loading and Capping   Drug Release

Fig. (2). Schematic illustration of GSH-sensitive MSNP-based system with MnO_2 nanosheets as gatekeepers in order to smart drug delivery to cancerous cells triggered by GSH

Despite the promising potential of redox-responsive DDSs in site-specific drug release, the clinical translation of these delivery devices is still challenging.

Unfortunately, it is noteworthy that unwanted drug release performance from redox-sensitive DDSs at non-targeted sites has been reported and resulted in unpopular side effects. Besides, a large number of therapeutic drugs still do not have adequate results in spite of the nanoscale size of redox-sensitive DDSs. However, redox-responsive systems may be enhanced for controlled drug delivery. Redox signals can be combined with other external or intracellular sensitive groups to develop smart systems with higher sensitivity that can be used as novel systems to overcome the limitations mentioned above. For instance, pH and redox dual-sensitive delivery systems can be used to deliver therapeutic drugs at the target site with higher efficiency, resulting in fewer side effects. Besides, the magnetic guidance can lead to the enhanced accumulation of carriers at the disease site. Moreover, enzyme sensitivity could not only accelerate the delivery of therapeutic drugs but also enhance the accumulation in diseased tissues (Li *et al.*, 2020a, Tang *et al.*, 2017).

7.3. OXIDATION-SENSITIVE DRUG DELIVERY

Reactive oxygen species (ROS) include a wide range of intermediate molecules with/without oxygen atoms in radical and non-radical forms. Radical species include superoxide anion ($O_2\bullet$), hydroxyl radical (HO$\bullet$), peroxyl radicals (ROO$\bullet$), organic radicals (R$\bullet$), alkoxyl radicals (RO$\bullet$), sulfonyl radicals (ROS$\bullet$), thiyl peroxyl radicals (RSOO$\bullet$) and thiyl radicals (RS$\bullet$). On the other hand, non-radical molecules include hydrogen peroxide (H_2O_2), hypochlorous acid (HOCl), organic hydroperoxides (ROOH), singlet oxygen ($1O_2$), and ozone/trioxygen (O_3). Different cells, such as endothelial cells, cancer-associated fibroblasts, and inflammatory cells, as well as angiogenesis and hypoxia, are involved in ROS generation. For example, cancer cells increase the ROS concentration up to 100 mM, which is 100 times higher than in normal conditions (Mirhadi *et al.*, 2020). Excess ROS levels can be considered markers of a wide range of diseases such as infections, diabetes, atherosclerosis, cardiovascular disease, and numerous cancers. These localized areas, are gaining considerable interest in designing drug-loaded carriers that can respond to ROS (Phillips and Gibson, 2014, Kamaly *et al.*, 2016).

In general, ROS-responsive delivery systems contain nano- or micro-sized polymers functionalized with chemical groups that respond to ROS. In an oxidative environment, these systems can swell to release therapeutic drugs progressively, or burst to discharge the entire drug all at once (Seetharaman *et al.*, 2017). A wide range of ROS-responsive small molecule linkers is investigated in the drug delivery field, including thioether, selenium/ tellurium (Se/Te), thioketal, boronic ester, polysaccharide, peroxalate ester, aminoacrylate, and polyproline

(Liang and Liu, 2016). For example, thioether is the most extensively investigated ROS-responsive bond due to its hydrophobic/ hydrophilic phase transition in response to the ROS. This phase transition occurs due to the conversion of thioether groups into sulfoxide and sulfones in response to the mild and strong oxidative conditions, respectively. In this regard, Gupta *et al.* synthesized a diblock polymer of propylene sulfide (PS) and N,N-dimethylacrylamide to form a ROS-sensitive micelle drug carrier (poly(PS74-b-DMA310)) that was then loaded with the Nile red and DiO as a model of drugs. This delivery system demonstrated smart delivery of hydrophobic drugs due to the solubility change and subsequent disassembly of the micelle in response to the H_2O_2, SIN-1, and peroxynitrite that are presented at the target sites of inflammation (Gupta *et al.*, 2012). Thioketal is another ROS-responsive bond that can be cleaved in response to the ROS and create acetone and two other thiol-containing fragments, which result in polymer chain scission and breakdown (Gao and Xiong, 2021). In this regard, Xu *et al.* designed a ROS-cleavable thioketal containing polyMTO-based nanoparticles to form ROS-Responsive polyprodrug nanoparticles for cancer therapy (Xu *et al.*, 2017). Selenium-containing polymers are another group of ROS-sensitive materials with the same mechanism of action as thioether. However, selenium-containing polymers have a more sensitive response to ROS compared to sulfur-containing polymers (Gao and Xiong, 2021). In this regard, Ma *et al.* synthesized a selenium-containing co-polymer (PEG-PUSe-PEG) with polymerization of toluene diisocyanate with monoselenide-containing diols and subsequent termination with PEG monomethylether. This delivery system exhibited ROS-sensitive release of therapeutic agents due to the formation of selenone groups in response to the mild oxidative environment, which enhanced the solubility of the system, leading to structural dissociation (Ma *et al.*, 2010).

Interestingly some surveys have been established to represent the design of MSN-based ROS-sensitive DDSs without employing ROS-sensitive bonds. In these systems, metal nanoparticles were employed as gatekeepers and were destabilized and removed from the MSNs in response to the ROS. In this regard, Faheem *et al.* designed a ROS-sensitive delivery system based on Ag NPs that cap the pores of drug-loaded MSNs. However, the presence of H_2O_2 etched the Ag nanolids, leading to the opening of pores and controlled release of therapeutic agents (Saravanakumar *et al.*, 2017, Muhammad *et al.*, 2015).

7.4. PH-SENSITIVE DRUG DELIVERY

pH-sensitive delivery systems can lead to the site-specific release of therapeutic drugs by varying the solubility of the delivery system or by cleaving pH-sensitive bonds upon pH gradient (Cicuéndez *et al.*, 2018). This pH gradient which was introduced at places (like tumor environment, blood vessels, vagina and gastrointestinal tract), can be used as an endogenous stimulus for designing smart delivery systems and controlling drug release (Gupta *et al.*, 2002).

So, conventional delivery systems can be replaced with these smart delivery systems. For instance, oral drug delivery has several limitations, such as poor stability in the gastric environment, low solubility, low bioavailability, drug expulsion *via* intestinal drug transport, and the continuous secretion of mucus which is known to prevent drug absorption and penetration (Mehta and Pawar, 2018, Herlem *et al.*, 2019, Mohammadzadeh and Javadzadeh, 2018, Ensign *et al.*, 2012). pH-sensitive delivery systems have a great potential for overcoming these limitations by improving the stability of drug delivery in the stomach and achieving controlled release in the intestines (Liu *et al.*, 2017). Numerous studies illustrate the benefits of pH-sensitive DDSs for the treatment of a wide range of diseases. This section discusses the applications of pH-sensitive systems in drug delivery and their drug release mechanism.

One of the main properties of solid tumors that have been widely studied is their extracellular lactic acidosis, caused by tumor response to hypoxia and the accumulation of acidic metabolic waste products in cancerous areas. Besides hypoxia, other complex metabolic processes, such as tumor respiration, H+ and HCO_3 − transport, and extracellular H+ venting, results in tumor acidity (Kashkooli *et al.*, 2020, Boedtkjer and Pedersen, 2020). According to the electrical and chemical probes, the recorded values of tumor extracellular fluid pH are in the range of 5.7–7.8. It is noteworthy that low pH has two aspects in cancer therapy: 1) increasing drug resistance by slowing the uptake of therapeutic drugs, such as DOX, leading to their poor effect of them on tumor tissue, and inducing vascular endothelial growth factor. 2) exploiting low pH as a stimulus to trigger payload release from pH-sensitive delivery systems (Shen *et al.*, 2008). The second aspect would be useful for localized delivery and triggered release of chemotherapeutic agents to tumor tissues. There is a wide range of pH-responsive delivery systems, such as pH-responsive scaffolds and pH-responsive nanostructures (Sang *et al.*, 2018, Li *et al.*, 2020b). In this context, a dual-drug-loaded pH-responsive scaffold was fabricated in Sang's work, in order to be sutured after tumor resection surgery and prevent cancer recurrence. In this delivery system, the ciprofloxacin-loaded shell was composed of a mixture of gelatin and sodium bicarbonate (added to provide pH sensitivity), and the Dox-loaded core was made up of poly(lactide-co-e-caprolactone). This smart implantable delivery system demonstrated a rapid and pH-responsive ciprofloxacin release, and sustained release of doxorubicin (Sang *et al.*, 2018). In addition to the pH-sensitive scaffolds, the pH-sensitive nanocarriers have also shown a significant potential for use in cancer targeting therapy. pH-sensitive nanostructure-based nanocarriers can be classified into three main categories; 1) polymeric nanocarriers, which are sub-divided into nanogels, micelles, polymer-drug conjugates, and core-shell polymeric NPs, 2) liposomes, and 3) inorganic NPs (Karimi *et al.*, 2016). In this regard, designing pH-sensitive nanocarriers with targeting ligands can provide better control over the delivery of therapeutic agents and increase cellular uptake while minimizing side effects. For instance, Bae *et al.* designed delivery micelles made from mixed block copolymers polyHis-PEG and PLLA-b-PEG-b- polyHis-biotin. In this study, pH variations, from physiological pH to acidic extracellular fluid of tumor tissues were used as a signal for ligand (biotin) exposure on the micelles. In other words, due to the pH-dependent water-solubility of poly (l-histidine) (polyHis), biotin was buried in the PEG shell in physiological pH, whereas in the acidic environment, the polyHis became soluble, leading to the binding of ligand biotin to its receptors (Shen *et al.*, 2008, Lee *et al.*, 2005).

However, using pH-sensitive delivery systems for cancer therapy has its own challenges: 1) acidic pH in perivascular areas is typically far away from the blood flow, which results in the lack of system response, 2) in most cases, the pH gradient does not significantly differ in healthy tissues and tumor tissues (Das *et al.*, 2020).

In addition to cancer treatment, pH-responsive delivery systems can be used for localized release of therapeutic agents against bacterial and viral infections. For example, Lin *et al.* prepared a delivery system based on parin-chitosan NPs, for localized delivery of antibiotics at the Helicobacter pylori infection site on the gastric epithelium. This system was able to protect the drug from destructive gastric acids due to the electrostatic interactions within the particles and its stable characteristic at pH 1.2–2.5. Upon contact with an H. pylori infection region on the gastric epithelium (pH ~7.4), the deprotonation of chitosan led to weakened electrostatic interactions and resulted in the collapse of the system and heparin release (Lin *et al.*, 2009).

pH-sensitive delivery systems can be used for tissue regeneration as well. Infections in tissues can slow regeneration processes, besides, the pH in infected tissues usually decreases due to the irregular angiogenesis or dysregulated metabolism, which results in a rapid shortage of oxygen and nutrients. The shortage of oxygen and nutrients further leads to a shift toward glycolytic metabolism (Municoy *et al.*, 2020). In this context, Cicuéndez *et al.* designed a levofloxacin (Levo)-loaded 3D scaffold for supporting tissue regeneration and management of bone infection with the ability to destroy bacterial biofilm without cytotoxic effects on human osteoblasts. This nanocomposite included a mesostructured glassy network with embedded hydroxyapatite nanoparticles. As a result, this smart system exhibited a significant release of levofloxacin (Levo) as an antibacterial agent at infection pH (6.7 and 5.5) due to the diverse interaction rate between different pH-dependent species of Levo and silanol groups of the mesoporous scaffold (Cicuéndez *et al.*, 2018).

pH-sensitive DDSs may be used in the prevention of sexually transmitted infections as well. For this purpose, it is necessary for the anti-HIV agents- or siRNA-loaded carriers to be released only during heterosexual intercourse in order to minimize side effects and avoid unnecessary exposure to therapeutic agents. It is noteworthy that vaginal pH can change from normal non-menstrual acidic conditions (pH 3.5-4.5) to neutral pH in the presence of the seminal fluid after heterosexual intercourse. Therefore, intravaginal rings can use this approach to release therapeutic agents with minimal side effects for prevention of sexually transmitted infections such as human immunodeficiency virus (HIV) (Kim *et al.*, 2018). In this regard, Kim *et al.* fabricated a smart delivery system that exhibited a smart switch between "on" and "off" for on-demand and regulation of drug release for the prevention of sexually transmitted infections. This research group used pH-responsive PU membranes, which can serve as membranes in reservoir-type intravaginal rings. The release of NaDF as an anti-HIV drug from this pH-sensitive delivery system occurs upon the change of pH from 4.5 to 7.0 during heterosexual intercourse. This phenomenon occurs due to the electrostatic interaction between the tertiary amines of the PU and anionic NaDF (which results in the reduced permeation of NaDF through the PU) at pH 4.5 and stops this interaction when pH=7 (Kim *et al.*, 2017).

As another application, pH-sensitive delivery systems can be used for wound healing when the wound has entered the inflammatory stage. (Banerjee *et al.*, 2012). In this context, Guo *et al.* prepared a pH-sensitive core-shell structure as a delivery system, including PCL as the core and CS/PEO as the shell for sequential dual-drug release in response to the different wound healing stages. In this study, lidocaine hydrochloride (Lid) was loaded in the shell that can be used as pain relief in the early stages of wound healing. Curcumin (Cur) was added into the core as an anti-inflammatory agent. Due to the pH-sensitivity of chitosan, upon acidic conditions, Lid was released because of the formation of $-NH_3$ + by protonation of $-NH_2$ on the chitosan molecular chains. Moreover, sodium bicarbonate (SB) was introduced to the core as a pH-responsive material to control curcumin release, when wound healing entered the inflammatory stage. (Guo *et al.*, 2020).

As shown in Fig. (**3**), there are three main strategies for achieving pH-sensitive delivery systems. An effective approach is using polymer building blocks with ionizable chemical groups that can change charge and/or hydrophilicity in response to the environment's pH changes. In this mechanism, the delivery carriers remain deprotonated/deionized at physiological pH, while an acidic environment permits protonation of the system. This leads to the disassembly or structural transformation of the system and results in the site-specific release of therapeutic agents at the target site. In general, an acidic environment causes distinct changes in cationic and anionic polymers, including hydrophobic/ hydrophilic phase transition for cationic polymers and hydrophilic-hydrophobic phase transition for the anionic polymers (Kanamala *et al.*, 2016).

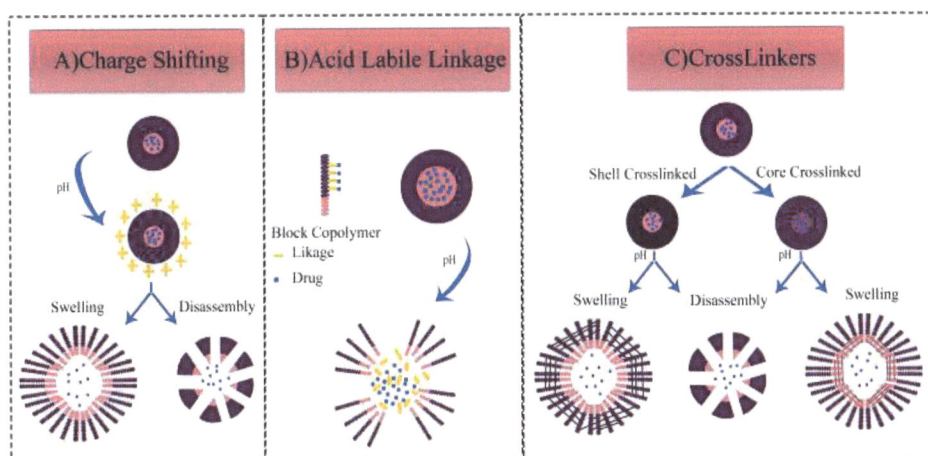

Fig. (3). Schematic illustration of three main approaches for designing pH-sensitive DDSSs, including **A)** using polymer building blocks with ionizable chemical groups that can change charge and/or hydrophilicity in response to pH, **B)** using acid-cleavable linkers, or **C)** using crosslinkers.

Cationic polymers are presented as the macromolecules with positive charges as a result of primary, secondary or tertiary amine functional groups, which can be either introduced in the polymer side chains and/or its backbone. These polymers can be protonated and become hydrophilic, disassembling the system in a specific environment at pH values smaller than their pKa, which makes them a great candidate for designing drug delivery systems for the treatment of a wide range of human diseases, and especially targeted cancer therapy. Generally, cationic polymers can be used for developing drug delivery systems because of their great loading efficacy, improved bioavailability, low toxicity, and enhanced release profile (Farshbaf *et al.*, 2018, Meléndez-Ortiz *et al.*, 2016, Chuang *et al.*, 2017).

According to the origins, cationic polymers are categorized into two groups, natural and synthetic. Poly (dimethylaminoethyl methacrylate) (PDMAEMA), poly(diethylaminoethyl methacrylate) (PDEAEMA), poly(ethyl pyrrolidine methacrylate) (PEP), and poly(ethyl piperazine acrylate) (PAcrNEP) are a number of pH-sensitive synthetic cationic polymers (Deen and Loh, 2018, Bawa *et al.*, 2009). Cationic gelatin, cationic chitosan, and cationic cellulose are some of the natural cationic polymers (Farshbaf *et al.*, 2018).

For example, Liang *et al.* used this strategy for designing a pH-sensitive delivery system to simultaneously lock/ release Dox and peptides. This research group used PEG-Dox conjugate and a poly(2-diisopropylaminoethyl methacrylate) (PDPA) homopolymer, with a custom-designed H4R4 peptide (added to take advantage of endosomal escape and pH-dependent properties which results in the enhancing localization of Dox into the nucleus) consisting of arginine (R) and histidine (H) groups. As a result, the system exhibited hydrophobic to hydrophilic transition due to the protonation of PDPA and H4R4 in acidic endosomal compartments, leading to the disassembly of the NPs and release of Dox (Liang *et al.*, 2014).

Another class of pH-sensitive polymers is anionic polymers. These polymers contain carboxylic groups such as PAA, PMAA, PEAA, PPAA, PBAA, NIPAM, and PGA. In an acidic environment, these anionic polymers become relatively hydrophobic; whilst, they are ionized and become hydrophilic in response to neutral pH or at higher pH values than their pKa (Liu *et al.*, 2014b, Meléndez-Ortiz *et al.*, 2016). It is worth to note that polymer dissolving pH can be controlled by modifying the amount of carboxyl or other substituent groups on these polymers. For instance, the carboxyl/ester ratio of poly(methacrylic acid-co-methyl methacrylate) _as an anionic polymer_ can be adjusted to control the pH value and the aqueous solubility of this polymer (Yoshida *et al.*, 2013).

So, we can conclude that cationic polymers (polybases) can be useful for achieving high bioavailability of drugs and taste-masking due to their high solubility in the stomach (pH 1 -- 3.5) and low water solubility in the oral cavity (pH 5.8 -- 7.4), respectively. On the other hand, anionic polymers (polyacids) with higher water solubility at neutral pH than acidic pH, are used for stably preserving drugs from acid degradation in the stomach (enteric DDS) or enzyme digestion in the intestine (colon drug delivery) (Yoshida *et al.*, 2013).

It is noteworthy that generally, cationic polymers present more toxicity than anionic polymers. On the other hand, the negative charge of anionic polymers may compromise cell uptake and endosomal escape due to charge repulsion. Therefore, the application of negative-to-positive charge reversal polymers is an interesting strategy to overcome these challenges (Kanamala *et al.*, 2016).

Another strategy for designing pH-sensitive drug delivery systems is the incorporation of acid-labile linkages into the polymer backbone. In this approach, nanoparticles composed of covalent pH-responsive linkages, stable under neutral pH but labile under an acidic environment, are used. This approach would be useful for designing drug-polymer conjugates which are stable under physiological conditions but can degrade and release therapeutic agents, specifically in tumor cells (Deirram *et al.*, 2019). In this regard, hydrazone bonds have been widely used as acid-cleavable linkers due to their responsive acuteness in drug release behavior. In addition to hydrazone/hydrazide bond, other acid-labile linkages such as acetal, oxime, and imine bonds can also be used for creating pH-sensitive delivery systems (Guo *et al.*, 2016). In this regard, a novel pH-sensitive micelle as a drug vehicle has been developed in Bae's work for controlling the systemic, local, and subcellular distribution of therapeutic agents. This carrier was composed of self-assembling amphiphilic block copolymers, PEG-poly- (aspartate hydrazone adriamycin). Dox was conjugated to the hydrophobic segments as an anticancer drug *via* pH-responsive hydrazone linkers. This delivery system may be used to protect Dox in body fluids (pH 7.4) and selectively release Dox in response to the endosomal/lysosomal intracellular pH. (pH 5-6) (Bae *et al.*, 2005).

Polymers with imine groups as acid-cleavable bonds have also been explored for the fabrication of pH-delivery systems. Imines are also known to be formed by condensation of primary amine with aldehydes or ketones. Imine-cleavable bonds can be hydrolyzed in the weak acidic environment (pH ~6.8, near the pH of solid tumors), but their stability under physiological conditions can be improved. The imine bond is liable to hydrolyze in an acidic environment which can be used for modifying the surface of the carriers and developing smart DDSs effectively. In this context, Xu *et al.* synthesized the Dox-loaded pentaerythritol tetra(3-mercaptopropionate)-allylurea-poly(ethylene glycol) (PETMP-AU-PEG) anchored with imide linkages. They confirmed that this delivery system was extremely stable in a neutral environment with reduced drug leakage. While in the weak acid environment, the system exhibited a selective release of DOX for treatment of cancer by local cleavage of imide bond (Zhuo *et al.*, 2020). In another study, imine-linked dextran (Dex)-DOX conjugates were synthesized successfully by oxidizing Dex into functionalized aldehyde and conjugating it with Dox. As a result, this system demonstrated localized delivery of Dox in tumor cells due to the fracturing of the imine bond in Dex−DOX in the acidic environment (Feng *et al.*, 2017).

Acetal bonds have also emerged as a successful linker for designing pH-sensitive systems. These bonds undergo pH-dependent hydrolysis to form biocompatible alcohol and aldehydes as hydrolyzed products. pH-responsive, acetal-linked polymeric micelle–drug conjugates were formed from acetal-bonded PEG block-polylactide copolymer, and were used to deliver Paclitaxel as a model of anticancer drug. In another research, a novel endosomal pH-sensitive PTX prodrug micelle was fabricated by (mPEG-PCL) diblock polymer linked *via* acid-cleavable acetal bound (mPEG-PCL-Ace-PTX) (Das *et al.*, 2020).

The amide bond is another acid-cleavable linker which may be hydrolyzed under acidic pH, but therapeutic agents and vehicles do not easily connect with amide bonds to attain targeted delivery. In this context, maleic acid derivatives, β-carboxylic amides, and *cis*-acotinyl amide can be employed effectively as an acid-cleavable linker (Cao *et al.*, 2019).

Oxime, as a rare acid-cleavable linker, is formed by condensation of aldehydes, ketones, or hydroxylamine. Oxime can hydrolyze into aldehydes, ketones, and hydroxylamines in an acidic environment. It should be mentioned that a great advantage of using oxime linkage for cancer-targeted nanosystems is the tunability of its acid lability by facile variation of the substituents (Zhuo *et al.*, 2020). In this regard, a novel pH-sensitive flower-like micelle formed from backbone-cleavable triblock copolymer (PCL-OPEG-PCL) was designed for the smart delivery of anticancer drugs. DOX was loaded into these micelles as a model of anticancer agent, with high efficiency. Based on *in vitro* studies, this nanosystem can be stable under physiological conditions, whereas it exhibits a fast release of DOX under a mildly acidic environment of 5.0, showing the pH-sensitive nature of the systems with oxime linkages (Liu *et al.*, 2014a).

The last strategy for designing pH-sensitive DDSs is using cross-linking to stabilize carriers to overcome poor circulation stability. Crosslinkers can either combine charge shifting polymers with non-cleavable linkages to create swellable carriers or acid-cleavable bonds, which result in pH-sensitive disassembly. In this context, reversible cross-linking enhances the ability to release drugs at the target site by allowing NPs to disassemble when the target site is reached (Deirram *et al.*, 2019).

For instance, Seetharaman *et al.* designed cross-linked prodrug micelles in which ibuprofen (Ibu) is tethered to carboxyl-terminated methoxy poly(ethylene glycol)-b-poly(propylene fumarate) (mPEG-PPF) diblock copolymers as a model of an anti-inflammatory drug, using an anhydride linkage. The PPF moieties were cross-linked with pH-sensitive crosslinker $N,N-$ dimethylaminoethyl methacrylate (DMAEMA). As a result, this pH-responsive mPEG-PPF prodrug micelle demonstrated effective and safe delivery of Ibu in the physiologically relevant acidic environment for the treatment of arthritis (Seetharaman *et al.*, 2017).

7.5. ENZYME-SENSITIVE DRUG DELIVERY

Enzyme-sensitive drug delivery systems can be effectively used for the treatment of a wide range of diseases. In these systems, several enzymes (such as proteases, phospholipases or glycosidases) which are found in pathological environments, such as inflammation or different types of cancers, can be exploited as a stimulus to trigger drug release from these smart systems at desired biological target (Majumder and Minko, 2021). There are a variety of implementations of enzyme-sensitive delivery systems for smart and controlled drug delivery. In this context, Fig. (**4**) illustrates 3 main approaches. 1) Therapeutic agents can be directly released from different types of systems *via* site-specific enzymatic cleavage. In this regard, therapeutic agents may be loaded into nanocarriers *via* covalent attachment or physical loading, involving a cross-linked matrix, a self-assembled system, or a caged porous structure. 2) Enzyme-sensitive delivery systems can be activated by enzymes to expose the targeting ligand for subsequent internalization into target cells. 3) Enzymes can play a critical role in the generation of particular products (such as creating an acidic condition), enhancing drug release from systems (Hu *et al.*, 2014).

It should be highlighted that the enzyme-active moieties can often be peptides, DNA, or synthetic sequences, and their cleavage in response to the presence of specific enzyme results in the release of therapeutic cargos due to the dissociation, changes in the amphiphilicity, or morphological transitions of carriers (Kamaly *et al.*, 2016).

It should be highlighted that proteases, phospoholipases, and oxidoreductases are the most investigated enzymes that can be used for enzyme-mediated drug release. In this regard, a wide range of enzyme-responsive delivery systems, such as polymer-based nanoparticles, liposomes, inorganic nanoparticles, hydrogels, *etc.*, has been designed. Protease overexpression is an ideal effector in smart delivery systems due to the imbalances in the expression and activity of particular proteases in the diseased sites (Hu *et al.*, 2014). Cathepsins are a class of proteases that are found in the lysosome. There is a wide range of cathepsins that are overexpressed in tumor cells. However, cathepsin B has an important role in various pathologies and oncogenic processes (Gondi and Rao, 2013). It is noteworthy that in most enzyme-responsive delivery systems, esters and short peptide sequences are cleaved by proteases. In this regard, Gly-Phe-Leu-Gly is cleaved in the lysosome as a common cleavable sequence, by cathepsin B, which is overexpressed in cancer cells (Kamaly *et al.*, 2016). Another class of proteases is metalloproteinases (MMPs). There are different types of matrices (MMPs), which are extracellular matrix-degrading enzymes, in numerous human diseases. For example, MMP-2 and MMP-9 are known to be involved in the progression and metastasis of various cancers (Kuang *et al.*, 2016). In this context, as shown in Fig. (**5a**), short peptide sequences which act as linkers between surface PEG chains and either TAT-functionalized liposomes can be cleavable by MMPS. In this study, after cleavage of the PEG shell in the tumor microenvironment, surface bioactive ligands were exposed, which enhanced intracellular penetration compared with nanocarriers without cleavable linkers (Mura *et al.*, 2013). Similarly, mesoporous silica nanoparticles can also be used for developing enzyme-sensitive delivery systems. In this regard, in another study, Lui *et al.* designed an enzyme-sensitive drug delivery system based on MSNs (MSNs-HSAPBA@ DOX) for smart and controlled *in vitro* and *in vivo* release of therapeutic agents, by employing HSA-PBA as an end-capping agent, functional polypeptide as an intermediate linker, and PBA as a targeting motif. As a result, this delivery system showed a significant sensitivity to MMP-2 for drug delivery, leading to cell apoptosis (Fig. **5b**) (Liu *et al.*, 2015).

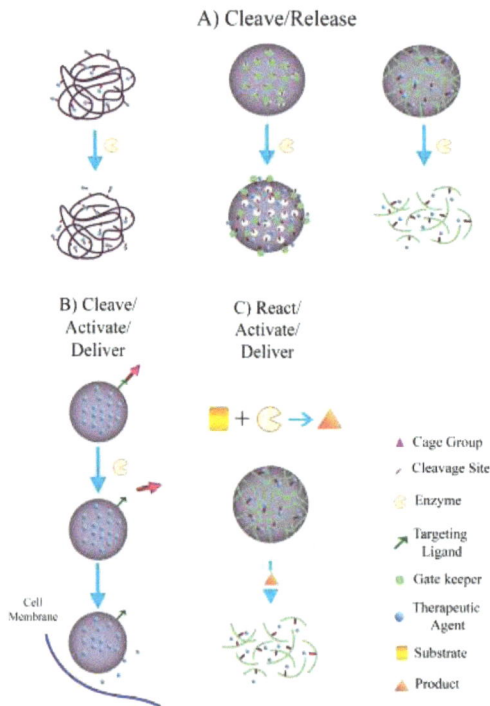

Fig. (4). A schematic illustrating 3 main implementations of enzyme-sensitive nanocarriers for smart and controlled release of therapeutic agents. (**A**) Therapeutic agents can be directly released from different types of systems *via* site-specific enzymatic cleavage. (**B**) Enzyme-sensitive delivery systems can be activated by enzymes to expose the targeting ligand for the subsequent internalization into target cells. (**C**) Enzymes can enhance the generation of particular products leading to the release of therapeutic cargos from nanocarriers.

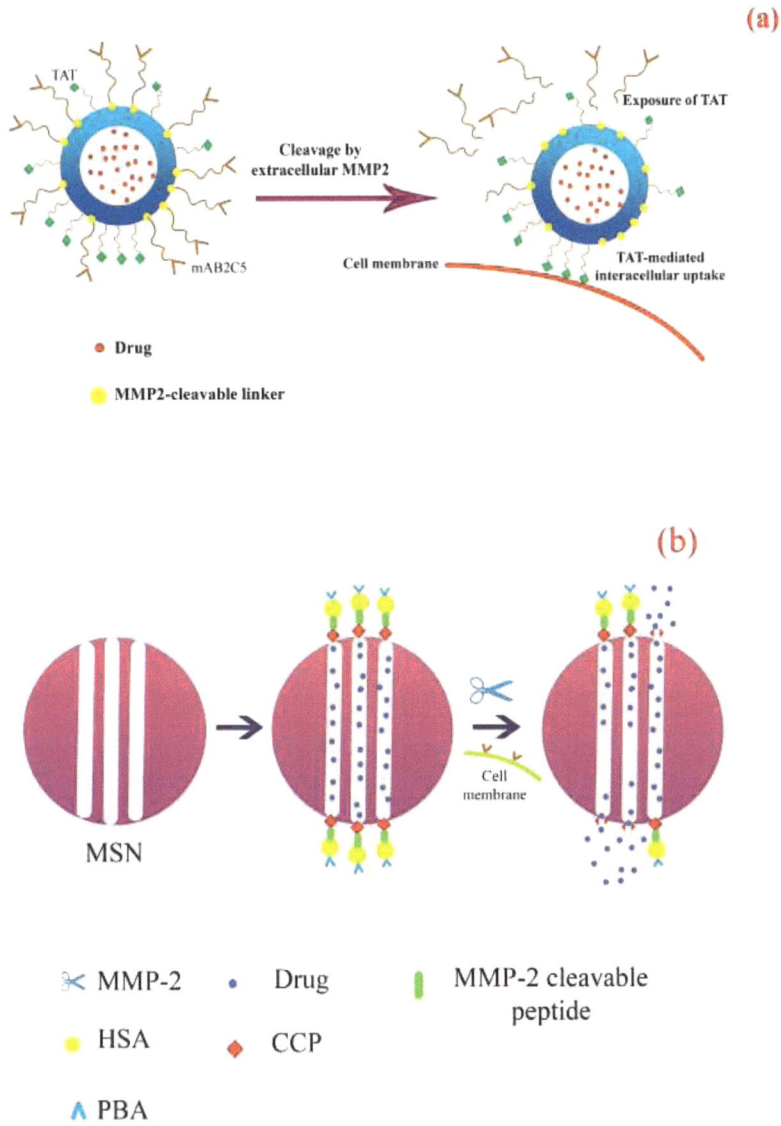

Fig. (5). Enzyme-sensitive drug delivery systems. (**a**) Multifunctional liposomal nanocarrier responsive to (MMP2) for drug delivery *via* TAT-mediated internalization. mAB 2C5; nucleosome-specific monoclonal antibody 2C5. (**b**) functionalization routes of enzyme-sensitive MSN-based drug delivery system.

Phospholipases such as phospholipase A2 (PLA2) are another important enzyme that is up-regulated in infectious and inflammatory diseases. In this regard, Antibiotics-loaded sPLA2-responsive delivery systems offer numerous benefits over other systems in the treatment of infections. These systems can release high concentrations of antibiotics at the target infection site where bacteria secrete sPLA2. Moreover, the overexpression of PLA2 was found in some advanced cancer stages such as prostate, breast, and pancreatic cancers (Shahriari *et al.*, 2019, Fouladi *et al.*, 2017). For example, Dox-loaded sPLA2 sensitive liposomes were designed in Mock's work for the treatment of prostate cancer (Mock *et al.*, 2013). In another study, Mumtaz Virk designed and created calcein-loaded unilanellar hybrid carriers with diameters of 100 nm by mixing polybutadiene-block-poly(ethylene oxide) and phosphocholine lipids using a combination of solvent inversion and sonication. As a result, PLA2 hydrolyzes lipids, resulted in the dissolution of lipid domains and release of calcein as pores. (Mumtaz Virk and Reimhult, 2018)

Another group of popular enzymes used in enzyme-mediated DDSs is oxidoreductases due to their central role in oxidative stress, which is related to diseases such as cancer and Alzheimer's. Besides, this group of enzymes is widely used as diagnostic tools, for instance, in the detection of glucose by glucose oxidase or as labels for immunodetection with horseradish peroxidase (De La Rica *et al.*, 2012). In this regard, Gu *et al.* designed an injectable nano-network for glucose-mediated insulin delivery. This delivery system included oppositely charged dextran NPs which encapsulated insulin and glucose-specific enzymes. The gel-like 3D scaffold dissociated and subsequently released insulin in a hyperglycemic condition (Gu *et al.*, 2013). In these systems, an increase in the blood glucose level causes glucose to penetrate into the membrane. The enclosing glucose oxidase catalyzes the glucose conversion to gluconic acid, causing degradation of the polymeric matrix and leading to the release of insulin (Sood *et al.*, 2016, Goldbart *et al.*, 2002). This delivery system can pave the way for both self-regulated and long-term diabetes management. It should be noted that all these examples demonstrate the great potential of enzyme-sensitive DDSs. However, the complexity and often the over-complexity of drug release from enzyme-sensitive delivery systems still remains a matter of concern, and a wide range of research and studies are needed to obtain precise information about the target enzyme levels at the desired site to fine-control cell uptake.

CONCLUSION

LCDDS has gained great interest in temporal-controlled and spatial-controlled drug delivery, tissue engineering and biomedicine. Smart stimuli-triggered materials/biomaterials establish the significant potential to improve the effectiveness of LCDDS-based therapy and minimize the side effects through specific local drug accumulation, demonstrating the adjustable release of therapeutic molecules/drugs and hybrid cure *via* integration of multifunctional and multimodal therapeutic regimes. These smart vehicles and devices require biocompatible materials/biomaterials that are responsive to a biological or chemical stimulus. Endogenous stimuli-sensitive carriers establish noteworthy benefits in increasing the therapeutic efficiency and decreasing the side effects of the cargo/therapeutic molecule loaded into the carrier/device. In this chapter, endogenous stimuli-responsive vehicles based on LCDDS were described and discussed. In this regard, ROS-, pH-, enzyme- and oxidation-responsive carriers were the most vehicles having endogenous stimuli and were extensively used in LCDD applications.

REFERENCES

Abdo, G.G., Zagho, M.M., Khalil, A. (2020). Recent advances in stimuli-responsive drug release and targeting concepts using mesoporous silica nanoparticles. *Emergent Materials, 3*(3), 407-425. [http://dx.doi.org/10.1007/s42247-020-00109-x]

Alsehli, M. (2020). Polymeric nanocarriers as stimuli-responsive systems for targeted tumor (cancer) therapy: Recent advances in drug delivery. *Saudi Pharm. J., 28*(3), 255-265. [http://dx.doi.org/10.1016/j.jsps.2020.01.004] [PMID: 32194326]

Askari, E., Naghib, S.M., Zahedi, A., Seyfoori, A., Zare, Y., Rhee, K.Y. (2021). Local delivery of chemotherapeutic agent in tissue engineering based on gelatin/graphene hydrogel. *J. Mater. Res. Technol., 12*, 412-422. [http://dx.doi.org/10.1016/j.jmrt.2021.02.084]

Askari, E., Seyfoori, A., Amereh, M., Gharaie, S.S., Ghazali, H.S., Ghazali, Z.S., Khunjush, B., Akbari, M. (2020). Stimuli-responsive hydrogels for local post-surgical drug delivery. *Gels, 6*(2), 14. [http://dx.doi.org/10.3390/gels6020014] [PMID: 32397180]

Bae, Y., Nishiyama, N., Fukushima, S., Koyama, H., Yasuhiro, M., Kataoka, K. (2005). Preparation and biological characterization of polymeric micelle drug carriers with intracellular pH-triggered drug release property: tumor permeability, controlled subcellular drug distribution, and enhanced *in vivo* antitumor efficacy. *Bioconjug. Chem., 16*(1), 122-130. [http://dx.doi.org/10.1021/bc0498166] [PMID: 15656583]

Banerjee, I., Mishra, D., Das, T., Maiti, T.K. (2012). Wound pH-responsive sustained release of therapeutics from a poly(NIPAAm-co-AAc) hydrogel. *J. Biomater. Sci. Polym. Ed., 23*(1-4), 111-132. [http://dx.doi.org/10.1163/092050610X545049] [PMID: 22133349]

Bawa, P., Pillay, V., Choonara, Y.E., du Toit, L.C. (2009). Stimuli-responsive polymers and their applications in drug delivery. *Biomed. Mater., 4*(2), 022001. [http://dx.doi.org/10.1088/1748-6041/4/2/022001] [PMID: 19261988]

Boedtkjer, E., Pedersen, S.F. (2020). The acidic tumor microenvironment as a driver of cancer. *Annu. Rev. Physiol., 82*(1), 103-126. [http://dx.doi.org/10.1146/annurev-physiol-021119-034627] [PMID: 31730395]

Cao, Z., Li, W., Liu, R., Li, X., Li, H., Liu, L., Chen, Y., Lv, C., Liu, Y. (2019). pH- and enzyme-triggered drug release as an important process in the design of anti-tumor drug delivery systems. *Biomed. Pharmacother., 118*, 109340. [http://dx.doi.org/10.1016/j.biopha.2019.109340] [PMID: 31545284]

Chang, S., Wang, Y., Zhang, T., Pu, X., Zong, L., Zhu, H., Zhao, L., Feng, B. (2019). Redox-responsive

disulfide bond-bridged mPEG-PBLA prodrug micelles for enhanced paclitaxel biosafety and antitumor efficacy. *Front. Oncol., 9*, 823.
[http://dx.doi.org/10.3389/fonc.2019.00823] [PMID: 31508374]

Chang, Y., Yang, K., Wei, P., Huang, S., Pei, Y., Zhao, W., Pei, Z. (2014). Cationic vesicles based on amphiphilic pillar[5]arene capped with ferrocenium: a redox-responsive system for drug/siRNA co-delivery. *Angew. Chem. Int. Ed., 53*(48), 13126-13130.
[http://dx.doi.org/10.1002/anie.201407272] [PMID: 25267331]

Chen, H., Liu, D., Guo, Z. (2016). Endogenous stimuli-responsive nanocarriers for drug delivery. *Chem. Lett., 45*(3), 242-249.
[http://dx.doi.org/10.1246/cl.151176]

Chen, L., Zhou, X., Nie, W., Zhang, Q., Wang, W., Zhang, Y., He, C. (2016). Multifunctional redox-responsive mesoporous silica nanoparticles for efficient targeting drug delivery and magnetic resonance imaging. *ACS Appl. Mater. Interfaces, 8*(49), 33829-33841.
[http://dx.doi.org/10.1021/acsami.6b11802] [PMID: 27960384]

Cho, H., Bae, J., Garripelli, V.K., Anderson, J.M., Jun, H.W., Jo, S. (2012). Redox-sensitive polymeric nanoparticles for drug delivery. *Chem. Commun. (Camb.), 48*(48), 6043-6045.
[http://dx.doi.org/10.1039/c2cc31463k] [PMID: 22575892]

Cho, M.H., Choi, E.S., Kim, S., Goh, S.H., Choi, Y. (2017). Redox-responsive manganese dioxide nanoparticles for enhanced MR imaging and radiotherapy of lung cancer. *Front Chem., 5*, 109.
[http://dx.doi.org/10.3389/fchem.2017.00109] [PMID: 29255705]

Chuang, C.H., Wu, P.C., Tsai, T.H., Fang, Y.P., Tsai, Y.H., Cheng, T.C., Huang, C.C., Huang, M.Y., Chen, F.M., Hsieh, Y.C., Lin, W.W., Tsai, M.J., Cheng, T.L. (2017). Development of pH-sensitive cationic PEGylated solid lipid nanoparticles for selective cancer-targeted therapy. *J. Biomed. Nanotechnol., 13*(2), 192-203.
[http://dx.doi.org/10.1166/jbn.2017.2338] [PMID: 29377649]

Cicuéndez, M., Doadrio, J.C., Hernández, A., Portolés, M.T., Izquierdo-Barba, I., Vallet-Regí, M. (2018). Multifunctional pH sensitive 3D scaffolds for treatment and prevention of bone infection. *Acta Biomater., 65*, 450-461.
[http://dx.doi.org/10.1016/j.actbio.2017.11.009] [PMID: 29127064]

Das, S.S., Bharadwaj, P., Bilal, M., Barani, M., Rahdar, A., Taboada, P., Bungau, S., Kyzas, G.Z. (2020). Stimuli-responsive polymeric nanocarriers for drug delivery, imaging, and theragnosis. *Polymers (Basel), 12*(6), 1397.
[http://dx.doi.org/10.3390/polym12061397] [PMID: 32580366]

de la Rica, R., Aili, D., Stevens, M.M. (2012). Enzyme-responsive nanoparticles for drug release and diagnostics. *Adv. Drug Deliv. Rev., 64*(11), 967-978.
[http://dx.doi.org/10.1016/j.addr.2012.01.002] [PMID: 22266127]

Deen, G., Loh, X. (2018). Stimuli-responsive cationic hydrogels in drug delivery applications. *Gels, 4*(1), 13.
[http://dx.doi.org/10.3390/gels4010013] [PMID: 30674789]

Deirram, N., Zhang, C., Kermaniyan, S.S., Johnston, A.P.R., Such, G.K. (2019). pH-responsive polymer nanoparticles for drug delivery. *Macromol. Rapid Commun., 40*(10), 1800917.
[http://dx.doi.org/10.1002/marc.201800917] [PMID: 30835923]

Duncan, B., Kim, C., Rotello, V.M. (2010). Gold nanoparticle platforms as drug and biomacromolecule delivery systems. *J. Control. Release, 148*(1), 122-127.
[http://dx.doi.org/10.1016/j.jconrel.2010.06.004] [PMID: 20547192]

Ensign, L.M., Cone, R., Hanes, J. (2012). Oral drug delivery with polymeric nanoparticles: The gastrointestinal mucus barriers. *Adv. Drug Deliv. Rev., 64*(6), 557-570.
[http://dx.doi.org/10.1016/j.addr.2011.12.009] [PMID: 22212900]

Farshbaf, M., Davaran, S., Zarebkohan, A., Annabi, N., Akbarzadeh, A., Salehi, R. (2018). Significant role of

cationic polymers in drug delivery systems. *Artif. Cells Nanomed. Biotechnol., 46*(8), 1872-1891.
[PMID: 29103306]

Feng, X., Li, D., Han, J., Zhuang, X., Ding, J. (2017). Schiff base bond-linked polysaccharide–doxorubicin conjugate for upregulated cancer therapy. *Mater. Sci. Eng. C, 76*, 1121-1128.
[http://dx.doi.org/10.1016/j.msec.2017.03.201] [PMID: 28482476]

Fouladi, F., Steffen, K.J., Mallik, S. (2017). Enzyme-responsive liposomes for the delivery of anticancer drugs. *Bioconjug. Chem., 28*(4), 857-868.
[http://dx.doi.org/10.1021/acs.bioconjchem.6b00736] [PMID: 28201868]

Gao, F., Xiong, Z. (2021). Reactive oxygen species responsive polymers for drug delivery systems. *Front Chem., 9*, 649048.
[http://dx.doi.org/10.3389/fchem.2021.649048] [PMID: 33968898]

Goldbart, R., Traitel, T., Lapidot, S.A., Kost, J. (2002). Enzymatically controlled responsive drug delivery systems. *Polym. Adv. Technol., 13*(10-12), 1006-1018.
[http://dx.doi.org/10.1002/pat.275]

Gondi, C.S., Rao, J.S. (2013). Cathepsin B as a cancer target. *Expert Opin. Ther. Targets, 17*(3), 281-291.
[http://dx.doi.org/10.1517/14728222.2013.740461] [PMID: 23293836]

Gong, C., Shan, M., Li, B., Wu, G. (2016). A pH and redox dual stimuli-responsive poly(amino acid) derivative for controlled drug release. *Colloids Surf. B Biointerfaces, 146*, 396-405.
[http://dx.doi.org/10.1016/j.colsurfb.2016.06.038] [PMID: 27388968]

Gong, C., Shan, M., Li, B., Wu, G. (2017). Injectable dual redox responsive diselenide-containing poly(ethylene glycol) hydrogel. *J. Biomed. Mater. Res. A, 105*(9), 2451-2460.
[http://dx.doi.org/10.1002/jbm.a.36103] [PMID: 28481038]

Gooneh-Farahani, S., Naghib, S.M., Naimi-Jamal, M.R. (2020). A novel and inexpensive method based on modified ionic gelation for pH-responsive controlled drug release of homogeneously distributed chitosan nanoparticles with a high encapsulation efficiency. *Fibers Polym., 21*(9), 1917-1926.
[http://dx.doi.org/10.1007/s12221-020-1095-y]

Gooneh-Farahani, S., Naimi-Jamal, M.R., Naghib, S.M. (2019). Stimuli-responsive graphene-incorporated multifunctional chitosan for drug delivery applications: a review. *Expert Opin. Drug Deliv., 16*(1), 79-99.
[http://dx.doi.org/10.1080/17425247.2019.1556257] [PMID: 30514124]

Gu, Z., Aimetti, A.A., Wang, Q., Dang, T.T., Zhang, Y., Veiseh, O., Cheng, H., Langer, R.S., Anderson, D.G. (2013). Injectable nano-network for glucose-mediated insulin delivery. *ACS Nano, 7*(5), 4194-4201.
[http://dx.doi.org/10.1021/nn400630x] [PMID: 23638642]

Guo, D., Huang, Y., Jin, X., Zhang, C., Zhu, X. (2021). A Redox-Responsive, *In-situ* polymerized polyplatinum (IV)-coated gold nanorod as an amplifier of tumor accumulation for enhanced thermo-chemotherapy. *Biomaterials, 266*, 120400.
[http://dx.doi.org/10.1016/j.biomaterials.2020.120400] [PMID: 33022477]

Guo, H., Tan, S., Gao, J., Wang, L. (2020). Sequential release of drugs form a dual-delivery system based on pH-responsive nanofibrous mats towards wound care. *J. Mater. Chem. B Mater. Biol. Med., 8*(8), 1759-1770.
[http://dx.doi.org/10.1039/C9TB02522G] [PMID: 32037408]

Guo, X., Cheng, Y., Zhao, X., Luo, Y., Chen, J., Yuan, W.E. (2018). Advances in redox-responsive drug delivery systems of tumor microenvironment. *J. Nanobiotechnology, 16*(1), 74.
[http://dx.doi.org/10.1186/s12951-018-0398-2] [PMID: 30243297]

Guo, X., Wang, L., Wei, X., Zhou, S. (2016). Polymer-based drug delivery systems for cancer treatment. *J. Polym. Sci. A Polym. Chem., 54*(22), 3525-3550.
[http://dx.doi.org/10.1002/pola.28252]

Gupta, M.K., Meyer, T.A., Nelson, C.E., Duvall, C.L. (2012). Poly(PS-b-DMA) micelles for reactive oxygen species triggered drug release. *J. Control. Release, 162*(3), 591-598.

[http://dx.doi.org/10.1016/j.jconrel.2012.07.042] [PMID: 22889714]

Gupta, P., Vermani, K., Garg, S. (2002). Hydrogels: from controlled release to pH-responsive drug delivery. *Drug Discov. Today, 7*(10), 569-579.
[http://dx.doi.org/10.1016/S1359-6446(02)02255-9] [PMID: 12047857]

Herlem, G., Picaud, F., Girardet, C., Micheau, O. (2019). Carbon nanotubes: synthesis, characterization, and applications in drug-delivery systems. *Nanocarriers for drug delivery,* 469-529.

Hu, Q., Katti, P.S., Gu, Z. (2014). Enzyme-responsive nanomaterials for controlled drug delivery. *Nanoscale, 6*(21), 12273-12286.
[http://dx.doi.org/10.1039/C4NR04249B] [PMID: 25251024]

Huo, M., Yuan, J., Tao, L., Wei, Y. (2014). Redox-responsive polymers for drug delivery: from molecular design to applications. *Polym. Chem., 5*(5), 1519-1528.
[http://dx.doi.org/10.1039/C3PY01192E]

Zeinali Kalkhoran, A.H., Naghib, S.M., Vahidi, O., Rahmanian, M. (2018). Synthesis and characterization of graphene-grafted gelatin nanocomposite hydrogels as emerging drug delivery systems. *Biomed. Phys. Eng. Express, 4*(5), 055017.
[http://dx.doi.org/10.1088/2057-1976/aad745]

Zeinali Kalkhoran, A.H., Vahidi, O., Naghib, S.M. (2018). A new mathematical approach to predict the actual drug release from hydrogels. *Eur. J. Pharm. Sci., 111*, 303-310.
[http://dx.doi.org/10.1016/j.ejps.2017.09.038] [PMID: 28962856]

Kamaly, N., Yameen, B., Wu, J., Farokhzad, O.C. (2016). Degradable controlled-release polymers and polymeric nanoparticles: mechanisms of controlling drug release. *Chem. Rev., 116*(4), 2602-2663.
[http://dx.doi.org/10.1021/acs.chemrev.5b00346] [PMID: 26854975]

Kanamala, M., Wilson, W.R., Yang, M., Palmer, B.D., Wu, Z. (2016). Mechanisms and biomaterials in pH-responsive tumour targeted drug delivery: A review. *Biomaterials, 85*, 152-167.
[http://dx.doi.org/10.1016/j.biomaterials.2016.01.061] [PMID: 26871891]

Karimi, M., Eslami, M., Sahandi-Zangabad, P., Mirab, F., Farajisafiloo, N., Shafaei, Z., Ghosh, D., Bozorgomid, M., Dashkhaneh, F., Hamblin, M.R. (2016). PH -Sensitive stimulus-responsive nanocarriers for targeted delivery of therapeutic agents. *Wiley Interdiscip. Rev. Nanomed. Nanobiotechnol., 8*(5), 696-716.
[http://dx.doi.org/10.1002/wnan.1389] [PMID: 26762467]

Moradi Kashkooli, F., Soltani, M., Souri, M. (2020). Controlled anti-cancer drug release through advanced nano-drug delivery systems: Static and dynamic targeting strategies. *J. Control. Release, 327*, 316-349.
[http://dx.doi.org/10.1016/j.jconrel.2020.08.012] [PMID: 32800878]

Kazemi, F., Naghib, S.M. (2020). *Smart controlled release of corrosion inhibitor from normal and stimuli-responsive micro/nanocarriers.. Corrosion Protection at the Nanoscale..* Elsevier.

Kim, S., Chen, Y., Ho, E.A., Liu, S. (2017). Reversibly pH-responsive polyurethane membranes for on-demand intravaginal drug delivery. *Acta Biomater., 47*, 100-112.
[http://dx.doi.org/10.1016/j.actbio.2016.10.006] [PMID: 27717914]

Kim, S., Traore, Y.L., Ho, E.A., Shafiq, M., Kim, S.H., Liu, S. (2018). Design and development of pH-responsive polyurethane membranes for intravaginal release of nanomedicines. *Acta Biomater., 82*, 12-23.
[http://dx.doi.org/10.1016/j.actbio.2018.10.003] [PMID: 30296620]

Kuang, T., Liu, Y., Gong, T., Peng, X., Hu, X., Yu, Z. (2015). Enzyme-responsive nanoparticles for anticancer drug delivery. *Curr. Nanosci., 12*(1), 38-46.
[http://dx.doi.org/10.2174/1573413711666150624170518]

Kumar, P., Liu, B., Behl, G. (2019). A Comprehensive Outlook of Synthetic Strategies and Applications of Redox-Responsive Nanogels in Drug Delivery. *Macromol. Biosci., 19*(8), 1900071.
[http://dx.doi.org/10.1002/mabi.201900071] [PMID: 31298803]

Le, C.M.Q., Thi, H.H.P., Cao, X.T., Kim, G.D., Oh, C.W., Lim, K.T. (2016). Redox-responsive core cross-

linked micelles of poly(ethylene oxide)- *b* -poly(furfuryl methacrylate) by Diels-Alder reaction for doxorubicin release. *J. Polym. Sci. A Polym. Chem.,* *54*(23), 3741-3750.
[http://dx.doi.org/10.1002/pola.28271]

Lee, E.S., Na, K., Bae, Y.H. (2005). Super pH-sensitive multifunctional polymeric micelle. *Nano Lett., 5*(2), 325-329.
[http://dx.doi.org/10.1021/nl0479987] [PMID: 15794620]

Li, R., Peng, F., Cai, J., Yang, D., Zhang, P. (2020). Redox dual-stimuli responsive drug delivery systems for improving tumor-targeting ability and reducing adverse side effects. *Asian journal of Pharmaceutical Sciences, 15*, 311-325.

Li, Z., Huang, J., Wu, J. (2020). pH-Sensitive nanogels for drug delivery in cancer therapy. *Biomater. Sci.*
[PMID: 33306076]

Liang, J., Liu, B. (2016). ROS-responsive drug delivery systems. *Bioeng. Transl. Med., 1*(3), 239-251.
[http://dx.doi.org/10.1002/btm2.10014] [PMID: 29313015]

Liang, K., Richardson, J.J., Ejima, H., Such, G.K., Cui, J., Caruso, F. (2014). Peptide-tunable drug cytotoxicity *via* one-step assembled polymer nanoparticles. *Adv. Mater., 26*(15), 2398-2402.
[http://dx.doi.org/10.1002/adma.201305002] [PMID: 24375889]

Lin, J.T., Du, J.K., Yang, Y.Q., Li, L., Zhang, D.W., Liang, C.L., Wang, J., Mei, J., Wang, G.H. (2017). pH and redox dual stimulate-responsive nanocarriers based on hyaluronic acid coated mesoporous silica for targeted drug delivery. *Mater. Sci. Eng. C, 81*, 478-484.
[http://dx.doi.org/10.1016/j.msec.2017.08.036] [PMID: 28888000]

Lin, Y.H., Chang, C.H., Wu, Y.S., Hsu, Y.M., Chiou, S.F., Chen, Y.J. (2009). Development of pH-responsive chitosan/heparin nanoparticles for stomach-specific anti-Helicobacter pylori therapy. *Biomaterials, 30*(19), 3332-3342.
[http://dx.doi.org/10.1016/j.biomaterials.2009.02.036] [PMID: 19299008]

Liu, B., Chen, H., Li, X., Zhao, C., Liu, Y., Zhu, L., Deng, H., Li, J., Li, G., Guo, F., Zhu, X. (2014). pH-responsive flower-like micelles constructed *via* oxime linkage for anticancer drug delivery. *RSC Advances, 4*(90), 48943-48951.
[http://dx.doi.org/10.1039/C4RA08719D]

Liu, J., Huang, Y., Kumar, A., Tan, A., Jin, S., Mozhi, A., Liang, X.J. (2014). pH-Sensitive nano-systems for drug delivery in cancer therapy. *Biotechnol. Adv., 32*(4), 693-710.
[http://dx.doi.org/10.1016/j.biotechadv.2013.11.009] [PMID: 24309541]

Liu, J., Zhang, B., Luo, Z., Ding, X., Li, J., Dai, L., Zhou, J., Zhao, X., Ye, J., Cai, K. (2015). Enzyme responsive mesoporous silica nanoparticles for targeted tumor therapy *in vitro* and *in vivo*. *Nanoscale, 7*(8), 3614-3626.
[http://dx.doi.org/10.1039/C5NR00072F] [PMID: 25633047]

Liu, L., Yao, W., Rao, Y., Lu, X., Gao, J. (2017). pH-Responsive carriers for oral drug delivery: challenges and opportunities of current platforms. *Drug Deliv., 24*(1), 569-581.
[http://dx.doi.org/10.1080/10717544.2017.1279238] [PMID: 28195032]

Lu, Y., Aimetti, A.A., Langer, R., Gu, Z. (2016). Bioresponsive materials. *Nat. Rev. Mater., 2*, 1-17.

Ma, N., Li, Y., Ren, H., Xu, H., Li, Z., Zhang, X. (2010). Selenium-containing block copolymers and their oxidation-responsive aggregates. *Polym. Chem., 1*(10), 1609-1614.
[http://dx.doi.org/10.1039/c0py00144a]

Majumder, J., Minko, T. (2021). Multifunctional and stimuli-responsive nanocarriers for targeted therapeutic delivery. *Expert Opin. Drug Deliv., 18*(2), 205-227.
[http://dx.doi.org/10.1080/17425247.2021.1828339] [PMID: 32969740]

Mehta, P.P., Pawar, V.S. (2018). Electrospun nanofiber scaffolds: technology and applications. *Applications of nanocomposite materials in drug delivery..* Elsevier.

[http://dx.doi.org/10.1016/B978-0-12-813741-3.00023-6]

Melendez-Ortiz, H.I., Varca, G., Zavala-Lagunes, E., Bucio, E. (2016). *State of the art of smart polymers: From fundamentals to final applications. Polymer Science: Research Advances, Practical Applications and Educational Aspects.* (pp. 476-487). Badajoz, Spain: Formatex Research Center.

Mi, P. (2020). Stimuli-responsive nanocarriers for drug delivery, tumor imaging, therapy and theranostics. *Theranostics, 10*(10), 4557-4588.
[http://dx.doi.org/10.7150/thno.38069] [PMID: 32292515]

Mirhadi, E., Mashreghi, M., Faal Maleki, M., Alavizadeh, S.H., Arabi, L., Badiee, A., Jaafari, M.R. (2020). Redox-sensitive nanoscale drug delivery systems for cancer treatment. *Int. J. Pharm., 589*, 119882.
[http://dx.doi.org/10.1016/j.ijpharm.2020.119882] [PMID: 32941986]

Mock, J.N., Costyn, L.J., Wilding, S.L., Arnold, R.D., Cummings, B.S. (2013). Evidence for distinct mechanisms of uptake and antitumor activity of secretory phospholipase A2 responsive liposome in prostate cancer. *Integr. Biol., 5*(1), 172-182.
[http://dx.doi.org/10.1039/c2ib20108a] [PMID: 22890797]

Mohammadzadeh, R., Javadzadeh, Y. (2018). An overview on oral drug delivery *via* nano-based formulations. *Pharmaceutical and Biomedical Research, 4*, 1-7.
[http://dx.doi.org/10.18502/pbr.v4i1.139]

Mollazadeh, S., Mackiewicz, M., Yazdimamaghani, M. (2021). Recent advances in the redox-responsive drug delivery nanoplatforms: A chemical structure and physical property perspective. *Mater. Sci. Eng. C, 118*, 111536.
[http://dx.doi.org/10.1016/j.msec.2020.111536] [PMID: 33255089]

Monteiro, P.F., Travanut, A., Conte, C., Alexander, C. (2021). Reduction-responsive polymers for drug delivery in cancer therapy—Is there anything new to discover? *Wiley Interdiscip. Rev. Nanomed. Nanobiotechnol., 13*(2), e1678.
[http://dx.doi.org/10.1002/wnan.1678] [PMID: 33155421]

Muhammad, F., Wang, A., Miao, L., Wang, P., Li, Q., Liu, J., Du, J., Zhu, G. (2015). Synthesis of oxidant prone nanosilver to develop H_2O_2 responsive drug delivery system. *Langmuir, 31*(1), 514-521.
[http://dx.doi.org/10.1021/la503922j] [PMID: 25486873]

Mumtaz Virk, M., Reimhult, E. (2018). Phospholipase A2-induced degradation and release from lipid-containing polymersomes. *Langmuir, 34*(1), 395-405.
[http://dx.doi.org/10.1021/acs.langmuir.7b03893] [PMID: 29231739]

Municoy, S., Álvarez Echazú, M.I., Antezana, P.E., Galdopórpora, J.M., Olivetti, C., Mebert, A.M., Foglia, M.L., Tuttolomondo, M.V., Alvarez, G.S., Hardy, J.G., Desimone, M.F. (2020). Stimuli-Responsive Materials for Tissue Engineering and Drug Delivery. *Int. J. Mol. Sci., 21*(13), 4724.
[http://dx.doi.org/10.3390/ijms21134724] [PMID: 32630690]

Mura, S., Nicolas, J., Couvreur, P. (2013). Stimuli-responsive nanocarriers for drug delivery. *Nat. Mater., 12*(11), 991-1003.
[http://dx.doi.org/10.1038/nmat3776] [PMID: 24150417]

Naghib, S.M., Zare, Y., Rhee, K.Y. (2020). A facile and simple approach to synthesis and characterization of methacrylated graphene oxide nanostructured polyaniline nanocomposites. *Nanotechnol. Rev., 9*(1), 53-60.
[http://dx.doi.org/10.1515/ntrev-2020-0005]

Pham, S.H., Choi, Y., Choi, J. (2020). Stimuli-Responsive Nanomaterials for Application in Antitumor Therapy and Drug Delivery. *Pharmaceutics, 12*(7), 630.
[http://dx.doi.org/10.3390/pharmaceutics12070630] [PMID: 32635539]

Phillips, D.J., Gibson, M.I. (2014). Redox-sensitive materials for drug delivery: targeting the correct intracellular environment, tuning release rates, and appropriate predictive systems. *Antioxid. Redox Signal., 21*(5), 786-803.
[http://dx.doi.org/10.1089/ars.2013.5728] [PMID: 24219144]

Rahmanian, M., seyfoori, A., Dehghan, M.M., Eini, L., Naghib, S.M., Gholami, H., Farzad Mohajeri, S., Mamaghani, K.R., Majidzadeh-A, K. (2019). Multifunctional gelatin–tricalcium phosphate porous nanocomposite scaffolds for tissue engineering and local drug delivery: *In vitro* and *in vivo* studies. *J. Taiwan Inst. Chem. Eng., 101*, 214-220.
[http://dx.doi.org/10.1016/j.jtice.2019.04.028]

Sang, Q., Li, H., Williams, G., Wu, H., Zhu, L.M. (2018). Core-shell poly(lactide-co-ε-caprolactone)-gelatin fiber scaffolds as pH-sensitive drug delivery systems. *J. Biomater. Appl., 32*(8), 1105-1118.
[http://dx.doi.org/10.1177/0885328217749962] [PMID: 29295656]

Saravanakumar, G., Kim, J., Kim, W.J. (2017). Reactive-oxygen-species-responsive drug delivery systems: promises and challenges. *Adv. Sci. (Weinh.), 4*(1), 1600124.
[http://dx.doi.org/10.1002/advs.201600124] [PMID: 28105390]

Seetharaman, G., Kallar, A.R., Vijayan, V.M., Muthu, J., Selvam, S. (2017). Design, preparation and characterization of pH-responsive prodrug micelles with hydrolyzable anhydride linkages for controlled drug delivery. *J. Colloid Interface Sci., 492*, 61-72.
[http://dx.doi.org/10.1016/j.jcis.2016.12.070] [PMID: 28068545]

Shahriari, M., Zahiri, M., Abnous, K., Taghdisi, S.M., Ramezani, M., Alibolandi, M. (2019). Enzyme responsive drug delivery systems in cancer treatment. *J. Control. Release, 308*, 172-189.
[http://dx.doi.org/10.1016/j.jconrel.2019.07.004] [PMID: 31295542]

Shen, Y., Tang, H., Radosz, M., Van Kirk, E., Murdoch, W.J. (2008). pH-responsive nanoparticles for cancer drug delivery. *Methods Mol. Biol., 437*, 183-216.
[http://dx.doi.org/10.1007/978-1-59745-210-6_10] [PMID: 18369970]

Sood, N., Bhardwaj, A., Mehta, S., Mehta, A. (2016). Stimuli-responsive hydrogels in drug delivery and tissue engineering. *Drug Deliv., 23*(3), 748-770.
[http://dx.doi.org/10.3109/10717544.2014.940091] [PMID: 25045782]

Sun, J., Wang, Z., Cao, A., Sheng, R. (2019). Synthesis of crosslinkable diblock terpolymers PDPA- *b* - P(NMS- *co* -OEG) and preparation of shell-crosslinked pH/redox-dual responsive micelles as smart nanomaterials. *RSC Advances, 9*(59), 34535-34546.
[http://dx.doi.org/10.1039/C9RA05082E] [PMID: 35529956]

Tang, M., Zhou, M., Huang, Y., Zhong, J., Zhou, Z., Luo, K. (2017). Dual-sensitive and biodegradable core-crosslinked HPMA copolymer–doxorubicin conjugate-based nanoparticles for cancer therapy. *Polym. Chem., 8*(15), 2370-2380.
[http://dx.doi.org/10.1039/C7PY00348J]

Torchilin, V. P. (2018). CHAPTER 1: Fundamentals of Stimuli-responsive Drug and Gene Delivery Systems. *Stimuli-responsive Drug Delivery Systems., 1-32.
[http://dx.doi.org/10.1039/9781788013536-00001]

Wen, H., Li, Y., Zhao, X. (2015). *Redox-Sensitive Polymeric Nanoparticles for Intracellular Drug Delivery.. Bio-Inspired Nanomaterials and Applications: Nano Detection, Drug/Gene Delivery, Medical Diagnosis and Therapy..* World Scientific.

Wu, G., Fang, Y.Z., Yang, S., Lupton, J.R., Turner, N.D. (2004). Glutathione metabolism and its implications for health. *J. Nutr., 134*(3), 489-492.
[http://dx.doi.org/10.1093/jn/134.3.489] [PMID: 14988435]

Xu, X., Saw, P.E., Tao, W., Li, Y., Ji, X., Bhasin, S., Liu, Y., Ayyash, D., Rasmussen, J., Huo, M., Shi, J., Farokhzad, O.C. (2017). ROS-responsive polyprodrug nanoparticles for triggered drug delivery and effective cancer therapy. *Adv. Mater., 29*(33), 1700141.
[http://dx.doi.org/10.1002/adma.201700141] [PMID: 28681981]

Yin, T., Wang, Y., Chu, X., Fu, Y., Wang, L., Zhou, J., Tang, X., Liu, J., Huo, M. (2018). Free adriamycin-loaded pH/reduction dual-responsive hyaluronic acid–adriamycin prodrug micelles for efficient cancer therapy. *ACS Appl. Mater. Interfaces, 10*(42), 35693-35704.

[http://dx.doi.org/10.1021/acsami.8b09342] [PMID: 30259743]

Yoshida, T., Lai, T.C., Kwon, G.S., Sako, K. (2013). pH- and ion-sensitive polymers for drug delivery. *Expert Opin. Drug Deliv., 10*(11), 1497-1513.
[http://dx.doi.org/10.1517/17425247.2013.821978] [PMID: 23930949]

Zhai, S., Hu, X., Hu, Y., Wu, B., Xing, D. (2017). Visible light-induced crosslinking and physiological stabilization of diselenide-rich nanoparticles for redox-responsive drug release and combination chemotherapy. *Biomaterials, 121*, 41-54.
[http://dx.doi.org/10.1016/j.biomaterials.2017.01.002] [PMID: 28068593]

Zhang, J., Sun, Y., Tian, B., Li, K., Wang, L., Liang, Y., Han, J. (2016). Multifunctional mesoporous silica nanoparticles modified with tumor-shedable hyaluronic acid as carriers for doxorubicin. *Colloids Surf. B Biointerfaces, 144*, 293-302.
[http://dx.doi.org/10.1016/j.colsurfb.2016.04.015] [PMID: 27107383]

Zhang, P., Zhang, H., He, W., Zhao, D., Song, A., Luan, Y. (2016). Disulfide-linked amphiphilic polymer-docetaxel conjugates assembled redox-sensitive micelles for efficient antitumor drug delivery. *Biomacromolecules, 17*(5), 1621-1632.
[http://dx.doi.org/10.1021/acs.biomac.5b01758] [PMID: 27018501]

Zhao, C., Shao, L., Lu, J., Zhao, C., Wei, Y., Liu, J., Li, M., Wu, Y. (2017). Triple Redox Responsive Poly(Ethylene Glycol)-Polycaprolactone Polymeric Nanocarriers for Fine-Controlled Drug Release. *Macromol. Biosci., 17*(4), 1600295.
[http://dx.doi.org/10.1002/mabi.201600295] [PMID: 27762492]

Zhao, S., Xu, M., Cao, C., Yu, Q., Zhou, Y., Liu, J. (2017). A redox-responsive strategy using mesoporous silica nanoparticles for co-delivery of siRNA and doxorubicin. *J. Mater. Chem. B Mater. Biol. Med., 5*(33), 6908-6919.
[http://dx.doi.org/10.1039/C7TB00613F] [PMID: 32264340]

Zhuo, S., Zhang, F., Yu, J., Zhang, X., Yang, G., Liu, X. (2020). pH-Sensitive Biomaterials for Drug Delivery. *Molecules, 25*(23), 5649.
[http://dx.doi.org/10.3390/molecules25235649] [PMID: 33266162]

CHAPTER 8

Nanoparticles-mediated Localized Controlled Drug Delivery Systems (LCDDSs)

Abstract: Nanoparticles (NPs) and nanostructures can facilitate multianalyte detection, imaging and selective targeting of therapeutic molecules to cancer cells. This method increases the drug dose and maximizes at the anticipated location, and the healthy cells/tissues and their environments are protected simultaneously. To develop the targeting potential of therapeutic molecules, the surface and size characteristics of NPs should be improved, thereby enhancing their targeting effectiveness and circulation time. Here, we have highlighted recent advances and progress in smart stimuli-sensitive nanocarriers synthesized to improve the efficiency and localization of drugs compared to unmodified drugs. Multifunctional NPs could enhance the controlled release and targeting ability of drugs/therapeutic agents/biomolecules. The smart multifunctionality establishes versatile NPs, moreover, localized controlled drug delivery systems (LCDDSs) are promising and considerably increase the efficiency of therapy and diagnosis (theranosis) in pharmaceutical and biomedical science/engineering.

Keywords: Cytotoxicity, Biocompatibility, Nanoparticles, Nanocarriers, Localized drug delivery, Triggered delivery.

8.1. INTRODUCTION

As mentioned in the previous chapters, one of the considerable challenges in typical drug delivery systems is to deliver the desired drug concentration at the specific organ, meanwhile reducing side effects, and preventing drug inefficiency. This negative aspect is a sensitive challenge, especially in tumor therapy, as cancer tissue can locally establish individual metastasis in numerous organs (Gooneh-Farahani *et al.*, 2020, Gooneh-Farahani *et al.*, 2019). The non-localized cytotoxicity effects of chemotherapeutic agents on both normal and cancerous cells limit the potential of chemotherapy. So local delivery systems and targeted drug delivery have been developed to release the drug at the target site in its therapeutic concentration with reduced local toxicity (De Jong and Borm, 2008, Askari *et al.*, 2021, Rahmanian *et al.*, 2019). Drug-loaded micro/nanoparticles may be exploited as drug/gene carriers for local/targeted delivery system, to reduce the degradation of the drug and the side effect, control the drug release profile, and increase patient compliance (Mandracchia and Tripodo, 2020, Sartipzadeh *et al.*, 2020, Kazemi and Naghib, 2020, Naghib and Kazemi, 2020). In general, the use of larger particles has inherent disadvantages such as poor bioavailability, poor absorption in the body, *in vivo* instability, and poor solubility. As well as the aforesaid challenges of macroscaled delivery systems, their ability to target the drugs in a specific site/cell and optimum effectiveness is still challenging (Patra *et al.*, 2018a). On the other hand, particles with larger sizes exhibit longer durations of nerve blockade because of numerous factors, such as longer time to degrade the carrier and release the therapeutic molecule, the potential for higher drug loading, and differences in clearance from tissues (Kohane, 2007). Using new delivery devices with specific and targeted drug release to the site of disease could be an opportunity that might solve these mentioned problems. In the past few decades, the development of nanoscale devices has represented a revolution in disease diagnosis and treatment (Singh and Lillard Jr, 2009).

Designing NPs as vehicles has been explored during the last 20 years for the purposes of drug delivery and modifying the therapeutic effect of the drugs. There are numerous types of nanostructures, including metallic NPs, polymeric core-shells, and micelles, that have been widely explored, especially in cancer therapy. (Latorre *et al.*, 2014). A nanoparticle is commonly defined as a solid colloidal particle that is between 1 and 100 nm in diameter. NPs can be used as drug vehicles for entrapping active drugs such as therapeutic agents or biologically active material. In this context, NPs can be functionalized by targeting moieties and binding to the desired target cells (Sung *et al.*, 2007).

The unique properties of NPs make them a good candidate for biomedical purposes. These features include their small size, which allows them to penetrate cell membranes and escape the endosome/lysosome system, a large surface that allows the attachment of many classes of therapeutic agents such as drugs, probes and proteins, and modulate drug release. Accordingly, nanoparticles may be used for the triggered release of drugs at the disease site and deliver several therapeutic agents simultaneously. Besides, NPs can move freely in the body environment in comparison with larger particles, which enhances the spatiotemporally controlled delivery of therapeutic agents (De Jong and Borm, 2008). Due to the unique features of NPs, they can lead to localized delivery and improve the pharmacokinetic profile of drugs (Gao *et al.*, 2018). Nanoscale formulations can attain therapeutic effects and minimize systemic side effects by using lower doses of the drug (Valente *et al.*, 2017). An NP-based localized delivery system usually requires bonding and protecting active drugs, biocompatibility, biodegradation, colloidal stability, and controlled-release kinetics (Adair *et al.*, 2010). The most widely used class of nanomaterials in the biomedical field include metallic NPs such as gold NPs, magnetic NPs, carbon nanotubes, graphene, polymeric micelles, liposomes and quantum dots. The exploitation of these NPs considerably enhances the drug efficiency and therapeutic results (Kong *et al.*, 2017, Seyfoori *et al.*, 2019, Kalkhoran *et al.*, 2018b, Kalkhoran *et al.*, 2018a). Numerous studies extensively discussed the drug release mechanisms in nano vehicles, including diffusion, solvent, chemical reaction, and stimuli-controlled release (Fig. **1**) (Patra *et al.*, 2018b).

Bottom-up and top-down techniques in nanotechnology offer novel paths for the generation of multi-functional local delivery systems with different sizes and compositions. It will be highly beneficial if the treatment site is recognized. In this context, using smart nano-materials is the desired selection to develop the smart LCDDSs that have been most widely used for inducing drug release and decreasing unwanted release. However, designing smart delivery systems with reproducibility, great quality, reliability, and high efficiency is still challenging (Bennet and Kim, 2014).

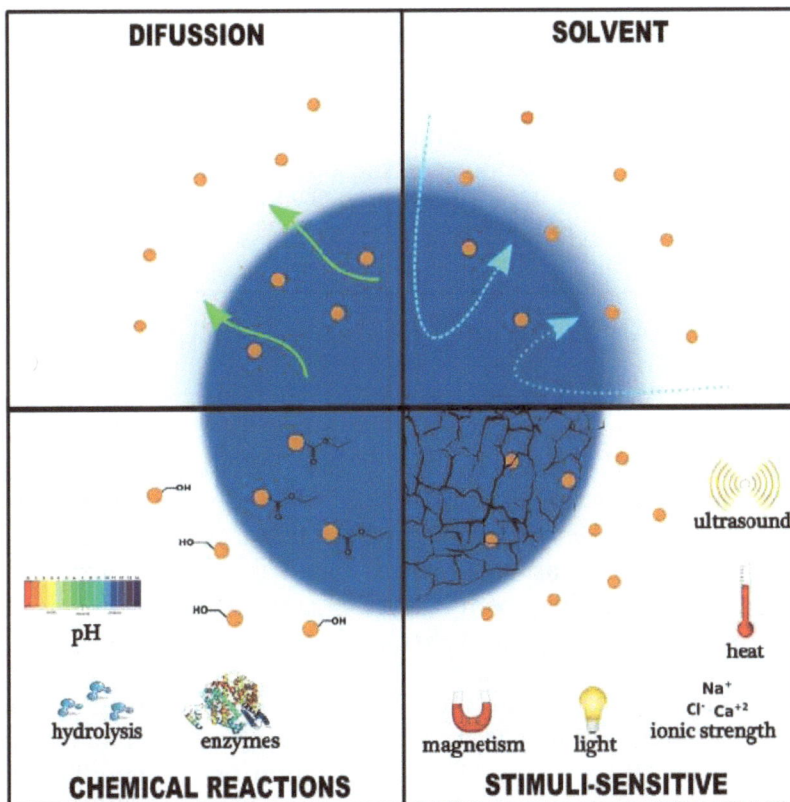

Fig. (1). The mechanisms of drug release using different types of nanocarriers (open access) (Patra *et al.*, 2018b).

So, in general, NP-based delivery carriers possess some important features to increase their efficiency and meet different tasks, such as (1) appropriate capacity and loading efficiency for loading sufficient therapeutic agents, (2) protection of drug bioactivity and good biocompatibility, (3) transfer of drugs to the targeted site at the appropriate time and less uptake by the normal tissue with the help of the NPs response to exogenous/endogenous stimulus, or by combining them with antibodies or targeting moieties that can bind them specifically to the diseased cells, (4) facile functionalization through reactive functional groups on the surface, in fact, NPs can be functionalized with organic agents (*e.g.*, lipid, polymer, and protein) or inorganic materials (*e.g.*, graphene oxide, silica, gold, and CNTs) as core materials, and (5) overcome the drug resistance (Dürr *et al.*, 2013, Huang *et al.*, 2016).

In contrast to the potential advantage of nanocarriers, there are also several concerns. First, all nano-based products need FDA approval for their safety, efficacy, quality, and environmental impact. Secondly, nanoscale formulations are very costly. Investigation costs alone are extraordinarily high, and advanced progresses are usually established by pharmaceutical corporations that cannot support themselves on current revenues (Emerich and Thanos, 2007).

In this chapter, we will focus on a range of NPs, including gold NPs, magnetic NPs, Calcium phosphate-based NPs, and mesoporous silica NPs that can be used as carriers for drug delivery. We will then discuss the mechanisms of drug release from the aforementioned NPs.

8.2. GOLD NANOPARTICLES IN TRIGGERED DRUG DELIVERY

In general, gold NPs (GNPs) exhibit unique chemical, physical, optical, and electronic properties and have been used in various fields, such as drug delivery applications (Ajnai *et al.*, 2014). Bulk gold and GNPs have different properties. For instance, bulk gold is a yellow solid, and it is inert in nature whilst GNPs are wine red solutions and are reported to be anti-oxidants. GNPs can be produced with various shapes, such as nanoprisms, nanotriangles, tetrahedral, irregular shape, multiple twined, icosahedral, decahedral, octahedral, sub-octahedral, nanorods, hexagonal platelets and spheres (Khan *et al.*, 2014).

GNPs are gaining interest as delivery systems due to their unique properties, including easy synthesis of their different shapes with a wide range of sizes from 1 nm to more than 100 nm, easy functionalization of GNPs with biomolecule moieties such as targeting ligands, drugs, and gene because of the existence of a negative charge on them, having macroscopic quantum tunneling effect, distinct surface effect, and the presence of surface plasmon resonance (SPR) bands. Based on all of these unique properties of GNPs, they have a significant potential for biomedical applications such as biosensors, imaging purposes, and drug delivery (Kong *et al.*, 2017). For instance, GNPs can be used as drug vehicles with high loading efficiency and the capacity to bind as many as 100 molecules onto the surface of a 2 nm gold core (Mishra *et al.*, 2013). Ghosh *et al.* demonstrated several applications and high potentials of GNPs in therapy (Ghosh *et al.*, 2008).

The conjugation of therapeutic drugs and targeting ligands to GNPs may enable specific interactions of GNPs with cells. The required motivation is delivering therapeutic agents to the target cells. Typically, targeted delivery systems are categorized into two main classes: 'active' and 'passive' targeting. The term 'passive targeting' has been defined as nanoparticle accumulation in diseased sites owing to the enhanced permeability and retention (EPR) effect. This phenomenon can lead to the deposition of therapeutic agents within target cells (Ajnai *et al.*, 2014). On the other hand, the term, 'active targeting' commonly refers to the nanoparticle that has been conjugated with targeting moieties to augment their homing toward desired target cells. It is noteworthy that surface modification and functionalization of the nanoparticle surface have a vital role in this kind of targeted delivery. In this context, therapeutic drugs or biomolecules can conjugate with GNPs *via* ionic or covalent bonding, or by physical absorption (Kong *et al.*, 2017). For instance GNPs can be conjugated with antibiotic agents during the synthesis process for bactericidal activity purposes (Saha *et al.*, 2007). In another study, Du *et al.* fabricated a targeted delivery system for neuroblastoma treatment. In this study, the research group functionalized the surface of GNPs with DNAs containing aptamer as a recognizer for the target protein on cancer cells. Uptake and intracellular localization of the GNP-DNA(Dox) were demonstrated in targeted human bone marrow neuroblastoma cells (Du *et al.*, 2014).

It is important to note the surface chemistry of NPs in the conjugation process. In other words, surface modification is a key parameter in developing NP-based drug delivery systems due to the binding to desired cells, preventing the aggregation of NPs and increasing the system stability, modifying the surface for decreasing cytotoxicity of NPs such as nanorods, and finally slowing the removal of the conjugate by the reticulo-endothelial system (RES) (Pissuwan *et al.*, 2011). For example, binding thiol terminated methoxypoly(ethylene glycol) to the surface of gold nanorods makes them stable in buffer solutions without a surfactant (Hafner and Liao, 2005).

There are numerous surface modification approaches for creating GNP-based delivery systems. The first is using a monolayer or bilayer of capping agents as a coating on GNP surface (Fig. **2a**). This approach may be used to separate hydrophobic agents from the aqueous environment. Another approach is producing a surface complex with reactive functional groups such as thiols or free amines in order to form Au–S or Au–N bonds (Fig. **2b**). A third strategy is creating drug attachment points on the GNP surface by using functional groups of capping agents resulting in drug-capping agent interactions (Fig. **2c**). Another approach is exploiting the electrostatic interactions between the capping agents on GNPs and payloads with opposite charges (Fig. **2d**). Finally, gold nanocages such as hollow structures have considerable potential as reservoirs. As shown in Fig. (**2e**), in this approach, temperature-responsive polymers which are disintegrated upon light irradiation can be used to release entrapped cargos due to the photo-thermal effect in GNPs (Fratoddi *et al.*, 2014, Jeong *et al.*, 2014).

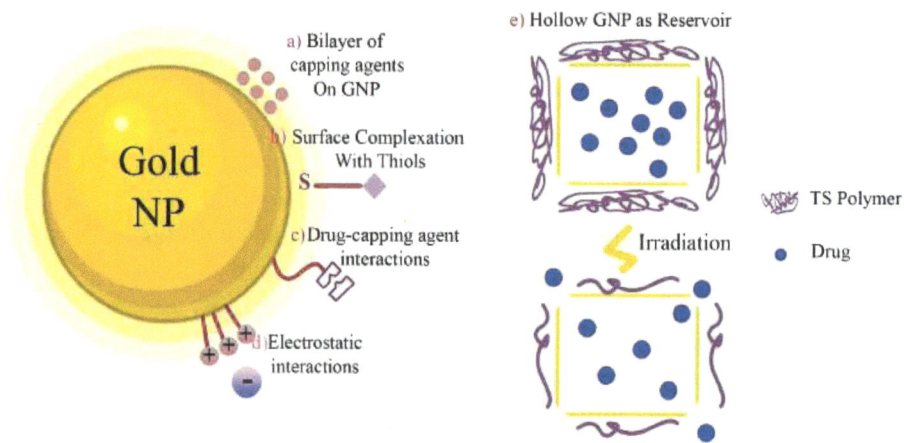

Fig. (2). Summary of the variety of approaches to loading and unloading therapeutic payloads into and from GNPs.

As mentioned before, GNPs can be used as smart delivery systems. In these systems, NPs can be designed to release the loaded drugs in response to endogenous biological stimuli, which are for diseased microenvironment (*e.g.,* glutathione (GSH), or pH) or exogenous stimuli which are manipulated from outside the body (*e.g.,* heat or light). The drug release mechanism of smart release systems has been previously discussed in Chapter 7 and 8. In this context, GNPs can be used as drug carriers for smart delivery systems due to their unique chemical and physical properties (Chen *et al.*, 2016, Raza *et al.*, 2019).

As mentioned before in Chapter 8, Glutathione (-glutamyl-cysteinyl-glycine; GSH) is a low-molecular-weight thiol. Glutathione (GSH)-mediated release systems represent a method in which therapeutic drugs can be released in a controlled manner. These systems are designed based on the big difference between intracellular GSH concentrations (2–10 mM) and extracellular concentrations (2-20 µM). In tumor cells, the GSH difference is four times higher than their counterparts in normal cells. Nano-carriers based on redox-sensitive components, such as disulfide linkages have been reported to take advantage of this method. In this regard, Disulfide-thiol exchange reactions can release prodrugs bound to the GNP. In fact, disulfide bonds can be easily broken down by reducing glutathione into sulfhydryl groups, and this phenomenon leads to the release of the loaded drugs (Duncan *et al.*, 2010, Han *et al.*, 2007a, Kamaly *et al.*, 2016, Wu *et al.*, 2004, Askari *et al.*, 2020, Guo *et al.*, 2018).

In this context, Hong *et al.* designed a GSH-responsive nanocarrier, using functionalized gold NPs with a mixed monolayer composed of tetra(ethylene glycol)ylated cationic ligands (TTMA), which facilitates the cellular uptake and thiolated Bodipy dye, HSBDP. In this system, the GSH is responsible for releasing BODIPY from the nanoparticle carrier due to the presence of thiol groups and place-exchange reaction (Fig. **3**) (Hong *et al.*, 2006).

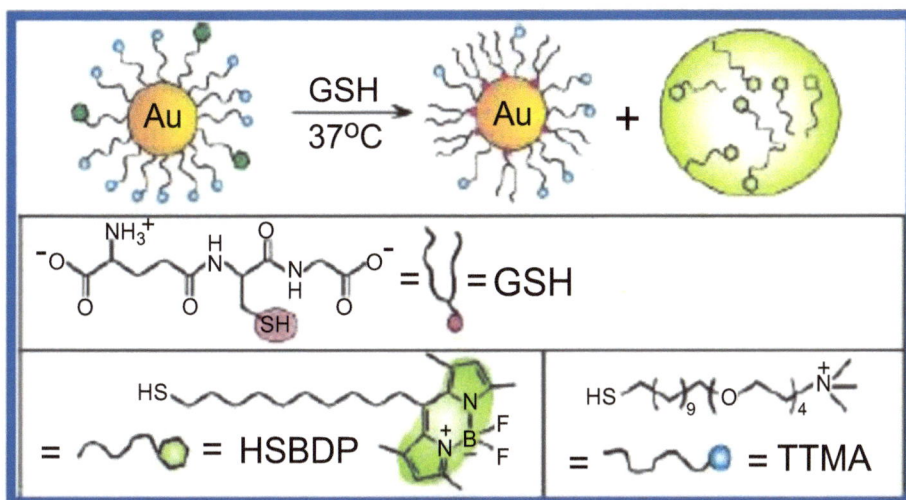

Fig. (3). Structure of the functionalized GNP carrier and GSH-mediated surface monolayer exchange reaction causes releasing a hydrophobic dye (Hong *et al.*, 2006).

Photochemical-induced releasing of payloads is another useful approach for developing GNP-based delivery systems. This mechanism represents numerous advantages, including great spatiotemporal control over drug release, noninvasive nature, and comfort of use (Linsley and Wu, 2017, Han *et al.*, 2007b). Photo-responsive polymers are composed of a photo-reactive moiety that converts the irradiation to a chemical signal through a photoreaction, such as isomerization, cleavage, and dimerization. These transformations control the shape, functionality, stiffness, and crosslinking degree of light-responsive materials (Tomatsu *et al.*, 2011). In this regard, light-induced anti-cancer 5- fluorouracil release from GNP was exploited. The functionalized GNPs with a mixed monolayer composed of photocleavable moieties and zwitterionic ligands have been used in this study. By using the zwitterionic ligand, it would be possible to achieve improved solubility and limited cellular uptake. Upon near-UV irradiation, with the wavelength of 365 nm, the 5-fluorouracil could be cleaved from the GNPs due to the photocleaving reaction of the orthonitrobenzyl group (Duncan *et al.*, 2010).

Plasmonic NPs have shown great potential in smart drug delivery applications, so it would be necessary to discuss plasmon, which is the basis of the photothermal effect. Metal-based NPs, such as GNPs with sizes smaller than the light wavelength, have a high localized surface plasmon that makes them excellent scatterers and absorbers of light at specific wavelengths and gives them their color. In this case, the electron oscillations induce an electric field around the nanoparticle that can be much larger than the incident light (Rivera *et al.*, 2012, García, 2011). Besides, the absorbed light produces local heating which is called the photothermal effect that can be used for selective treatment. There are four main methods that have been employed in designing photothermal-induced drug release of NPs: 1) the therapeutic agents can be loaded in a polymeric matrix and local heating upon irradiation will loosen the matrix, causing drug release; 2) the drugs and nanoparticles can be embedded in liposomes and local heating will break the liposomes, resulting in drug release; 3) covalent conjugation of drug to the heat-cleavable functional molecules which is bound to the NP, upon irradiation and local heating this bound will break, causing drug release, and 4) therapeutic dosages can be loaded in a matrix surrounding the particle and attached by noncovalent interactions, in this case, the local heating facilitates drug release (Guerrero *et al.*, 2014).

GNPs with various sizes and shapes display a great surface plasmon resonance and photothermal conducting property. This method offers excellent spatiotemporal control over the release of therapeutic agents (Poon *et al.*, 2010). In this regard, hollow gold nanospheres (HGNS) are a novel class of GNPs that can be widely used in biomedical applications such as delivery and imaging due to their unique properties such as high and adjustable absorption band (520–950 nm), and small diameter (30-50 nm) (You *et al.*, 2012). As an example, You *et al.* have embedded DOX onto HGNS coated with polyethylene glycol (PEG). This DOX@PEG-HGNS system demonstrated rapid DOX release upon laser irradiation (You *et al.*, 2010). The generated heat upon light irradiation can be used as a stimulus to trigger the release of drugs from thermo-responsive polymers. In this context, Ou *et al.* designed a delivery system for triple-negative breast cancer treatment. They combined PEG-coated multibranched gold nano-antennas with Dox-low-thermoresponsive liposomes (LTSLs). NIR light-to-heat conversion permits successful delivery of DOX from the LTSLs in breast cancer cells (Ou *et al.*, 2016).

There are several methods for the synthesis of GNPs. Some of these methods can precisely control the size, shape, and stability of products. In general, the synthesis method of GNPs can be divided into biological and physicochemical approaches. Ultraviolet (UV) radiation method, γ-irradiation, microwave (MW) irradiation, sonochemical method, laser ablation, photochemical process, and thermolytic process are considered physical methods. On the other hand, in chemical procedures such as the Turkevitch method, chemical reactions are performed in an aqueous medium by a reduction agent. Citrate and sodium borohydride is the most known reducing agents in this approach. Biological methods known as the favorable environment are another route of synthesis. In this method, green chemistry of NP synthesis *via* biological procedures using plant extracts, bacteria, fungi, algae, yeast, and viruses, aims to reduce hazardous generated wastes (Elahi *et al.*, 2018).

Despite the many advantages of GNPs in developing DDSs, numerous studies have investigated the effect of GNP size on cytotoxicity. As an instance, 1.4 nm gold nanoclusters have been exhibited to irreversibly and selectively bind to the major grooves of B-DNA and cause enhanced toxicity (Galvin *et al.*, 2012). On the other hand, less toxicity has been reported from 3.7 nm NPs, whereas they both entered the cell nucleus. There is a direct correlation between cytotoxicity and the concentration of GNPs. In this regard, low concentration (1 ppm) of 2-20 nm GNPs did not exhibit toxicity to murine macrophage cell line, whilst concentrations higher than 10 ppm induced apoptosis of cells and upregulation of pro-inflammatory genes. However, it is worth noting that surface modifications can prevent the cytotoxic effects of NPs (Das *et al.*, 2011).

8.3. MAGNETIC NANOPARTICLES IN TRIGGERED DRUG DELIVERY

As mentioned in the previous section, the main purpose to develop novel delivery devices is to get the desired drug concentration at the specific site and at the appropriate time. Many traditional delivery systems cannot penetrate into diseased sites; for instance, in case of cancer treatment, typical tumor treatments that work by blocking cell division are not able to treat cancer tissues within hypoxic regions. One approach for overcoming this limitation is triggered drug release by the magnetic field. In this context, magnetic NPs (MNPs) can be used to minimize toxicity, increase drug efficiency, and enhance local concentrations (Mody *et al.*, 2014, Misra, 2008).

Recent studies have introduced several excellent MNPs such as gadolinium, Prussian blue, cobalt and nickel, but magnetic iron oxide (usually maghemite γ-Fe_2O_3 or magnetite Fe_3O_4) NPs have already been broadly studied, due to their great MRI contrast feature and low systemic toxicity which makes them an ideal selection for cancer theranostics (Mukherjee *et al.*, 2020, Vallabani and Singh, 2018).

Drug-conjugated MNPs can release the drug at the target by applying a magnetic field (Arruebo *et al.*, 2007). A great feature of an MNP carrier is superparamagnetism which is the ability to align magnetic moments along the applied field and lose the magnetization once the field is turned off (Sensenig *et al.*, 2012). Superparamagnetic iron oxide NPs (SPIONs) are the most considerably scrutinized inorganic systems for magnetic resonance imaging (MRI) and targeted drug delivery. SPIONs can be employed to induce local heating in diseased targets. Localized hyperthermia can trigger the release of entrapped drugs and cause cell death by thermo-induced apoptosis (Chee *et al.*, 2018). MNPs have been utilized for a wide range of purposes including one or more of the following groups:

1. Contrast agents for MRI, which would allow the combination of therapy and diagnostic.
2. Immunoassays, where MNPs bounded to antibodies are used to detect and quantify antigens in biological samples.
3. Hyperthermia agents, where the MNPs are employed to induce local heating for the site-specific delivery of therapeutic drugs or killing diseased cells.
4. Magnetic vectors that can be directed by applying magnetic field gradients towards a specific site (Estelrich *et al.*, 2015).

The use of MNPs for drug delivery applications was pioneered by Widder, Senyi, and colleagues in the late 1970s. Therapeutic drugs can be attached to, or entrapped within MNPs. These systems may have magnetic cores that can be coated with biocompatible materials loaded with payloads *via* linking to functional groups or may compose of porous polymers that contain MNPs (McBain *et al.*, 2008). In this context, the most relevant drug/gene loading mechanisms include direct encapsulation or adsorption of the payloads through physical interactions (*e.g.*, hydrophobic or electrostatic interaction) between the MNPs and the therapeutic drugs; or chemical reactions (*e.g.*, covalent bonding through active groups) between the surface functional groups of MNPs and drug payloads. It is noteworthy that the MNPs should be coated and functionalization to prevent particle agglomeration, improve drug pharmacokinetics, enhance colloidal stability, allow covalent or electrostatic binding of therapeutic agents, target moieties, and/or additional imaging probes, control the interactions with non-targeted cells, minimize non-specific protein adsorption, reduce systemic toxicity, improve sustained drug release, *etc.* Different approaches to attaching polymers onto the surface of MNPs are summarized in Fig. (**4**) (Huang *et al.*, 2016, Bucak *et al.*, 2012, Mukherjee *et al.*, 2020).

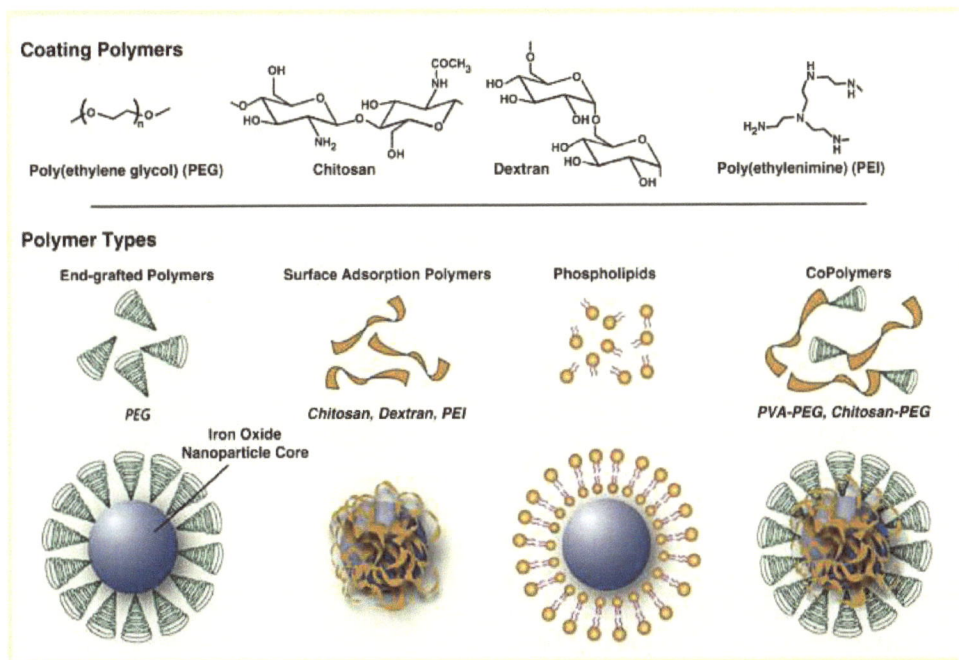

Fig. (4). different MNPs coating resulting in different assembly of polymers (open access) (Bucak *et al.*, 2012).

As we said before, there are several methods allowing the increase of the drug release at the site of treatment from NP-based delivery systems, such as functionalization or using responsiveness of NPs. Combining NPs with antibodies or targeting agents can bind them specifically to the disease biomarkers *via* ligand-receptor or antigen-antibody interactions. This phenomenon enables the MNPs to accumulate at diseased parts, thus enhancing their therapeutic effects (Vangijzegem *et al.*, 2019, Kempe *et al.*, 2011). It is a well-established fact that folic acid (FA) as a ligand, has a high affinity for the FA receptor protein, which is commonly overexpressed in a variety of tumors. FA can be tagged to an NP carrier and used for active targeting to FA receptors on the surface of tumor cells (Bucak *et al.*, 2012). Angelopoulou *et al.* used this approach for a highly selective release of (DOX) to cancer cells of solid tumors. In this study, Alginate-coated magnetic iron oxide nanoassemblies (MIONs) were synthesized, then Poly(ethylene glycol) (OH-PEG-NH2) was conjugated to the carboxylic acid end group of alginate, and FA was conjugated to the hydroxyl terminal group of PEG. The DOX-loaded (Mag-Alg-PEG-FA) exhibited increased apoptosis and cytotoxicity against the MDA-MB-231 cell line, overexpressing the folate receptor. Besides, this delivery system can accumulate at the site of treatment by applying an external magnetic field to the tumor area (Angelopoulou *et al.*, 2019).

MNPs can be used for gene therapy. In this method, the SPIO must be coated with cationic polymers, such as polyethylenimine (PEI), which promotes DNA transfection into cells due to its high positive charge. As an instance, Kumar *et al.* designed an MN-EPPT-siBIRC5 system which was composed of SPIO, peptides (EPPT), and a synthetic siRNA that targets the tumor-specific antiapoptotic gene BIRC5. The uptake of this nano-drug by breast cancer cells and delivery of siRNA to tumor cells resulted in a considerable downregulation of BIRC5 and an increase in necrosis and apoptosis in tumor cells (Ahmed and Douek, 2013).

The heat energy which is emitted from superparamagnetic NPs has shown great promise for biomedical and pharmaceutical applications and can be used to 1) induce hypothermic shock and apoptosis, particularly in tumor cells; 2) cause structural rearrangements and swelling/ deswelling of the nanoparticle shells, enhancing the diffusion-controlled release of carrier agents; and 3) induce local heating for the site-specific burst release and delivery of therapeutic payloads due to the thermal decomposition of the shell itself. It should be noted that the latter mechanism can be used for heat-induced decomposition of covalent linkers, and release of covalently bound therapeutic agents (Kumar and Mohammad, 2011, Norris *et al.*, 2019).

In general, hyperthermia is classified into three main groups, including local, regional and whole-body hyperthermia, based on the tumor size. Whole-body hyperthermia heats the entire body using several mechanisms such as hot water blankets, electric blankets, and hot wax. In the regional hyperthermia approach, heat is applied to a smaller part of the body, such as the entire organ or limb, using external arrays of applicators, and regional perfusion. In local hyperthermia, heat is applied to a very small area and is typically used for small tumor regions using electromagnetic waves such as ultrasound, microwaves and radio waves. According to the location of cancer, the applicators are placed at the surface or under the skin of superficial cancer or implanted inside the targeted area. In contrast to the benefits of local hyperthermia, such as control over the site-specificity and a better heat uniformity, this method had two main disadvantages: (a) it was extremely invasive for deep tumor areas and (b) a low penetration depth of only a few centimeters. Nanotechnology is a helpful solution for eliminating these two problems of local hyperthermia and making it a noninvasive approach with fewer side effects for targeting deep tumoral cells. In this regard, MNPs that are delivered only to the tumor region can be employed as hyperthermia agents to induce local heating by applying an alternating magnetic field (AMF) (Obaidat *et al.*, 2019).

In this regard, thermo-responsive polymers may be used for developing MNP-based delivery systems. Cheon and coworkers synthesized the SPION-based system with a 4,4-azobis(4-cyanovaleric acid) as a thermo-responsive covalent-linker to release geldanamycin to breast cancer cells after the thermal cleavage of azo-linker. In this study, an external alternating magnetic field was applied with a transducer, and the tumor temperature was maintained at 43 °C for 30 minutes. Geldanamycin caused heat shock protein inhibition and induced tumor cell hyperthermia and apoptosis, with complete removal of the cancerous tissue after 8 days of treatment (Norris *et al.*, 2019).

Hayashi *et al.* proposed a tailorable and on-demand drug release with more control by simultaneously using the hyperthermia effect and targeted delivery system. This research group used Superparamagnetic iron oxide with folate conjugate as a targeting ligand for breast tumoral cells. Applying a high-frequency magnetic field (HFMF) resulted in a hyperthermic effect as a driving force to release the Chemotherapeutic drugs incorporated in the beta-Cyclodextrin. It is noteworthy that this delivery system can be controlled by switching the HFMF on and off (Hayashi *et al.*, 2010). In the same study, Shen and coworkers used thermo-responsive polymer PNIPAm to optimize drug adsorption and delivery. This research group developed Fe_3O_4/PNIPAM/5-Fu@$mSiO_2$–CHI/R6G nanocomposites with the ability to generate heat under a magnetic field, which can be used for hyperthermia therapy (Shen *et al.*, 2016).

In another study, Campbell *et al.* designed an injectable hydrogel-thermo responsive microgel-SPION system containing SPIONs and temperature-sensitive hydrazide-functionalized PNIPAM (PNIPAM-Hzd) crosslinked with aldehyde-functionalized dextranas as *in situ*-gelling hydrogel matrix, p(NIPAM-NIPMAM) as temperature-sensitive microgels, and 4 kDa fluoresceinlabeled dextran as a model drug (Fig. **5**). When an alternating magnetic field (AMF) is applied, the temperature-responsive microgel can be driven to deswell due to the heat generated by SPIONs which increases the local temperature of the microgels above their volume phase transition temperature. This phenomenon generates free volume within the nanocomposite system, leading to increased drug diffusion through the matrix. On the other hand, removing the AMF decreases the release rate of drugs due to the microgels reswelling and refilling the pores. So the high-low pulsatile release performance of therapeutic agents is possible in this system (Campbell *et al.*, 2015).

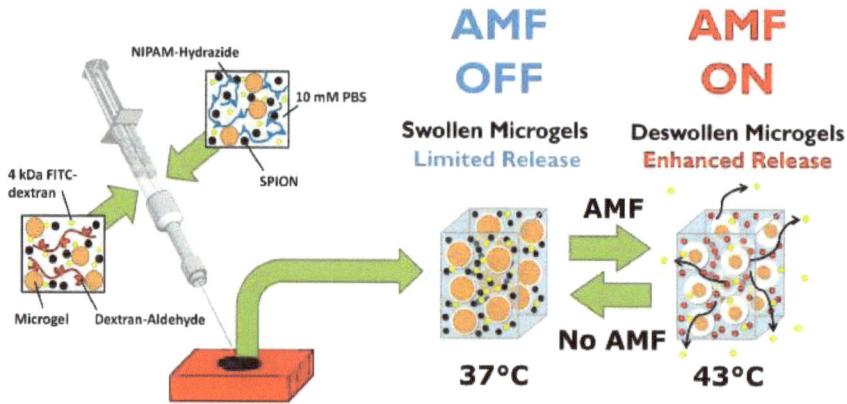

Fig. (5). Fabrication of smart delivery system and its high-low pulsatile release of therapeutic agents by switching the AMF on and off (Campbell *et al.*, 2015).

Using an external magnetic field can be problematic in drug delivery. One reason is its complex process and expensive proposal, particularly for daily administration of therapeutics for a long period of time. To overcome this challenge, Ge *et al.* developed a magnetite Fe_3O_4/poly(lactic-co-glycolic acid) nanocomposite as an implantable scaffold for targeted drug delivery purposes. Under the effect of such magnetic scaffolds, the injected magnetic nanodrugs can be effectively delivered to the implant location. Such magnetic scaffolds have shown great potential as implants for the treatment of bone cancer, obesity, and deafness (Price *et al.*, 2018, Ge *et al.*, 2017).

MNPs can be used for developing dual responsive nanocarriers. In this context, Yu *et al.* developed a pH and magnetic dual-responsive delivery system by combining $Fe_3O_4@SiO_2$ NPs with imidazole group-modified PEG-polypepide (mPEG-poly(l-Asparagine)) to form superparamagnetic core-pH-sensitive shell-hydrophilic corona. DOX was successfully loaded into the aforementioned nanocarrier as a model drug. This drug-loaded nanocarrier exhibited super-paramagnetic property with a pH-responsive drug release behavior (Yu *et al.*, 2013).

There are several parameters that need to be considered in the effective use of MNPs for drug delivery. Some of these factors include the target tissue depth, the size and magnetism of the MNPs, field strength and geometry, blood flow rate, and vascular supply. It should be highlighted that the size of NPs must be small so that they can be superparamagnetic in order to prevent agglomeration in the absence of a magnetic field and to remain in systemic circulation without being removed and filtered through the patient's natural filters such as liver or immune system (Chomoucka *et al.*, 2010). Another approach for overcoming the accumulation of MNPs leading to toxicity at multiple sites is using poly(ethylene glycol) (PEG) as an FDA-approved polymer that has become the most extensively investigated "stealth" polymer in biomedical applications. Owing to the flexible and hydrophilic nature of PEG, on NP surfaces, it can form a dynamic hydration barrier, which avoids the plasma proteins binding on the surface of the particles and clearance by the mononuclear phagocytic system, (Sanadgol and Wackerlig, 2020).

However, there are still several concerns about the accumulation of MNPs in the body environment. For instance, intravenously injected MNPs have a tendency to agglomerate in the liver and spleen, leading to the lack of sufficient tumor accumulation for an effective treatment. For the *in-situ* localized cancer therapy, intra-tumor injection of ferrofluid can be theoretically reasonable. When MNPs are injected directly inside the solid tumors, the small particulate size and the high osmotic pressure across the solid malignant tumor make them easily leak out along the syringe needle and escape from the target site during the long period of treatment. Using *in-situ* gelation of delivery systems is a considerable strategy for overcoming this problem. In this context, a magnetic nanoemulsion hydrogel was injected directly into the target site, which could be transformed into solid-state in the body environment with no leakage after feeling the physiological temperature (37°C) (Wu *et al.*, 2017).

For example, Murali *et al.* designed a thermoresponsive injectable delivery system that can be used for sustained drug delivery, hyperthermia treatment, and long-term theranostic ability. This injectable MNP incorporated a hydrogel system including biocompatible aminated guar gum (AGG) as a gelling agent, doxorubicin hydrochloride as the model drug, and Fe_3O_4-ZnS core-shell as the imaging agent. This delivery system exhibited gel formation at the physiological temperature (37°C) that was stable over a wide temperature and pH range. The in-vitro de-gelation and drug release of up to 90% can be achieved after 20 days of incubation. Besides, the magnetic core-shell NPs can be released slowly from the hydrogel system to provide a diagnosis of the diseased site (Murali *et al.*, 2014).

Numerous methods have been devised to synthesize MNPs covering a wide range of compositions and tunable sizes, such as coprecipitation, sol-gel syntheses, flow injection synthesis, hydrothermal and high-temperature reactions, polyol processes, aerosol technologies such as spray and laser pyrolysis, electrochemical methods, and sonolysis. It should be noted that the synthesis of high-quality

MNPs with a reproducible process resulting in a monodisperse population of magnetic grains is still challenging. However, the most common technique for the fabrication of MNPs is the chemical coprecipitation of iron salts (Laurent *et al.*, 2008).

Clearly, the toxicity of the MNP-based therapeutics is another important challenge that needs further investigation. The degree of toxicity depends on several elements such as dose and size, shape and structure, administration method, chemical composition, biodegradability, biocompatibility, solubility, surface chemistry, biodistribution, *etc.* So, it is not simple to report precise nanoparticle toxicity. Another considerable challenge in MNP-based delivery systems is the ability to administer them directly to the disease target site. As mentioned before, using an external magnetic field is not ideal in drug delivery, besides, the magnetic field from permanent magnets can only penetrate into a tissue depth of 8–12 cm, so, this method is not suitable for deeper solid tumors. In this regard, one approach for improving MNP-based localized drug delivery is using magnetic implantable scaffolds, which can attract MNPs if needed (Tran and Webster, 2010).

8.4. CALCIUM PHOSPHATE-BASED NANOPARTICLES IN TRIGGERED DRUG DELIVERY

In the past few decades, many researchers have focused on the fabrication of high-quality calcium phosphates (CaPs)-based nanocoatings and thin-film nanolaminates for biomedical applications (Ben-Nissan *et al.*, 2016). So, it is worth highlighting and discussing the potential of this material in drug delivery.

Calcium phosphate NPs (CaPNPs) have achieved considerable interest in pharmaceutics due to their high biocompatibility and good biodegradability, as calcium phosphate is the inorganic mineral of human bone and teeth (Epple *et al.*, 2010). Besides CaPs could be prepared in nanoform with a wide range of morphologies using simple and eco-friendly precipitation processes (Desai and Uskoković, 2013).

In the case of polymeric NPs, the acidic or degradation byproducts have gained more concerns due to their adverse interaction with the therapeutic agents or tissue as they come in contact during circulation. Ca^{2+} and PO_4^{3-} which are the degradation byproducts of CaPs are already inherent to the body, and are found in the bloodstream in relatively high concentrations (1–5 mM). This natural occurrence of CaPs is one of the substantial advantages over conventional synthetic dosage forms, which might trigger an immunogenic response. Besides, as we said before, the success of a DDS relies on its effective delivery of the desired drug concentration to the specific organ. Regardless of the Ca/P ratio, phase and crystallinity, CaPs are negligibly soluble at a physiological pH of 7.4; whilst, their dissolution is accelerated in an acidic environment, *e.g.*, a pH below 6.5. On the other hand, despite the organic or polymeric DDSs, CaPs are not prone to enzymatic degradation in the physiological environment. Therefore, these unique features of CaPs, including non-immunogenic response, non-toxic degradation byproducts, and pH-dependent solubility, make them a good choice for developing novel drug delivery systems (Bose and Tarafder, 2012, Huang *et al.*, 2018, Wang *et al.*, 2017). In this regard, CaPs can be used as pH-responsive drug carriers for selectively delivering therapeutic agents in response to an acidic tumor environment. So the CaPs can enhance the local effect of chemotherapeutic agents in cancer therapy (Zhang *et al.*, 2020, Levingstone *et al.*, 2019). CaPs can be found in several individual phases with varying properties, such as different crystalline structures, composition and Ca/P ratio, solubility degree and bioresorbability. Some of these phases include hydroxyapatite (HAp), amorphous calcium phosphate (ACP), tricalcium phosphate (TCP), tetracalcium phosphate (TTCP), octacalcium phosphate (OCP), monetite (M), and brushite (B). Besides, the development of multiphasic systems has gained increasing interest recently (Turon *et al.*, 2017). Among the numerous CaPs, increasing attention is given to the development of hydroxyapatite NPs (HANPs) in the drug delivery field due to their biocompatible, osteoconductive, and noninflammatory properties (Choi and Ben-Nissan, 2015, Bose *et al.*, 2011). So in the following sections, we will focus on HANP-based delivery systems in triggered drug delivery.

Many Researchers have used HANPs to deliver drugs, therapeutic factors, and genetic cargoes (Yang *et al.*, 2013). As an instance, Bharath *et al.* designed a novel pH-sensitive nanocarrier based on HA with mesoporous nanoplates (HAp PNPs) and by using Andrographolide as a model anticancer drug. This delivery system exhibited effective Andrographolide release into A431 cell lines at a pH of 4.4 (Bharath *et al.*, 2019). In another study, Curtin *et al.* combined BMP-2-loaded HANPs with collagen for developing bioactive and biodegradable delivery scaffolds that act as a gene-activated matrix for plasmid-DNA (pDNA) encoding bone morphogenetic protein 2 (BMP2) delivery. As a result of the transfection of mesenchymal stem cells, enhanced osteogenesis and high levels of calcium production were observed (Curtin *et al.*, 2012).

HA nanoprobes can be combined with targeting moieties such as amino acids like arginine, proteins like albumin, and vitamins like folic acid and *etc*. These targeting moieties can be attached through surface coating of the HANPs with poly acrylic acid (PAA), poly lactic acid (PLA), poly ethylene glycol (PEG) or poly ethylene imine (PEI) (Syamchand and Sony, 2015). In a study, the FA conjugated DOX-loaded HA nanorods were designed as a powerful nanocarrier for tumor-targeted drug delivery. In this study, DOX@HAP-FA can target folate receptor (FR)-overexpressing tumor cells and then the therapeutic agents can be delivered to the tumoral cells without affecting healthy cells. (Ghiasi *et al.*, 2019).

Localized delivery of antimicrobial agents to the infection site, can improve the specificity of antibiotic drugs and the treatment efficacy without the risk of undesired side effects. As an instance, in the treatment of osteomyelitis, combining HA coating with the antibiotic agent is a considerable method, which may guarantee bone implant integration without bacterial adhesion. In this context, Geuli *et al.* focused on coating antibiotic-loaded HANPs on titanium implants. It is noteworthy that the use of drug-loaded CaP-based coating, such as HA, and bioglass provides additional values as osteoconductivity in addition to the antibacterial properties (Geuli *et al.*, 2017).

Synthesis of CaP NPs is an intimate part of drug loading or incorporation processes. There are numerous techniques for the synthesis of nano-sized HA, that include: solid state reaction, sol-gel microwave processes, flame spray pyrolysis, spray-drying, and wet chemical. In general, Wet chemical method has several advantages over the other fabrication approaches, including, cost-effectiveness, low processing temperature, fabrication of highly pure products, and simplicity. Besides, this approach is able to produce nanocrystalline powders, bulk amorphous NPs, and thin films (Jafari and Adibkia, 2015, Bose and Tarafder, 2012).

Ultimately CaPNP-based delivery systems have their own disadvantages, including their lower loading efficiency and capacity in comparison to hollow organic NPs or liposomes, their higher accumulation in aqueous suspensions, which leads to the prevention of their penetration into cells, or an instant macrophage capture and clearance, and their fast surface degradation that resulted in a burst release of the therapeutic cargoes in the organism. All of these drawbacks could hinder the use of CaPNPs for biomedical applications which require a more sustained and prolonged release. In this context, surface decoration of CaPNPs with ionic organic molecules can stabilize them in their colloidal form. Besides, to overcome the burst release effect in CaPNP-based delivery systems, they can be engineered to encapsulate the drug within the crystalline matrix (Degli Esposti *et al.*, 2018).

8.5. MESOPOROUS SILICA

Silica was approved by the FDA as "Generally Recognized Safe". Recently, silica NPs in the form of Cornell dots (Cdots) were approved by the FDA for stage I human clinical trial for targeted molecular imaging. Mesoporous silica NPs

(MSNs) exhibited a three-stage degradation behavior in simulated body fluid, suggesting that MSNs might degrade after administration. This feature of MSNs, make them a good choice for developing drug delivery systems (Zhou *et al.*, 2018).

Among inorganic-based materials, MSNs are gaining tremendous attention in biomedical applications. MSNs are solid materials with a porous honeycomb-like structure composed of hundreds of empty channels that are able to absorb or encapsulate therapeutic drugs. In contrast to the other amorphous silica materials that exhibit low biocompatibility, MSNs have extensive biocompatibility at concentrations adequate for drug delivery applications (Vivero-Escoto *et al.*, 2010, Rajani *et al.*, 2020).

MSNs possess some unique characteristics which offer advantages that may allow clinically applicable nanoformulations for the treatment of various diseases:

1. Tunable particle size. The particle size of MSN can be easily engineered between 50 and 300 nm allowing facile endocytosis by living animal and plant cells without any significant cytotoxicity.

2. Uniform and tunable pore size. The pore diameter of MSN can be engineered from 2 to 6 nm. This feature permits adjusting the loading efficiency and capacity and to study the kinetics of drug release with great accuracy.

3. Stable and rigid framework. MSN is more resistant to heat, pH, mechanical stress, and hydrolysis-induced degradations, in comparison with other polymer-based delivery systems.

4. Large surface area and high pore volume. The total surface area (N900 m2/g) and pore volume (N0.9 cm3/g) are very large, which permit high drug-loading capacity (Slowing *et al.*, 2008).

The most unique feature of the MSNs is their internal mesopore structure which can be controlled by the initial reagents or the surfactant. As mentioned previously, mesopores are not randomly distributed, but rather specifically aligned with hundreds of empty channels. The channels have considerable potential as a reservoir of therapeutic agents without interconnections between channels. It should be highlighted that MSNs have unique surface properties and a high density of surface silanol groups, which can be modified with numerous organic functional groups: (a) to control the surface charge of MSNs, (b) to chemically link with functional molecules, (c) to control the size of pore entrance for loading therapeutic cargoes in the nanopores, (d) to improve the colloidal stability of the MSNs, and (e) to prevent the binding of non-specific serum proteins and avoiding early clearance from the circulation. In general, there are three main approaches of surface functionalization of MSNs including co-condensation, post-synthesis grafting, and surfactant displacement methods (Kwon *et al.*, 2013, Selvarajan *et al.*, 2020).

The use of silica mesostructures for drug delivery applications was pioneered in the late 1983s. Numerous studies have been carried out demonstrating the high potential of MSNs in delivering a wide range of therapeutic agents such as proteins, small molecules, photosensitized molecules, ribonucleic acids, deoxyribonucleic acids, *etc.* It is noteworthy that MSNs can be used to protect these therapeutic agents from degradation and designing zero-premature payload release systems while carrying therapeutics to the target site with no leakage and on-demand release of drugs (Mirzaei *et al.*, 2020).

Both passive and active targeting can be used for the fabrication of novel MSN-based nanocarriers for targeted drug delivery (Sun, 2012). For instance, MSNs can easily accumulate in the cancer region and represent promising delivery nanocarriers, due to the enhanced permeation and retention (EPR) effect as a result of the leaky vasculature and the lack of lymphatic drainage of small structures by solid tumors. To this end, Lee *et al.* have shown proficient treatment by passive targeting of DOX-loaded to the tumor site in a melanoma model (Barui and Cauda, 2020, Lee *et al.*, 2010).

Another explored strategy for enhancing drug delivery with MSNs is active targeting and decorating the outermost surface of MSNs with moieties able to interact selectively with specific membrane receptors predominantly expressed in diseased cells, in vascular structures, or in the nuclear membrane. As shown in (Fig. **6**), numerous targeting molecules, including peptides, antibodies, aptamers, small molecules, saccharides, and proteins, can be added to the MSNs' surface (Vallet-Regí *et al.*, 2018, Watermann and Brieger, 2017).

As an instance, Zhou *et al.* conjugated rituximab (as a chimeric monoclonal antibody) to the DOX-loaded MSNs for developing a targeted drug delivery system. These nanocarriers could selectively adhere to the surface of lymphoma B cells *via* targeting the CD20 antigen (Zhou *et al.*, 2017).

Designing a "smart" delivery nanocarrier that can respond to the stimuli from the environment to open the pores is another strategy for controlling drug release from MSN-based DDSs (Castillo *et al.*, 2019).

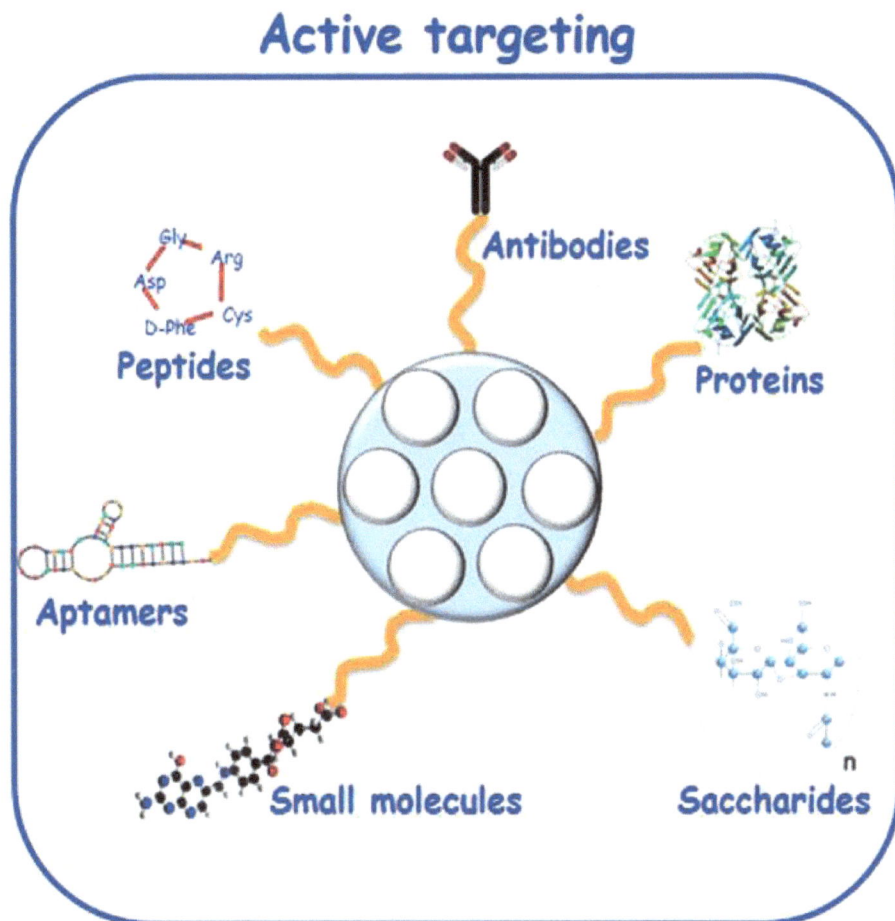

Fig. (6). Schematic depiction of active targeting possibilities on MSNs (open access) (Vallet-Regí *et al.*, 2018).

Both exogenous stimuli (temperature, light, magnetic and electric field, or ultrasound) and endogenous stimuli (pH, reactive oxygen species, enzyme, etc.) can be employed for designing gatekeepers that can be used to maintain the "zero release" of the therapeutic cargoes inside the MSNs and trigger on-demand payload release from these nanocarriers (Iturrioz-Rodríguez *et al.*, 2019). Among the smart MSN-based delivery systems, gatekeeper systems with pH-responsive linkers are one of the most commonly used systems. These linkers are cleaved in an acidic environment, triggering the release of the therapeutic agents from the MSN-based carriers. Acetal bonds, hydrazine bonds, hydrazone bonds or ester bonds are the most commonly explored pH-responsive linkers (Iturrioz-Rodríguez *et al.*, 2019). However, there are numerous stimuli- cleavable gatekeepers to keep the loaded drug in the MSN pores in on-demand drug release nanodevices. For instance, Lin and Zink reported a series of nano-caps as gatekeepers for MSN-based DDSs, including CdS, Au, Fe_3O_4, and PAMAM NPs, which were uncovered under exogenous stimuli by redox, light, or magnetism leading to the release of loaded therapeutic agents (He and Shi, 2011). In another study, Karimi reported a series of linkers, such as disulfide bonds, reversible boronate ester linkers, and Gly-Phe-Leu-Gly (GFLG) peptide that can respond to redox, pH, and enzyme, respectively (Karimi *et al.*, 2016).

The preparation of MSN-based delivery systems with both stimuli-sensitive and targeting abilities has two methods. One includes developing a multifunctional targeting moiety that acts as both a targeting and a capping agent to achieve MSN-based controlled and targeted drug delivery. The second method includes designing a stimuli-responsive gatekeeper that is further modified with a target molecule to achieve multifunctional drug delivery (Wang *et al.*, 2015).

Silica NPs are usually synthesized through hydrolytic sol–gel process, which includes the hydrolysis and condensation of silicon alkoxide precursors under acidic or basic catalysis (Manzano and Vallet-Regí, 2020). Surfactants such as cetyltrimethylammonium bromide (also known as CTAB) have been used in the case of MSNPs synthesis. Typically, at a concentration more than the critical micelle concentration, the surfactant will self-aggregate into micelles. Afterward, the silica precursors can be condensed to form MSNs on the surface of the micelles. At the end of the process, the template surfactant can be eliminated either by solvent extraction or by calcination to establish the pores. Fig. (**7**) illustrates the MSNs synthetic procedure (Carvalho *et al.*, 2020). In this regard, the characteristics of MSNs such as the pore structure, pore size, morphology and size of MSNs can be rationally engineered for biomedical applications which require accurate control over particle properties (Tang *et al.*, 2012).

MSNs exhibited remarkably lower cell toxicity towards inflammatory cells and phagocytes *in vitro* in comparison with amorphous colloidal silica NPs. Some researchers demonstrated that the surface modification of MSNs increases their cellular uptake, the pore diameter enhances the adsorption capacity, and the various shapes and the particles geometry can disturb normal cell functions. Therefore different parameters in the design path of the MSNs should be taken into consideration to reduce possible toxicity (Karimi *et al.*, 2016).

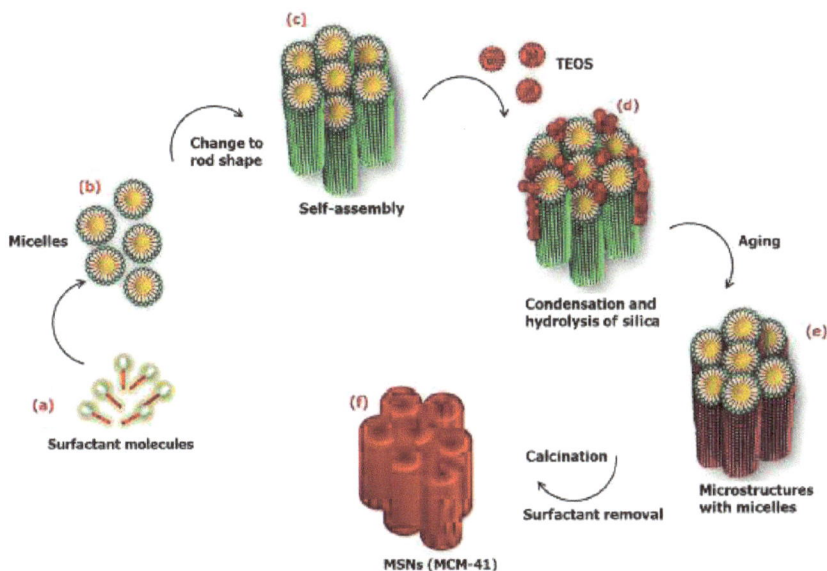

Fig. (7). Schematic representation of the MSNs synthetic path (open access) (Murugan *et al.*, 2020).

CONCLUSION

This chapter studied NPs used in LCDDS for the delivery of therapeutic molecules. Drugs and cancer chemotherapeutics have several side effects and acquired drug resistance that establishes LCDDS is greatly necessary. Several efforts have been established for LCDDS-based NPs through various approaches that are able to overcome the problems often related to conventional therapy. In spite of possessing remarkable clinical outcomes taken from numerous tools and technologies, more developments are needed to amend targeted LCDDS to reduce harmful influences, and consequently improve the life expectancy of the patients. Some remarkable developments have been considered for LCDDS by nanocarriers, nanospheres and nanocapsules (such as graphene, magnetic NPs, colloidal gold NPs, CNT, and stimuli-responsive NPs), which are designed, synthesized and engineered to release the drug in specialized states of the cell environment. However, there are still some challenges in the specificity and selectivity of NPs in the body. Therefore, some critical studies need to address these challenges and drawbacks and improve new/alternative techniques for conquering them. Recently, multifunctional bioagents for LCDDS are being significantly developed for personalized medicine. Incorporating peptides/ligands into other tools and technologies such as immunoliposomes which precisely bind to tumor cells/stem cells and cancer blood vessels, have served a promising function in developing nano-based LCDDSs and controlling the tumor growth.

REFERENCES

Adair, J.H., Parette, M.P., Altınoğlu, E.İ., Kester, M. (2010). Nanoparticulate alternatives for drug delivery. *ACS Nano, 4*(9), 4967-4970.
[http://dx.doi.org/10.1021/nn102324e] [PMID: 20873786]

Ahmed, M., Douek, M. (2013). The role of magnetic nanoparticles in the localization and treatment of breast cancer. *BioMed Res. Int., 2013*, 1-11.
[http://dx.doi.org/10.1155/2013/281230] [PMID: 23936784]

Ajnai, G., Chiu, A., Kan, T., Cheng, C.C., Tsai, T.H., Chang, J. (2014). Trends of gold nanoparticle-based drug delivery system in cancer therapy. *J. Exp. Clin. Med., 6*(6), 172-178.
[http://dx.doi.org/10.1016/j.jecm.2014.10.015]

Angelopoulou, A., Kolokithas-Ntoukas, A., Fytas, C., Avgoustakis, K. (2019). Folic acid-functionalized, condensed magnetic nanoparticles for targeted delivery of doxorubicin to tumor cancer cells overexpressing the folate receptor. *ACS Omega, 4*(26), 22214-22227.
[http://dx.doi.org/10.1021/acsomega.9b03594] [PMID: 31891105]

Arruebo, M., Fernández-Pacheco, R., Ibarra, M.R., Santamaría, J. (2007). Magnetic nanoparticles for drug delivery. *Nano Today, 2*(3), 22-32.
[http://dx.doi.org/10.1016/S1748-0132(07)70084-1]

Askari, E., Naghib, S.M., Zahedi, A., Seyfoori, A., Zare, Y., Rhee, K.Y. (2021). Local delivery of chemotherapeutic agent in tissue engineering based on gelatin/graphene hydrogel. *J. Mater. Res. Technol., 12*, 412-422.
[http://dx.doi.org/10.1016/j.jmrt.2021.02.084]

Askari, E., Seyfoori, A., Amereh, M., Gharaie, S.S., Ghazali, H.S., Ghazali, Z.S., Khunjush, B., Akbari, M. (2020). Stimuli-responsive hydrogels for local post-surgical drug delivery. *Gels, 6*(2), 14.
[http://dx.doi.org/10.3390/gels6020014] [PMID: 32397180]

Barui, S., Cauda, V. (2020). Multimodal decorations of mesoporous silica nanoparticles for improved cancer therapy. *Pharmaceutics, 12*(6), 527.
[http://dx.doi.org/10.3390/pharmaceutics12060527] [PMID: 32521802]

Ben-Nissan, B., Macha, I., Cazalbou, S., Choi, A.H. (2016). Calcium phosphate nanocoatings and nanocomposites, part 2: thin films for slow drug delivery and osteomyelitis. *Nanomedicine (Lond.), 11*(5), 531-544.
[http://dx.doi.org/10.2217/nnm.15.220] [PMID: 26891748]

Bennet, D., Kim, S. (2014). Polymer nanoparticles for smart drug delivery. *Application of nanotechnology in drug delivery, 257*

Bharath, G., Rambabu, K., Banat, F., Anwer, S., Lee, S., BinSaleh, N., Latha, S., Ponpandian, N. (2019). Mesoporous hydroxyapatite nanoplate arrays as pH-sensitive drug carrier for cancer therapy. *Mater. Res. Express, 6*(8), 085409.
[http://dx.doi.org/10.1088/2053-1591/ab2348]

Bose, S., Tarafder, S. (2012). Calcium phosphate ceramic systems in growth factor and drug delivery for bone tissue engineering: A review. *Acta Biomater., 8*(4), 1401-1421.
[http://dx.doi.org/10.1016/j.actbio.2011.11.017] [PMID: 22127225]

Bose, S., Tarafder, S., Edgington, J., Bandyopadhyay, A. (2011). Calcium phosphate ceramics in drug delivery. *J. Miner. Met. Mater. Soc., 63*(4), 93-98.
[http://dx.doi.org/10.1007/s11837-011-0065-7]

Bucak, S., Yavuztürk, B., Demir, A. (2012). Magnetic nanoparticles: synthesis, surface modifications and

application in drug delivery. *Recent Advances in Novel Drug Carrier Systems, 2*, 165-200.
[http://dx.doi.org/10.5772/52115]

Campbell, S., Maitland, D., Hoare, T. (2015). Enhanced pulsatile drug release from injectable magnetic hydrogels with embedded thermosensitive microgels. *ACS Macro Lett., 4*(3), 312-316.
[http://dx.doi.org/10.1021/acsmacrolett.5b00057] [PMID: 35596334]

Carvalho, G.C., Sábio, R.M., de Cássia Ribeiro, T., Monteiro, A.S., Pereira, D.V., Ribeiro, S.J.L., Chorilli, M. (2020). Highlights in Mesoporous Silica Nanoparticles as a Multifunctional Controlled Drug Delivery Nanoplatform for Infectious Diseases Treatment. *Pharm. Res., 37*(10), 191.
[http://dx.doi.org/10.1007/s11095-020-02917-6] [PMID: 32895867]

Castillo, R.R., Lozano, D., González, B., Manzano, M., Izquierdo-Barba, I., Vallet-Regí, M. (2019). Advances in mesoporous silica nanoparticles for targeted stimuli-responsive drug delivery: an update. *Expert Opin. Drug Deliv., 16*(4), 415-439.
[http://dx.doi.org/10.1080/17425247.2019.1598375] [PMID: 30897978]

Chee, C.F., Leo, B.F., Lai, C.W. (2018). *Superparamagnetic iron oxide nanoparticles for drug delivery. Applications of Nanocomposite Materials in Drug Delivery.*. Elsevier.

Chen, H., Liu, D., Guo, Z. (2016). Endogenous stimuli-responsive nanocarriers for drug delivery. *Chem. Lett., 45*(3), 242-249.
[http://dx.doi.org/10.1246/cl.151176]

Choi, A.H., Ben-Nissan, B. (2015). Calcium phosphate nanocoatings and nanocomposites, part I: recent developments and advancements in tissue engineering and bioimaging. *Nanomedicine (Lond.), 10*(14), 2249-2261.
[http://dx.doi.org/10.2217/nnm.15.57] [PMID: 26119630]

Chomoucka, J., Drbohlavova, J., Huska, D., Adam, V., Kizek, R., Hubalek, J. (2010). Magnetic nanoparticles and targeted drug delivering. *Pharmacol. Res., 62*(2), 144-149.
[http://dx.doi.org/10.1016/j.phrs.2010.01.014] [PMID: 20149874]

Curtin, C.M., Cunniffe, G.M., Lyons, F.G., Bessho, K., Dickson, G.R., Duffy, G.P., O'Brien, F.J. (2012). Innovative collagen nano-hydroxyapatite scaffolds offer a highly efficient non-viral gene delivery platform for stem cell-mediated bone formation. *Adv. Mater., 24*(6), 749-754.
[http://dx.doi.org/10.1002/adma.201103828] [PMID: 22213347]

Das, M., Shim, K.H., An, S.S.A., Yi, D.K. (2011). Review on gold nanoparticles and their applications. *Toxicol. Environ. Health Sci., 3*(4), 193-205.
[http://dx.doi.org/10.1007/s13530-011-0109-y]

de Jong, W.H., Borm, P.J. (2008). Drug delivery and nanoparticles: Applications and hazards. *Int. J. Nanomedicine, 3*(2), 133-149.
[http://dx.doi.org/10.2147/IJN.S596] [PMID: 18686775]

Degli Esposti, L., Carella, F., Adamiano, A., Tampieri, A., Iafisco, M. (2018). Calcium phosphate-based nanosystems for advanced targeted nanomedicine. *Drug Dev. Ind. Pharm., 44*(8), 1223-1238.
[http://dx.doi.org/10.1080/03639045.2018.1451879] [PMID: 29528248]

Desai, T.A., Uskoković, V. (2013). Calcium phosphate nanoparticles: a future therapeutic platform for the treatment of osteomyelitis? *Ther. Deliv., 4*(6), 643-645.
[http://dx.doi.org/10.4155/tde.13.33] [PMID: 23738660]

Du, Y.Q., Yang, X.X., Li, W.L., Wang, J., Huang, C.Z. (2014). A cancer-targeted drug delivery system developed with gold nanoparticle mediated DNA–doxorubicin conjugates. *RSC Advances, 4*(66), 34830-34835.
[http://dx.doi.org/10.1039/C4RA06298A]

Duncan, B., Kim, C., Rotello, V.M. (2010). Gold nanoparticle platforms as drug and biomacromolecule delivery systems. *J. Control. Release, 148*(1), 122-127.
[http://dx.doi.org/10.1016/j.jconrel.2010.06.004] [PMID: 20547192]

Dürr, S., Janko, C., Lyer, S., Tripal, P., Schwarz, M., Zaloga, J., Tietze, R., Alexiou, C. (2013). Magnetic nanoparticles for cancer therapy. *Nanotechnol. Rev., 2*(4), 395-409.
[http://dx.doi.org/10.1515/ntrev-2013-0011]

Elahi, N., Kamali, M., Baghersad, M.H. (2018). Recent biomedical applications of gold nanoparticles: A review. *Talanta, 184*, 537-556.
[http://dx.doi.org/10.1016/j.talanta.2018.02.088] [PMID: 29674080]

Emerich, D.F., Thanos, C.G. (2007). Targeted nanoparticle-based drug delivery and diagnosis. *J. Drug Target., 15*(3), 163-183.
[http://dx.doi.org/10.1080/10611860701231810] [PMID: 17454354]

Epple, M., Ganesan, K., Heumann, R., Klesing, J., Kovtun, A., Neumann, S., Sokolova, V. (2010). Application of calcium phosphatenanoparticles in biomedicine. *J. Mater. Chem., 20*(1), 18-23.
[http://dx.doi.org/10.1039/B910885H]

Estelrich, J., Escribano, E., Queralt, J., Busquets, M. (2015). Iron oxide nanoparticles for magnetically-guided and magnetically-responsive drug delivery. *Int. J. Mol. Sci., 16*(12), 8070-8101.
[http://dx.doi.org/10.3390/ijms16048070] [PMID: 25867479]

Fratoddi, I., Venditti, I., Cametti, C., Russo, M.V. (2014). Gold nanoparticles and gold nanoparticle-conjugates for delivery of therapeutic molecules. Progress and challenges. *J. Mater. Chem. B Mater. Biol. Med., 2*(27), 4204-4220.
[http://dx.doi.org/10.1039/C4TB00383G] [PMID: 32261559]

Galvin, P., Thompson, D., Ryan, K.B., McCarthy, A., Moore, A.C., Burke, C.S., Dyson, M., MacCraith, B.D., Gun'ko, Y.K., Byrne, M.T., Volkov, Y., Keely, C., Keehan, E., Howe, M., Duffy, C., MacLoughlin, R. (2012). Nanoparticle-based drug delivery: case studies for cancer and cardiovascular applications. *Cell. Mol. Life Sci., 69*(3), 389-404.
[http://dx.doi.org/10.1007/s00018-011-0856-6] [PMID: 22015612]

Gao, W., Chen, Y., Zhang, Y., Zhang, Q., Zhang, L. (2018). Nanoparticle-based local antimicrobial drug delivery. *Adv. Drug Deliv. Rev., 127*, 46-57.
[http://dx.doi.org/10.1016/j.addr.2017.09.015] [PMID: 28939377]

García, M.A. (2011). Surface plasmons in metallic nanoparticles: fundamentals and applications. *J. Phys. D Appl. Phys., 44*(28), 283001.
[http://dx.doi.org/10.1088/0022-3727/44/28/283001]

Ge, J., Zhang, Y., Dong, Z., Jia, J., Zhu, J., Miao, X., Yan, B. (2017). Initiation of targeted nanodrug delivery *in vivo* by a multifunctional magnetic implant. *ACS Appl. Mater. Interfaces, 9*(24), 20771-20778.
[http://dx.doi.org/10.1021/acsami.7b05009] [PMID: 28557411]

Geuli, O., Metoki, N., Zada, T., Reches, M., Eliaz, N., Mandler, D. (2017). Synthesis, coating, and drug-release of hydroxyapatite nanoparticles loaded with antibiotics. *J. Mater. Chem. B Mater. Biol. Med., 5*(38), 7819-7830.
[http://dx.doi.org/10.1039/C7TB02105D] [PMID: 32264383]

Ghiasi, B., Sefidbakht, Y., Rezaei, M. (2019). *Hydroxyapatite for biomedicine and drug delivery. Nanomaterials for Advanced Biological Applications..* Springer.

Ghosh, P., Han, G., De, M., Kim, C., Rotello, V. (2008). Gold nanoparticles in delivery applications. *Adv. Drug Deliv. Rev., 60*(11), 1307-1315.
[http://dx.doi.org/10.1016/j.addr.2008.03.016] [PMID: 18555555]

Gooneh-Farahani, S., Naghib, S.M., Naimi-Jamal, M.R. (2020). A novel and inexpensive method based on modified ionic gelation for pH-responsive controlled drug release of homogeneously distributed chitosan nanoparticles with a high encapsulation efficiency. *Fibers Polym., 21*(9), 1917-1926.
[http://dx.doi.org/10.1007/s12221-020-1095-y]

Gooneh-Farahani, S., Naimi-Jamal, M.R., Naghib, S.M. (2019). Stimuli-responsive graphene-incorporated multifunctional chitosan for drug delivery applications: a review. *Expert Opin. Drug Deliv., 16*(1), 79-99.

[http://dx.doi.org/10.1080/17425247.2019.1556257] [PMID: 30514124]

Guerrero, A.R., Hassan, N., Escobar, C.A., Albericio, F., Kogan, M.J., Araya, E. (2014). Gold nanoparticles for photothermally controlled drug release. *Nanomedicine (Lond.), 9*(13), 2023-2039. [http://dx.doi.org/10.2217/nnm.14.126] [PMID: 25343351]

Guo, X., Cheng, Y., Zhao, X., Luo, Y., Chen, J., Yuan, W.E. (2018). Advances in redox-responsive drug delivery systems of tumor microenvironment. *J. Nanobiotechnology, 16*(1), 74. [http://dx.doi.org/10.1186/s12951-018-0398-2] [PMID: 30243297]

Liao, H., Hafner, J.H. (2005). Gold nanorod bioconjugates. *Chem. Mater., 17*(18), 4636-4641. [http://dx.doi.org/10.1021/cm050935k]

Han, G., Ghosh, P., Rotello, V. M. (2007). Functionalized gold nanoparticles for drug delivery. [http://dx.doi.org/10.2217/17435889.2.1.113]

Han, G., Ghosh, P., Rotello, V. M. (2007). Multi-functional gold nanoparticles for drug delivery. *Bio-applications of Nanoparticles, 48*

Hayashi, K., Ono, K., Suzuki, H., Sawada, M., Moriya, M., Sakamoto, W., Yogo, T. (2010). High-frequency, magnetic-field-responsive drug release from magnetic nanoparticle/organic hybrid based on hyperthermic effect. *ACS Appl. Mater. Interfaces, 2*(7), 1903-1911. [http://dx.doi.org/10.1021/am100237p] [PMID: 20568697]

He, Q., Shi, J. (2011). Mesoporous silica nanoparticle based nano drug delivery systems: synthesis, controlled drug release and delivery, pharmacokinetics and biocompatibility. *J. Mater. Chem., 21*(16), 5845-5855. [http://dx.doi.org/10.1039/c0jm03851b]

Hong, R., Han, G., Fernández, J.M., Kim, B., Forbes, N.S., Rotello, V.M. (2006). Glutathione-mediated delivery and release using monolayer protected nanoparticle carriers. *J. Am. Chem. Soc., 128*(4), 1078-1079. [http://dx.doi.org/10.1021/ja056726i] [PMID: 16433515]

Huang, J.L., Chen, H.Z., Gao, X.L. (2018). Lipid-coated calcium phosphate nanoparticle and beyond: a versatile platform for drug delivery. *J. Drug Target., 26*(5-6), 398-406. [http://dx.doi.org/10.1080/1061186X.2017.1419360] [PMID: 29258343]

Huang, J., Li, Y., Orza, A., Lu, Q., Guo, P., Wang, L., Yang, L., Mao, H. (2016). Magnetic nanoparticle facilitated drug delivery for cancer therapy with targeted and image-guided approaches. *Adv. Funct. Mater., 26*(22), 3818-3836. [http://dx.doi.org/10.1002/adfm.201504185] [PMID: 27790080]

Iturrioz-Rodríguez, N., Correa-Duarte, M.A., Fanarraga, M.L. (2019). Controlled drug delivery systems for cancer based on mesoporous silica nanoparticles. *Int. J. Nanomedicine, 14*, 3389-3401. [http://dx.doi.org/10.2147/IJN.S198848] [PMID: 31190798]

Jafari, S., Adibkia, K. (2015). Application of hydroxyapatite nanoparticle in the drug delivery systems. *J. Mol. Pharm. Org. Process Res., 3*(1), 1-2. [http://dx.doi.org/10.4172/2329-9053.1000e118]

Jeong, E.H., Jung, G., Hong, C.A., Lee, H. (2014). Gold nanoparticle (AuNP)-based drug delivery and molecular imaging for biomedical applications. *Arch. Pharm. Res., 37*(1), 53-59. [http://dx.doi.org/10.1007/s12272-013-0273-5] [PMID: 24214174]

Kamaly, N., Yameen, B., Wu, J., Farokhzad, O.C. (2016). Degradable controlled-release polymers and polymeric nanoparticles: mechanisms of controlling drug release. *Chem. Rev., 116*(4), 2602-2663. [http://dx.doi.org/10.1021/acs.chemrev.5b00346] [PMID: 26854975]

Karimi, M., Mirshekari, H., Aliakbari, M., Sahandi-Zangabad, P., Hamblin, M.R. (2016). Smart mesoporous silica nanoparticles for controlled-release drug delivery. *Nanotechnol. Rev., 5*(2), 195-207. [http://dx.doi.org/10.1515/ntrev-2015-0057]

Kazemi, F., Naghib, S.M. (2020). *Smart controlled release of corrosion inhibitor from normal and stimuli-responsive micro/nanocarriers. Corrosion Protection at the Nanoscale.*. Elsevier.

Kempe, H., Kates, S.A., Kempe, M. (2011). Nanomedicine's promising therapy: magnetic drug targeting. *Expert Rev. Med. Devices, 8*(3), 291-294.
[http://dx.doi.org/10.1586/erd.10.94] [PMID: 21542699]

Khan, A.K., Rashid, R., Murtaza, G., Zahra, A. (2014). Gold nanoparticles: synthesis and applications in drug delivery. *Trop. J. Pharm. Res., 13*(7), 1169-1177.
[http://dx.doi.org/10.4314/tjpr.v13i7.23]

Kohane, D.S. (2007). Microparticles and nanoparticles for drug delivery. *Biotechnol. Bioeng., 96*(2), 203-209.
[http://dx.doi.org/10.1002/bit.21301] [PMID: 17191251]

Kong, F.Y., Zhang, J.W., Li, R.F., Wang, Z.X., Wang, W.J., Wang, W. (2017). Unique roles of gold nanoparticles in drug delivery, targeting and imaging applications. *Molecules, 22*(9), 1445.
[http://dx.doi.org/10.3390/molecules22091445] [PMID: 28858253]

Kumar, C.S.S.R., Mohammad, F. (2011). Magnetic nanomaterials for hyperthermia-based therapy and controlled drug delivery. *Adv. Drug Deliv. Rev., 63*(9), 789-808.
[http://dx.doi.org/10.1016/j.addr.2011.03.008] [PMID: 21447363]

Kwon, S., Singh, R.K., Perez, R.A., Abou Neel, E.A., Kim, H.W., Chrzanowski, W. (2013). Silica-based mesoporous nanoparticles for controlled drug delivery. *J. Tissue Eng., 4*
[http://dx.doi.org/10.1177/2041731413503357] [PMID: 24020012]

Latorre, A., Couleaud, P., Aires, A., Cortajarena, A.L., Somoza, Á. (2014). Multifunctionalization of magnetic nanoparticles for controlled drug release: A general approach. *Eur. J. Med. Chem., 82*, 355-362.
[http://dx.doi.org/10.1016/j.ejmech.2014.05.078] [PMID: 24927055]

Laurent, S., Forge, D., Port, M., Roch, A., Robic, C., Vander Elst, L., Muller, R.N. (2008). Magnetic iron oxide nanoparticles: synthesis, stabilization, vectorization, physicochemical characterizations, and biological applications. *Chem. Rev., 108*(6), 2064-2110.
[http://dx.doi.org/10.1021/cr068445e] [PMID: 18543879]

Lee, J.E., Lee, N., Kim, H., Kim, J., Choi, S.H., Kim, J.H., Kim, T., Song, I.C., Park, S.P., Moon, W.K., Hyeon, T. (2010). Uniform mesoporous dye-doped silica nanoparticles decorated with multiple magnetite nanocrystals for simultaneous enhanced magnetic resonance imaging, fluorescence imaging, and drug delivery. *J. Am. Chem. Soc., 132*(2), 552-557.
[http://dx.doi.org/10.1021/ja905793q] [PMID: 20017538]

Levingstone, T.J., Herbaj, S., Dunne, N.J. (2019). Calcium phosphate nanoparticles for therapeutic applications in bone regeneration. *Nanomaterials (Basel), 9*(11), 1570.
[http://dx.doi.org/10.3390/nano9111570] [PMID: 31698700]

Linsley, C.S., Wu, B.M. (2017). Recent advances in light-responsive on-demand drug-delivery systems. *Ther. Deliv., 8*(2), 89-107.
[http://dx.doi.org/10.4155/tde-2016-0060] [PMID: 28088880]

Mandracchia, D., Tripodo, G. (2020). Micro and nano-drug delivery systems. In: Bari, E., Perteghella, S., Torre, M.L., (Eds.), *Silk-based Drug Delivery Systems.* RSC Publishing.
[http://dx.doi.org/10.1039/9781839162664-00001]

Manzano, M., Vallet-Regí, M. (2020). Mesoporous silica nanoparticles for drug delivery. *Adv. Funct. Mater., 30*(2), 1902634.
[http://dx.doi.org/10.1002/adfm.201902634]

McBain, S.C., Yiu, H.H., Dobson, J. (2008). Magnetic nanoparticles for gene and drug delivery. *Int. J. Nanomedicine, 3*(2), 169-180.
[PMID: 18686777]

Mirzaei, M., Zarch, M.B., Darroudi, M., Sayyadi, K., Keshavarz, S.T., Sayyadi, J., Fallah, A., Maleki, H. (2020). Silica Mesoporous Structures: Effective Nanocarriers in Drug Delivery and Nanocatalysts. *Appl. Sci. (Basel), 10*(21), 7533.

[http://dx.doi.org/10.3390/app10217533]

Mishra, D., Hubenak, J.R., Mathur, A.B. (2013). Nanoparticle systems as tools to improve drug delivery and therapeutic efficacy. *J. Biomed. Mater. Res. A, 101*(12), 3646-3660.
[http://dx.doi.org/10.1002/jbm.a.34642] [PMID: 23878102]

Misra, R.D.K. (2008). Magnetic nanoparticle carrier for targeted drug delivery: perspective, outlook and design. *Mater. Sci. Technol., 24*(9), 1011-1019.
[http://dx.doi.org/10.1179/174328408X341690]

Mody, V.V., Cox, A., Shah, S., Singh, A., Bevins, W., Parihar, H. (2014). Magnetic nanoparticle drug delivery systems for targeting tumor. *Appl. Nanosci., 4*(4), 385-392.
[http://dx.doi.org/10.1007/s13204-013-0216-y]

Mukherjee, S., Liang, L., Veiseh, O. (2020). Recent advancements of magnetic nanomaterials in cancer therapy. *Pharmaceutics, 12*(2), 147.
[http://dx.doi.org/10.3390/pharmaceutics12020147] [PMID: 32053995]

Murali, R., Vidhya, P., Thanikaivelan, P. (2014). Thermoresponsive magnetic nanoparticle – Aminated guar gum hydrogel system for sustained release of doxorubicin hydrochloride. *Carbohydr. Polym., 110*, 440-445.
[http://dx.doi.org/10.1016/j.carbpol.2014.04.076] [PMID: 24906777]

Murugan, B., Sagadevan, S., J, A.L., Fatimah, I., Fatema, K.N., Oh, W.C., Mohammad, F., Johan, M.R. (2020). Role of mesoporous silica nanoparticles for the drug delivery applications. *Mater. Res. Express, 7*(10), 102002.
[http://dx.doi.org/10.1088/2053-1591/abbf7e]

Naghib, S.M., Kazemi, F. (2020). pH-responsive controlled release of corrosion inhibitor from nanocarriers/nanocapsules. *Corrosion Protection at the Nanoscale..* Elsevier.

Norris, M.D., Seidel, K., Kirschning, A. (2019). Externally induced drug release systems with magnetic nanoparticle carriers: an emerging field in nanomedicine. *Adv. Ther. (Weinh.), 2*(1), 1800092.
[http://dx.doi.org/10.1002/adtp.201800092]

Obaidat, I.M., Narayanaswamy, V., Alaabed, S., Sambasivam, S., Muralee Gopi, C.V.V. (2019). Principles of Magnetic Hyperthermia: A Focus on Using Multifunctional Hybrid Magnetic Nanoparticles. *Magnetochemistry, 5*(4), 67.
[http://dx.doi.org/10.3390/magnetochemistry5040067]

Ou, Y.C., Webb, J.A., Faley, S., Shae, D., Talbert, E.M., Lin, S., Cutright, C.C., Wilson, J.T., Bellan, L.M., Bardhan, R. (2016). Gold nanoantenna-mediated photothermal drug delivery from thermosensitive liposomes in breast cancer. *ACS Omega, 1*(2), 234-243.
[http://dx.doi.org/10.1021/acsomega.6b00079] [PMID: 27656689]

Patra, J., Das, G., Fraceto, L., Campos, E.V.R., Rodriguez-Torres, M.P., Acosta-Torres, L.S., Diaz-Torres, L.A., Grillo, R., Swamy, M.K., Sharma, S., Habtemariam, S., Shin, H.S. (2018). Nano based drug delivery systems: Recent developments and Future Prospects. 16, 71.

Patra, J.K., Das, G., Fraceto, L.F., Campos, E.V.R., Rodriguez-Torres, M.P., Acosta-Torres, L.S., Diaz-Torres, L.A., Grillo, R., Swamy, M.K., Sharma, S., Habtemariam, S., Shin, H.S. (2018). Nano based drug delivery systems: recent developments and future prospects. *J. Nanobiotechnology, 16*(1), 71.
[http://dx.doi.org/10.1186/s12951-018-0392-8] [PMID: 30231877]

Pissuwan, D., Niidome, T., Cortie, M.B. (2011). The forthcoming applications of gold nanoparticles in drug and gene delivery systems. *J. Control. Release, 149*(1), 65-71.
[http://dx.doi.org/10.1016/j.jconrel.2009.12.006] [PMID: 20004222]

Poon, L., Zandberg, W., Hsiao, D., Erno, Z., Sen, D., Gates, B.D., Branda, N.R. (2010). Photothermal release of single-stranded DNA from the surface of gold nanoparticles through controlled denaturating and Au-S bond breaking. *ACS Nano, 4*(11), 6395-6403.
[http://dx.doi.org/10.1021/nn1016346] [PMID: 20958080]

Price, P.M., Mahmoud, W.E., Al-Ghamdi, A.A., Bronstein, L.M. (2018). Magnetic drug delivery: Where the

field is going. *Front Chem., 6,* 619.
[http://dx.doi.org/10.3389/fchem.2018.00619] [PMID: 30619827]

Rahmanian, M., seyfoori, A., Dehghan, M.M., Eini, L., Naghib, S.M., Gholami, H., Farzad Mohajeri, S., Mamaghani, K.R., Majidzadeh-A, K. (2019). Multifunctional gelatin–tricalcium phosphate porous nanocomposite scaffolds for tissue engineering and local drug delivery: *In vitro* and *in vivo* studies. *J. Taiwan Inst. Chem. Eng., 101,* 214-220.
[http://dx.doi.org/10.1016/j.jtice.2019.04.028]

Rajani, C., Borisa, P., Karanwad, T., Borade, Y., Patel, V., Rajpoot, K., Tekade, R.K. (2020). Cancer-targeted chemotherapy: Emerging role of the folate anchored dendrimer as drug delivery nanocarrier. *Pharmaceutical Applications of Dendrimers..* Elsevier.

Raza, A., Rasheed, T., Nabeel, F., Hayat, U., Bilal, M., Iqbal, H. (2019). Endogenous and exogenous stimuli-responsive drug delivery systems for programmed site-specific release. *Molecules, 24*(6), 1117.
[http://dx.doi.org/10.3390/molecules24061117] [PMID: 30901827]

Rivera, V., Ferri, F., Marega, E., jr (2012). Localized surface plasmon resonances: noble metal nanoparticle interaction with rare-earth ions. *Plasmonics-Principles and Applications., 283,* 312.

Saha, B., Bhattacharya, J., Mukherjee, A., Ghosh, A., Santra, C., Dasgupta, A.K., Karmakar, P. (2007). *In vitro* structural and functional evaluation of gold nanoparticles conjugated antibiotics. *Nanoscale Res. Lett., 2*(12), 614.
[http://dx.doi.org/10.1007/s11671-007-9104-2]

Sanadgol, N., Wackerlig, J. (2020). Developments of Smart Drug-Delivery Systems Based on Magnetic Molecularly Imprinted Polymers for Targeted Cancer Therapy: A Short Review. *Pharmaceutics, 12*(9), 831.
[http://dx.doi.org/10.3390/pharmaceutics12090831] [PMID: 32878127]

Sartipzadeh, O., Naghib, S.M., Shokati, F., Rahmanian, M., Majidzadeh-A, K., Zare, Y., Rhee, K.Y. (2020). Microfluidic-assisted synthesis and modelling of monodispersed magnetic nanocomposites for biomedical applications. *Nanotechnol. Rev., 9*(1), 1397-1407.
[http://dx.doi.org/10.1515/ntrev-2020-0097]

Selvarajan, V., Obuobi, S., Ee, P.L.R. (2020). Silica Nanoparticles—A Versatile Tool for the Treatment of Bacterial Infections. *Front Chem., 8,* 602.
[http://dx.doi.org/10.3389/fchem.2020.00602] [PMID: 32760699]

Sensenig, R., Sapir, Y., MacDonald, C., Cohen, S., Polyak, B. (2012). Magnetic nanoparticle-based approaches to locally target therapy and enhance tissue regeneration *in vivo. Nanomedicine (Lond.), 7*(9), 1425-1442.
[http://dx.doi.org/10.2217/nnm.12.109] [PMID: 22994959]

Seyfoori, A., Ebrahimi, S.A.S., Omidian, S., Naghib, S.M. (2019). Multifunctional magnetic $ZnFe_2O_4$-hydroxyapatite nanocomposite particles for local anti-cancer drug delivery and bacterial infection inhibition: An *in vitro* study. *J. Taiwan Inst. Chem. Eng., 96,* 503-508.
[http://dx.doi.org/10.1016/j.jtice.2018.10.018]

Shen, B., Ma, Y., Yu, S., Ji, C. (2016). Smart multifunctional magnetic nanoparticle-based drug delivery system for cancer thermo-chemotherapy and intracellular imaging. *ACS Appl. Mater. Interfaces, 8*(37), 24502-24508.
[http://dx.doi.org/10.1021/acsami.6b09772] [PMID: 27573061]

Singh, R., Lillard, J.W., Jr (2009). Nanoparticle-based targeted drug delivery. *Exp. Mol. Pathol., 86*(3), 215-223.
[http://dx.doi.org/10.1016/j.yexmp.2008.12.004] [PMID: 19186176]

Slowing, I., Viveroescoto, J., Wu, C., Lin, V. (2008). Mesoporous silica nanoparticles as controlled release drug delivery and gene transfection carriers. *Adv. Drug Deliv. Rev., 60*(11), 1278-1288.
[http://dx.doi.org/10.1016/j.addr.2008.03.012] [PMID: 18514969]

Sun, X. (2012). Mesoporous silica nanoparticles for applications in drug delivery and catalysis. *Graduate*

Theses and Dissertations., 12812.
[http://dx.doi.org/10.31274/etd-180810-1595]

Sung, J.C., Pulliam, B.L., Edwards, D.A. (2007). Nanoparticles for drug delivery to the lungs. *Trends Biotechnol., 25*(12), 563-570.
[http://dx.doi.org/10.1016/j.tibtech.2007.09.005] [PMID: 17997181]

Syamchand, S.S., Sony, G. (2015). Multifunctional hydroxyapatite nanoparticles for drug delivery and multimodal molecular imaging. *Mikrochim. Acta, 182*(9-10), 1567-1589.
[http://dx.doi.org/10.1007/s00604-015-1504-x]

Tang, F., Li, L., Chen, D. (2012). Mesoporous silica nanoparticles: synthesis, biocompatibility and drug delivery. *Adv. Mater., 24*(12), 1504-1534.
[http://dx.doi.org/10.1002/adma.201104763] [PMID: 22378538]

Tomatsu, I., Peng, K., Kros, A. (2011). Photoresponsive hydrogels for biomedical applications. *Adv. Drug Deliv. Rev., 63*(14-15), 1257-1266.
[http://dx.doi.org/10.1016/j.addr.2011.06.009] [PMID: 21745509]

Tran, N., Webster, T.J. (2010). Magnetic nanoparticles: biomedical applications and challenges. *J. Mater. Chem., 20*(40), 8760-8767.
[http://dx.doi.org/10.1039/c0jm00994f]

Turon, P., del Valle, L., Alemán, C., Puiggalí, J. (2017). Biodegradable and biocompatible systems based on hydroxyapatite nanoparticles. *Appl. Sci. (Basel), 7*(1), 60.
[http://dx.doi.org/10.3390/app7010060]

Valente, F., Astolfi, L., Simoni, E., Danti, S., Franceschini, V., Chicca, M., Martini, A. (2017). Nanoparticle drug delivery systems for inner ear therapy: An overview. *J. Drug Deliv. Sci. Technol., 39*, 28-35.
[http://dx.doi.org/10.1016/j.jddst.2017.03.003]

Vallabani, N. S., Singh, S. (2018). Recent advances and future prospects of iron oxide nanoparticles in biomedicine and diagnostics. *3 Biotech, 8*, 1-23.

Vallet-Regí, M., Colilla, M., Izquierdo-Barba, I., Manzano, M. (2017). Mesoporous silica nanoparticles for drug delivery: current insights. *Molecules, 23*(1), 47.
[http://dx.doi.org/10.3390/molecules23010047] [PMID: 29295564]

Vangijzegem, T., Stanicki, D., Laurent, S. (2019). Magnetic iron oxide nanoparticles for drug delivery: applications and characteristics. *Expert Opin. Drug Deliv., 16*(1), 69-78.
[http://dx.doi.org/10.1080/17425247.2019.1554647] [PMID: 30496697]

Vivero-Escoto, J.L., Slowing, I.I., Trewyn, B.G., Lin, V.S.Y. (2010). Mesoporous silica nanoparticles for intracellular controlled drug delivery. *Small, 6*(18), 1952-1967.
[http://dx.doi.org/10.1002/smll.200901789] [PMID: 20690133]

Wang, X., Zhang, M., Zhang, L., Li, L., Li, S., Wang, C., Su, Z., Yuan, Y., Pan, W. (2017). Designed Synthesis of Lipid-Coated Polyacrylic Acid/Calcium Phosphate Nanoparticles as Dual pH-Responsive Drug-Delivery Vehicles for Cancer Chemotherapy. *Chemistry, 23*(27), 6586-6595.
[http://dx.doi.org/10.1002/chem.201700060] [PMID: 28218434]

Wang, Y., Zhao, Q., Han, N., Bai, L., Li, J., Liu, J., Che, E., Hu, L., Zhang, Q., Jiang, T., Wang, S. (2015). Mesoporous silica nanoparticles in drug delivery and biomedical applications. *Nanomedicine, 11*(2), 313-327.
[http://dx.doi.org/10.1016/j.nano.2014.09.014] [PMID: 25461284]

Watermann, A., Brieger, J. (2017). Mesoporous silica nanoparticles as drug delivery vehicles in cancer. *Nanomaterials (Basel), 7*(7), 189.
[http://dx.doi.org/10.3390/nano7070189] [PMID: 28737672]

Wu, G., Fang, Y.Z., Yang, S., Lupton, J.R., Turner, N.D. (2004). Glutathione metabolism and its implications for health. *J. Nutr., 134*(3), 489-492.

[http://dx.doi.org/10.1093/jn/134.3.489] [PMID: 14988435]

Wu, H., Song, L., Chen, L., Huang, Y., Wu, Y., Zang, F., An, Y., Lyu, H., Ma, M., Chen, J., Gu, N., Zhang, Y. (2017). Injectable thermosensitive magnetic nanoemulsion hydrogel for multimodal-imaging-guided accurate thermoablative cancer therapy. *Nanoscale, 9*(42), 16175-16182.
[http://dx.doi.org/10.1039/C7NR02858J] [PMID: 28770920]

Yang, Y.H., Liu, C.H., Liang, Y.H., Lin, F.H., Wu, K.C.W. (2013). Hollow mesoporous hydroxyapatite nanoparticles (hmHANPs) with enhanced drug loading and pH-responsive release properties for intracellular drug delivery. *J. Mater. Chem. B Mater. Biol. Med., 1*(19), 2447-2450.
[http://dx.doi.org/10.1039/c3tb20365d] [PMID: 32261043]

You, J., Zhang, G., Li, C. (2010). Exceptionally high payload of doxorubicin in hollow gold nanospheres for near-infrared light-triggered drug release. *ACS Nano, 4*(2), 1033-1041.
[http://dx.doi.org/10.1021/nn901181c] [PMID: 20121065]

You, J., Zhang, R., Zhang, G., Zhong, M., Liu, Y., Van Pelt, C.S., Liang, D., Wei, W., Sood, A.K., Li, C. (2012). Photothermal-chemotherapy with doxorubicin-loaded hollow gold nanospheres: A platform for near-infrared light-trigged drug release. *J. Control. Release, 158*(2), 319-328.
[http://dx.doi.org/10.1016/j.jconrel.2011.10.028] [PMID: 22063003]

Yu, S., Wu, G., Gu, X., Wang, J., Wang, Y., Gao, H., Ma, J. (2013). Magnetic and pH-sensitive nanoparticles for antitumor drug delivery. *Colloids Surf. B Biointerfaces, 103*, 15-22.
[http://dx.doi.org/10.1016/j.colsurfb.2012.10.041] [PMID: 23201714]

Zeinali Kalkhoran, A.H., Naghib, S.M., Vahidi, O., Rahmanian, M. (2018). Synthesis and characterization of graphene-grafted gelatin nanocomposite hydrogels as emerging drug delivery systems. *Biomed. Phys. Eng. Express, 4*(5), 055017.
[http://dx.doi.org/10.1088/2057-1976/aad745]

Zeinali Kalkhoran, A.H., Vahidi, O., Naghib, S.M. (2018). A new mathematical approach to predict the actual drug release from hydrogels. *Eur. J. Pharm. Sci., 111*, 303-310.
[http://dx.doi.org/10.1016/j.ejps.2017.09.038] [PMID: 28962856]

Zhang, J., Zhang, H., Jiang, J., Cui, N., Xue, X., Wang, T., Wang, X., He, Y., Wang, D. (2020). Doxorubicin-loaded carbon dots lipid-coated calcium phosphate nanoparticles for visual targeted delivery and therapy of tumor. *Int. J. Nanomedicine, 15*, 433-444.
[http://dx.doi.org/10.2147/IJN.S229154] [PMID: 32021189]

Zhou, S., Wu, D., Yin, X., Jin, X., Zhang, X., Zheng, S., Wang, C., Liu, Y. (2017). Intracellular pH-responsive and rituximab-conjugated mesoporous silica nanoparticles for targeted drug delivery to lymphoma B cells. *J. Exp. Clin. Cancer Res., 36*(1), 24.
[http://dx.doi.org/10.1186/s13046-017-0492-6] [PMID: 28166836]

Zhou, Y., Quan, G., Wu, Q., Zhang, X., Niu, B., Wu, B., Huang, Y., Pan, X., Wu, C. (2018). Mesoporous silica nanoparticles for drug and gene delivery. *Acta Pharm. Sin. B, 8*(2), 165-177.
[http://dx.doi.org/10.1016/j.apsb.2018.01.007] [PMID: 29719777]

CHAPTER 9

Additive Manufacturing in Developing Localized Controlled Drug Delivery Systems (LCDDSs)

Abstract: Patients may show various defects to medications depending on race, gender, fitness, age, pharmacokinetic and health conditions. To address this challenge, there is a need to establish personalized, on-demand, programable and smart carriers that can control drug release with new and robust techniques. Additive manufacturing (AM) is the key sustenance of digital technology that has been developing and growing recently. AM offers several opportunities in localized controlled drug delivery systems (LCDDS), including materials recycling as well as on-site manufacturing, design freedom and full customization. Moreover, the industrial, biomedical and academic requests for AM for LCDDS have been continually rising, demonstrating significant marks for an extensive range of products. This chapter outlines AM approaches and their functions for LCDDS and describes AM technologies, such as recent advances in controlled drug release, as well as their processed materials and working principles. Furthermore, the benefits of 3D printing in the progressions of the LCDDS, the advantages of 4D printing, the impression of designing and material selection in these techniques are discussed. Finally, the potentials of AM approaches and their LCDD applications that designate a promising healthcare future are described.

Keywords: 3D printing, 4D printing, Additive manufacturing, Localized drug delivery, Smart delivery, Stimuli-responsive material.

9.1. INTRODUCTION

Many studies have been conducted for designing drug delivery systems (Kalkhoran *et al.*, 2018, Zeinali Kalkhoran *et al.*, 2018) and manufacturing (Askari *et al.*, 2021b) methods with the aim of increasing drug efficiency and possessing high-quality delivery systems (Agrawal and Gupta, 2019, Gooneh-Farahani *et al.*, 2019a, Gooneh-Farahani *et al.*, 2020, Gooneh-Farahani *et al.*, 2019b). Today, conventional manufacturing methods of delivery systems, including formative (molds) or subtractive (machining) techniques, are not efficient due to their high cost and multiple steps. Therefore, these common methods cannot be used for designing localized drug delivery systems with complex geometries. 3D printing or additive manufacturing (AM) techniques which have been developed over the past four decades, can effectively pave the

Seyed Morteza Naghib, Samin Hoseinpour & Shadi Zarshad

way for the fabrication of complex localized drug delivery systems in a cost-effective and timely manner (Ahangar *et al.*, 2019, Askari *et al.*, 2021a, Rahmanian *et al.*, 2019). 3D printing uses a 3D-digital model and a 3D printer to print one or more materials layer-by-layer. Actually, this method fabricates complex structures by adjusting the shape of each individual layer. The main advantages of this method include a fast, facile, and cost-effective manufacturing process, precise and high control over the shape of the structure, high reproducibility, individualized productions, and no restrictions on the spatial arrangement of the products, making it superior to other methods (Ghilan *et al.*, 2020).

Therefore, 3D printing plays an important role in the fabrication of systems used in the biomedical field, such as complex tissue constructs, customized DDS, soft robots, *etc*. This method enabled researchers to develop high-resolution biomedical systems with multi-material design by combining machine learning and topological optimization algorithms (Tetsuka and Shin, 2020). The attention to the use of 3D printing technology in developing DDSs has increased since 2015 when the Food and Drug Administration (FDA) approved the first printed drug Spritam® as an anti-epileptic tablet with high porosity and ultra-fast dissolving by the patient saliva (Algahtani *et al.*, 2018). In addition to the aforementioned advantages, 3D printing permits the researchers to create delivery systems with accurate dosing, flexible design, and high drug loading capacity compared to the conventional methods. The use of 3D printing in the fabrication of drug delivery systems is apparently cost-effective due to the minimum waste of raw materials, besides the equipment required for this method fits in a small space (Jacob *et al.*, 2020). Therefore, it can be said that the use of 3D printing in developing specifically localized drug delivery systems would maximize the clinical outcome in patients.

Despite numerous advantages of 3D printing, this method also has its challenges and disadvantages, which have to be considered. One of the most important challenges is the fabrication speed. Besides having the appropriate material selection, such as thermoplastic pharmaceutical and medical-grade filaments in 3D printing, it is a challenging process and has its own limitation (Wallis *et al.*, 2020).

In this chapter, the benefits of using 3D printing in the development of the pharmaceutical industry are described. Then 4D printing and the importance of designing and material selection in this method are discussed.

9.2. 3D PRINTING METHODS

Numerical strategies focused on biomedical manufacturing, such as solvent casting, electrospinning, lyophilization, 3D printing, *etc.* (Eltom *et al.*, 2019). "3Dprinting" or additive manufacturing (AM) attempts to build constructs using a computer-controlled layer-by-layer manner. Building 3D biomedical devices includes 4 main steps: 1) creating a digital model obtained from computed tomography (CT) scan or magnetic resonance imaging (MRI), 2) building a CAD model by software, 3) fabricating the construction by adding materials(sometimes including biological agents, cells and growth factors) layer by layer, and 4) post-printing process such as cell seeding (Ventola, 2014).

A better understanding of common 3D printing strategies is the first step in developing and exploiting this method in the context of drug delivery. Generally, inkjet-based printing (IBP), extrusion-based printing (EBP) and light-based printing (LBP) are the three most commonly used printing strategies. Inkjet-based printing (IBP) is a non-contact method in which the printing photo resin or glue is jetted out through the thousands of small print heads. Once the material comprising low-viscosity droplets is solidified, the platform supporting the structure will be lowered, enabling a new layer to be printed on top. This method offers the compositional control of structures and enables the fabrication of heterogeneous and multi-material systems (Zhou *et al.*, 2020). IBP technique uses thermal or piezoelectric actuators, and could be categorized into three main groups: continuous-inkjet printing, electro-hydrodynamic jet printing, and the most common category, drop-on-demand inkjet printing (Derakhshanfar *et al.*, 2018). In thermal inkjet printers, the small printer heads are heated electrically to jet the printing droplets out of the nozzle. The Piezoelectric printer is another type of inkjet printer. During the printing process, a voltage is applied to the piezoelectric crystal inside the printer head, which leads to a quick change in shape to disrupt the bioink into droplets from the nozzle at certain intervals and then cured to form a solid structure (Xie *et al.*, 2020). It is noteworthy that the bio-ink used in IBP must be a liquid with low viscosity (3.5–12 mPa s) (Zhang *et al.*, 2019).

This 3D printing method enables designing DDSs with complex drug release kinetics and entrapping of multi-drug into a single system. Another advantage of IBP is its cost-effectiveness and minimum waste at a high processing rate. Nevertheless, more studies are needed to industrialize this method in the pharmaceuticals field (Pandey *et al.*, 2020).

Another 3D printing method is based on extrusion. This method uses a piston, pneumatic actuator, or screw to feed material into a cartridge and through a nozzle. The range of materials used in this EBP method is wide, but all feature a curing chemical or photoactivated step. The actuators control and regulate the position of the nozzle and material deposition in three dimensions. This method uses supports for printing complex shapes, and manually removing this support material can be problematic. The EBP uses multi-head or multi-nozzle printers for printing multi-material shapes with minimal user input aside from geometry and materials (Placone and Engler, 2018). Fused deposition modeling (FDM) and direct ink writing (DIW) are the most known of the EBP category (Wang *et al.*, 2018).

DIW uses viscoelastic inks in a liquid state, and squeezes them out of the nozzle by pressure. It should be highlighted that the ink properties such as shear thinning and shear strength are critically important because these properties affect the fluid passing through the nozzle and shape stability after ink printing onto the tray. FDM also needs a nozzle and moving platform to create the 3D construction. However, unlike DIW, FDM relies on an extra heater to soften raw material. Besides, the solidifying rate of molten thermoplastic materials is controlled by the fan, located at the end of the nozzle (Liu and Yan, 2018). FDM has gained much attention in pharmaceutical industries, especially in 3D-printed tablets (Uziel *et al.*, 2019). Besides, FDM can be effectively used for printing local drug delivery systems (Yi *et al.*, 2016).

Another main group of 3D printing methods is based on photo-curable polymers and the capability to selectively photo-polymerize them upon laser emissions or projections of light. Based on how the unpolymerized polymer is going to cure, this method is classified as Stereolithography (SLA), two-photon polymerization (TPP), and Digital Light Processing (DLP), (Economidou *et al.*, 2018). SLA is a fast and accurate fabrication method that uses ultraviolet (UV) or visible light to polymerize light-exposed photosensitive polymers in a layer-by-layer manner. This nozzle-free method removes the undesirable properties of shear pressure which exist in nozzle-based printing. It should be noted that photoinitiator (PI) molecules in the uncured resin react to irradiated light, and locally trigger the chemical polymerization response and only treat and solidify desirable areas (Kačarević *et al.*, 2018). The application of SLA method in drug delivery has been studied recently. Some of these systems include drug-loaded scaffolds, torus-shaped tablets, patches, and microneedles. It should be noted that for manufacturing DDSs with higher drug content, the active pharmaceutical ingredient must be sufficiently soluble in the polymer, limiting SLA usage for higher drug loading systems (Palo *et al.*, 2017). In TPP, unlike SLA, the response of the PI in the vat of liquid resin, and thereby activation of the polymerization response, does not occur in the entire illumination pathway of the laser, and only happens in the area of its focal point, named as the volume pixel or voxel. In this method, the molecules absorb two photons simultaneously upon high-intensity femtosecond pulsed laser irradiation, and instead of conventional UV light, a laser such as titanium-sapphire laser with twice the wavelength of near-infrared has been employed (Schmidleithner and Kalaskar, 2018). The advent of the high-resolution TPP method allowed for the fabrication of complex constructs having dimensions in the millimeter scale for drug delivery systems and biomedical applications, without the necessity of laborious and complex fabrication methods (Moussi *et al.*, 2020). Another light-based 3D printing method is DLP which uses a projector to project the image of the cross-section of the desired structure into a photo-curable resin. In DLP, the whole layer is printed simultaneously, so, this method is typically faster than SLA (Knowlton *et al.*, 2017, Quan *et al.*, 2020). Generally, light-based 3D printing is a high-resolution method with no nozzle clogging problem and can be used for making complex fabrications (Vikram Singh *et al.*, 2019). Nonetheless, there are several limitations in SLA, such as the lack of biocompatible and biodegradable polymeric resins, destructive effects of remaining toxic photocuring agents, the inability to entirely remove the supporting materials, and the inability to form horizontal gradients in the fabrications (Li *et al.*, 2016). Fig. (**1**) shows these three bioprinting strategies.

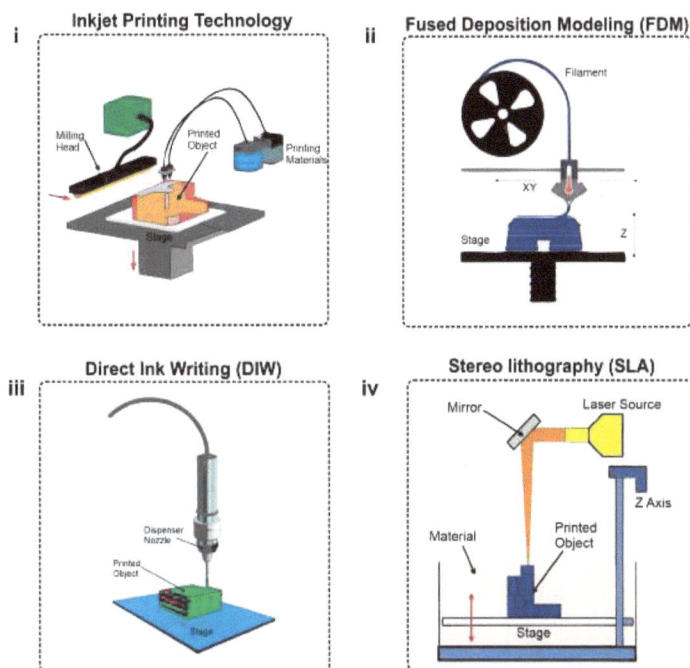

Fig. (1). Schematic of three bioprinting methods. (i) IBP with a thermal or piezoelectric printer; (ii,iii) EBP, (ii) FDM for depositing melted polymers, and (iii) DIW for printing polymer solution, (iv) LBP, including SLA (Gul *et al*, 2018).

In summary, each of the 3D printing methods requires its own conditions and materials. For example, LBP methods utilize photo-sensitive resins with PI, and a cautious choice needs to be made between the emitted wavelength from the light source and how the PI absorbs light and dissolves into the prepolymer resin formulation. Whilst most of the EBP methods utilize thermoplastic filaments. Therefore, the material and printing method selections are important keys in the pharmaceutical field, and the material properties such as stability, biocompatibility, biodegradability, mechanical properties, melting point, glass transition temperature, and non-reactivity with the drug are of great importance (Bird *et al.*, 2019). Table **1** demonstrates a wide range of pharmaceutical formulations that are fabricated by 3D printing methods.

Table 1. Different pharmaceutical formulations synthesized by 3D printing methods.

Type of the 3D Printing Method	Dosage Form	Active Materials	References
FDM and HME	Tablet	Dipyridamole/polyvinylpyrrolidone	(Okwuosa *et al.*, 2016)
FDM	Tablet	Prednisolone/ poly(vinyl alcohol)	(Skowyra *et al.*, 2015)
FDM and HME	Core-shell gastric-resistant tablets	Polyvinylpyrrolidone (PVP) and methacrylic acid co-polymer	(Okwuosa *et al.*, 2017)
SLA	Patch with nose-shape	Salicylic acid/ PEGDA and PEG	(Goyanes *et al.*, 2016)
FDM	Biodegradable microneedle	Polylactic acid	(Luzuriaga *et al.*, 2018)
Inkjet printing	Transdermal microneedles	5-fluororacil, curcumin and cisplatin/ co-polymer of polyvinyl caprolactam–polyvinyl acetate–polyethylene glycol	(Uddin *et al.*, 2015)
FDM	Patch	5-fluororacil /poly(lactide-co-glycolide), polycaprolactone	(Yi *et al.*, 2016)
SLA	Implantable bladder device	Lidocaine hydrochloride/elastic resin	(Xu *et al.*, 2021)
Inkjet printing	Tablet	Fenofibrate/ beeswax	(Kyobula *et al.*, 2017)
SLA	Tablet	4-aminosalicylic acid and paracetamol (acetaminophen)/ PEGDA	(Wang *et al.*, 2016)
DLP	Transdermal microneedles	Diclofenac sodium/ PEGDA	(Kundu *et al.*, 2020)
FDM and HME	Tablet	HPC, Eudragit® RL PO, and PEG	(Tan *et al.*, 2020)

9.3   THE   ROLE   OF   3D   PRINTING   IN   DEVELOPING   AND FABRICATING DDSS

Table **1** demonstrates a wide range of pharmaceutical formulations that are fabricated by 3D printing methods. As mentioned before, 3D printing is an effective method with significant advantages for developing and fabricating drug delivery systems, due to its high speed of fabrication, accuracy, and the possibility of creating versatile and complex constructs. In addition, this method allows the preparation of DDSs according to the patient's needs, such as implantable drug delivery devices. Conventional manufacturing methods are unable to create tailored dosage forms with adjusted release profiles, besides they can lead to constructs with disparate properties, whilst the three-dimensional method can result in the final products with similar qualities such as similar release profile of drugs, drug dosage, and the stability of the drug. So, 3D printing paves the way for overcoming disadvantages in conventional manufacturing methods. The extrusion-based techniques still excel compared to the other printing methods (Horst, 2018). 3D-printed shell-core enteric tablets use CAD software to create a digital model of the tablet structure and export it into STL files. The printer used in this study is composed of dual FDM 3D with two diverse filaments for the enteric shell and the core. Theophylline with great solubility in acidic conditions was utilized as a model drug (Okwuosa *et al.*, 2017).

Numerous dosage forms such as transdermal, implantable, oral, rectal, vaginal, suppositories, intrauterine devices, and surgical stents are used to provide drugs for local and systemic therapeutic effects. The traditional manufacturing procedures need greatly skilled techniques for fabricating the above-mentioned drug delivery systems, especially for complex implantable systems, where the resulting construct needs to be able to exactly fit within the physiological structure. Using CAD software in the 3D printing method leads to devices with precise dimensional requirements to fit within the patient's anatomy or body cavity. So 3D printing would be a reliable and helpful method for designing localized drug delivery systems (Beg *et al.*, 2020). 3D printing as a fast and accurate method has a great future in controlling oral tablets to be personalized in a different structure. In this context, 3D printing can be employed for modifying the dose of tablets by changing the software setting. For people who have swallowing difficulties and the pediatric population, there is a specific requirement for a wide range of doses and shapes. Additive manufacturing techniques can engineer the oral medication according to the patient's requirement and propose more flexibility for treatments (Kotta *et al.*, 2018, Mohammed *et al.*, 2020).

3D printing can be employed for developing transdermal systems to deliver the drug through the skin. These systems are used for patients with chronic diseases such as diabetes and can be beneficial to escape first-pass metabolism and/or pH-mediated degradation. Additive manufacturing could be exploited for the fabrication of multilayered transdermal patches and drug-loaded microneedles for transdermal delivery. Drug-loaded microneedles are commonly less than 500 mm in height and are expected to enter the stratum corneum (10–15 mm) to release the drugs (Prasad and Smyth, 2016, Camović *et al.*, 2019). As an instance, Luzuriaga *et al.* utilized the FDM method for 3D printing of drug-loaded microneedles using PLA as a thermoplastic, biodegradable, and FDA-approved polymer. They showed how the height of the printed microneedle may be adjusted by exploiting post-treatment chemical etching, to produce needles with tip with sizes in the range of 1 – 55 μm. These drug-loaded microneedles can successfully penetrate and break off into porcine skin, and their degradability allows them to release drugs over time (Luzuriaga *et al.*, 2018).

Additive manufacturing can also be used to fabricate implantable drug delivery systems with modified drug release profiles (Moussi *et al.*, 2019). Scaffolds are the min group of implantable delivery systems which deliver high drug concentrations to the target site. As an example, scaffold-based delivery systems are used to stimulate the recovery of bone conditions and prevent infections. Generally, drug release from implantable systems can be categorized into physical & chemical systems. The physical-based delivery system works by absorption of the drugs through a particular polymeric matrix or coating. As an instance, stents with drug-loaded coatings are employed as drug delivery systems. In these devices, the thickness of the coating regulates the drug release profile. On the other hand, chemical systems are based on methods such as degradation, swallowing vehicles, or splitting chemically bound drugs. The swelling ratio of chemical-based delivery systems such as hydrogels is modified with the change in environmental features such as temperature and pH (Mohammed *et al.*, 2020). Implantable DDSs can be designed in precise architecture to deliver high concentrations of drugs to the target site for a long time (Elkasabgy *et al.*, 2020, Huang *et al.*, 2007). As an instance, Wang *et al.* printed poly L-lactic acid (PLLA)-based implant as a localized drug delivery system for sustained release of anticancer drugs to treat osteosarcoma. This research group used 3D printing to create a biodegradable, and biocompatible implant with favorable physical properties. (Wang *et al.*, 2020). In another study, Sun *et al.* used DIW for the fabrication of the degradable calcium phosphate scaffold. This Porous delivery system is loaded with berberine as an antibacterial agent, and used for the regeneration of jaw bone. This research group proposed 3D printing to customize the physical properties of this implantable system, such as porosity, shape, and size. The antimicrobial release kinetics in this berberine-loaded scaffold was adjusted by the cross-linking degree of the scaffold (Sun *et al.*, 2020).

Additive manufacturing can be used for printing the vaginal drug delivery systems in different shapes and medication concentrations for delivering hormones to the vagina. Fu *et al.* used FDM for printing progesterone-loaded vaginal rings in different "O", "Y" or "M"-shapes. This localized delivery system was used for the sustained release of progesterone for more than 7 days with diffusion-controlled release performance (Fu *et al.*, 2018).

3D printing is also proposed for developing drug-loaded stents. One of the key advantages of 3D printed stents, in contrast to the other ones, is the customized construction based on the patient's needs. Patient-specific 3D printed stents are designed according to the airway anatomy with precise size and shape to prevent issues with regular stents (Cheng *et al.*, 2017). In a study, an antibiotic-loaded stent was designed precisely according to the patient's anatomy to treat obstructive salivary gland disease. In this process, PCL and AMOX/CTX were mixed successfully as the base material and antibiotic agents, respectively, and the stent was printed precisely using CAD software. In this study, the antibiotic agents did not lose their activity during the printing process, and each of the antibacterial agents was successfully released from the system in a prolonged controlled manner (Kim *et al.*, 2019).

Additive manufacturing permits the fabrication of small self-emulsifying suppositories composed of a precise dose of the medication with a desired size and shape for rectal drug delivery purposes (Seoane-Viaño *et al.*, 2020). As an instance, Persaud *et al.* fabricated a rectal suppository, consisting of a polyvinylalcohol (PVA) shell filled with a PEG/artesunate mixture. This research group designed the above-mentioned localized delivery system using the FDM 3D printer (Persaud *et al.*, 2020). Additive manufacturing is also practicable in the manufacture of drug-loaded patches with customized flexibility, geometry, and release profile, Yi *et al.* fabricated an anticancer-loaded patch for localized drug delivery to the target site of a tumor. The introduced 3D printed patch contained a combination of poly(lactide-co-glycolide), polycaprolactone, and 5-fluorouracil for sustained drug release over four weeks (Yi *et al.*, 2016).

As mentioned, additive manufacturing can be exploited for drug-loaded devices with customized geometry and size for every patient. This strategy may be used to create personalized systems for localized drug delivery. For instance, Muwaffak *et al.* used a 3D scanner to scan a patient's nose and design a personalized wound dressing including zinc, silver, and copper as anti-microbial agents. This custom-made wound dressing remained in the wound position and had many advantages compared to flat dressings (Trenfield *et al.*, 2019).

3D printing can be successfully used to fabricate colonic drug delivery systems with multi-layered polymeric materials. These systems commonly use the covalent linkage of a medication with a vehicle, and the drug release at the target site occurs due to the changing of pH-dependent solubility, swelling or erosion, and degradation of vehicles by the colonic enzymes. In colonic drug delivery systems, the material selection, manufacturing process, and multiple coating layers are the key parameters to prevent drug release in undesired gastrointestinal tract sites (Jacob *et al.*, 2020). As an instance, for delivering budesonide to the upper small intestine and to the colon, Goyanes *et al.* used FDM 3D printing, hot-melt extrusion, and fluid bed coating to create budesonide-loaded PVA filaments. The functionality of the mentioned tablets was compared with the default preparation like Entocort. It was shown that 3D-printed tablets provide sustained release of the drug till it reaches the colon (Charbe *et al.*, 2017). This method can be effectively used to produce the colon-drug delivery system with gastro-resistant properties by coating the drug-loaded tablet with a polymer like Eudragit L100A (Goyanes *et al.*, 2015). Further, Mohammed *et al.* demonstrated the different types of 3D printed dosage forms (Mohammed *et al.*, 2020).

9.4. FROM 3D PRINTING TO 4D PRINTING

Despite the promising advantages of 3D printing, the 3D printed constructs have a static and inanimate nature with no functional variation across directions or time (Lui *et al.*, 2019, Morouço *et al.*, 2017). Thus, it is required to create 3D printed constructs with dynamic properties, which allows us to produce complex structures for different applications. To this end, four-dimensional (4D) printing uses stimuli-responsive materials (also referred as "intelligent," "smart," "stimuli-sensitive," or "environmentally sensitive") as bio-ink to produce biologically dynamic constructs with the ability to change their physical and/or chemical properties in response to a specific trigger (Morouço *et al.*, 2017).

4D printing is an extension of the 3D printing concept with the addition of "time" as a fourth dimension. The transformation over time exhibited excellent functionality for biomedical applications. In other words, this approach could be potentially useful for creating constructs capable of changing shape and functionality over time after being triggered by external stimuli, such as temperature, moisture, electrical and magnetic fields, light, pH, or a combination of these stimuli. Stimuli-responsive materials with the ability to respond to a trigger have a great potential to be used as bioinks in 4D-bioprinting. The printability and biocompatibility of these materials are the key parameters for having a successful 4D bio-printing process (Ashammakhi *et al.*, 2018). 4D bioprinting has a good future in developing complex structures in the field of tissue engineering, drug delivery, and consumer products, besides 4D printing does not need any support materials during the printing process (Saritha and Boyina, 2021, Bajpai *et al.*, 2020). 4D printing has shown interesting promise in developing implantable systems with great shape control after printing by using stimuli-responsive materials. This approach successfully promoted seamless integration and minimally invasive surgery during implantation. Thus, material selection and the designing process are two key parameters in the 4D printing technology. Fig. (**1**) shows 4D printing basics and its process (Pei *et al.*, 2017).

It should be highlighted that both 3D printing and 4D printing utilize additive manufacturing principles to create constructs in a layer-by-layer manner. However, the shape, size, and functionality of the 4D printed constructs can be engineered by the use of smart components, environment condition, and designing processes that are programmed for scheduled transformation (*e.g.*, swelling, folding, bending, or twisting) over time after printing. Whilst the 3D printed constructs were composed of static materials that were located at the predefined positions during the fabrication process (Lui *et al.*, 2019). There is a big interest in designing smart drug delivery systems with the ability to release drugs to the target site at a specific time. 4D printing paves the way for creating smart constructs that can change their own spatial dissemination for entrapping and release of drug/gene in a programmable manner. As an example, drugs can be encapsulated into an unfolded construct, and the structure can self-fold/self-unfold for the protection/release of drugs in response to micro-environmental changes (Lukin *et al.*, 2019).

As mentioned before, material selection is a key parameter in developing 4D printing. Shape memory polymers (SMP) are one of the most applicable materials in 4D printing (Layani *et al.*, 2018). Shape memory polymers are a subset of smart materials capable of being deformed from programmed shape ("temporary shape") to the remembered shape ("permanent shape"). The temporary shape is obtained by mechanical deformation and subsequent fixation of that deformation. Transformation or reversion to the initial shape occurs when the SMP is subjected to external stimuli like heat or light. (Behl and Lendlein, 2000).

Thermo-induced SMPs are the most investigated polymers in 4D bio-printing. The programming of these polymers has 4 steps, including 1) increasing the temperature above the critical temperature such as glass transition temperature, 2) applying external force and deformation, 3) fixing the temporary shape followed by cooling down, and 4) removing the external force. SMPs consist of two segments, netpoints and molecular switches as hard and soft segments, respectively. The basic role of net points in SMPs is storing the permanent shape. This segment can have a chemical or physical nature like covalent cross-links or crystalline domains, whilst the switching segments actuate transformation. It is noteworthy that the shape memory effect may not be activated in the body environment if the transition temperature is higher than the body temperature (Wang *et al.*, 2017, Kan *et al.*, 2018). SMPs can play an important role in developing biomedical devices such as implantable systems. In these systems, the transition temperature must be around body temperature (37 °C), and programming occurs before implantation. The new orientation of the polymer chains reduces the entropy of the system, so the new shape is at a higher energy level. The polymer chains are rigid; therefore, the construct does not return to its relaxed shape below the transition temperature. But after implantation, the programmed shape will recover its remembered shape due to the heating in the body environment and entropic recovery of the net points (Hasan *et al.*, 2016). There is a strong interest in using SMPs for a variety of biomedical applications such as medical devices like self-tightening surgical sutures, the regeneration of damaged tissue by self-deploying structures, micro-grippers in drug delivery, and more (Hearon *et al.*, 2015, Liu *et al.*, 2007, Zhang *et al.*, 2014).

In recent years, drug-loaded stents were developed as a system for localized drug delivery (Tsuji *et al.*, 2003). There is a strong interest in using SMPs for developing 4D printed stents. 4D printing is introduced to recover the defects in ordinary stents like stent migration and stent fracture. As an example, Zarek *et al.* fabricated a polycaprolactone dimethacrylate (PCL) based endoluminal stent using SLA printing. The printed stent enters the body in its temporary form and recovers its permanent shape, matching trachea anatomy, within 14 seconds at normal body temperature (Zarek *et al.*, 2017).

SMPs can be used for printing smart systems with complicated roles in the body environment, and this concept would be useful for designing complicated drug delivery systems. In this context, Miao *et al.* created a thermally actuated nerve guidance conduit composed of graphene hybrid for entubulation and guiding axonal regrowth purposes. This 4D reprogrammable conduit exhibited flat-rolling transformation at body temperature and would be useful for wrapping damaged nerves and facilitating surgical operations (Miao *et al.*, 2018b).

Natural SMPs as novel biocompatible inks have gained a high tendency in recent years. Miao *et al.* demonstrated that an SOEA-based cardiac patch with significant cardiomyogenesis could be realized by employing a novel photolithographic-stereolithographic tandem strategy. This shape-memory patch would be useful for applications requiring minimally invasive procedures and seamless integration with damaged tissues. Besides, the above-mentioned patch could be loaded with drugs for localized drug delivery purposes (Miao *et al.*, 2018a).

Therefore SMPs can be widely used in developing localized drug delivery systems with a self-anchoring property that could self-deploy at the desired location and release the drug at the target site. Besides, there is no migration of the drug carrier in such systems (Wischke and Lendlein, 2010).

We have already talked about stimuli-responsive materials in Chapter 7. Using these materials converts the 3D printing to 4D printing, and one of the most important materials in this group is thermo-responsive materials such as Poly(Nisopropylacrylamide) (PNIPAm) as a famous thermo-responsive polymer with huge volume phase transition (Chung *et al.*, 1999). The temperature of diseased regions is typically higher than other parts because of the inflammation, therefore, drug-loaded systems with a base of PNIPAm or other thermo-responsive polymers can be printed, and these 4D systems can release the drug molecules at the diseased site due to their shrinkage induced by temperature increase. Yoshida *et al.* studied the release of drug agents surrounded by a printed PNIPAm gel capsule in response to temperature change. The 4D-printed device possessing drug agents move through blood vessels and release the drug at a specific site (Yoshida *et al.*, 2020).

Many kinds of research investigate the potential use of liquid responsive materials in 4D printing. These printed materials would be efficient at various fabrication processes like the formation of complex cell/drug/gene-loaded geometries from flat constructs after submersion in water. This phenomenon has also attracted much interest in many applications such as targeted drug delivery, biosensors, smart valves, and 3D culture (Kwag *et al.*, 2016, Lui *et al.*, 2019). For instance, 3D printing is not able to create hollow tubular structures with small internal diameters for manufacturing canal-like shapes. This challenge was recently addressed by using 4D printing in Kirillova's work. He printed hyaluronic acid-based hydrogel that could be cross-linked with green light and then folded into a tubular form in the presence of water or media culture. The reason for folding the printed films lies in the cross-linking gradient in the films, as the top layer of the film absorbs more light than the bottom layers (Kirillova *et al.*, 2017).

This phenomenon has also attracted much interest in many applications such as drug delivery. For instance, Jamal *et al.* engineered a cell-laden hollow cylinder with patterned holes in the exterior surface. Bilayer poly(ethylene glycol) (PEG) with two different molecular weights has been employed as bioink for encapsulating insulin-secreting beta TC-6. The Self-folding structure is driven by the differential swelling ratio of the two PEG bilayers in aqueous media. This research group demonstrated that the unique topographical feature of this 4D-printed structure has led to enhanced cell viability and insulin release in response to glucose in comparison to the planar counterpart. (Jamal *et al.*, 2013).

Making use of photo-responsive materials is another way to develop 4D bio-printing. As mentioned before in Chapter 7, photo-responsive polymers are composed of a photo-reactive moiety that converts the irradiation to a chemical signal through a photoreaction such as isomerization, cleavage, and dimerization. These transformations control the shape, functionality, stiffness, and cross-linking degree of light-responsive materials as a suitable choice for 4D bio-printing (Tomatsu *et al.*, 2011). Light-responsive materials help us with printing carriers with spatiotemporal control over drug release. Meanwhile, properties such as low cost and being contact-free make light an ideal stimulus (Li *et al.*, 2019). In this regard, Gupta and his colleagues printed a 4D drug carrier with a core/shell structure. According to Fig. (**2**), this structure is composed of an aqueous core that can be formulated to maintain the activity of therapeutic agents and poly (lactic-co-glycolic) acid-containing gold nanorods as a shell. The mentioned capsule is able to release therapeutic agents followed by laser irradiation with a specific wavelength and bursting of the capsule due to the plasmonic effect in gold nanorods. This example shows the great potential of 4D printing in designing localized drug delivery systems with precise control over drug release (Gupta *et al.*, 2015).

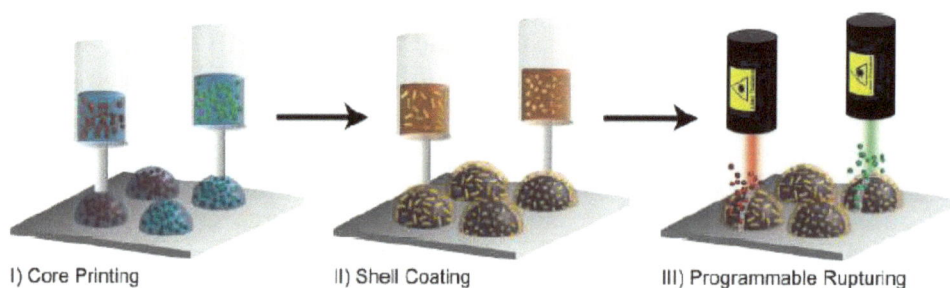

I) Core Printing   II) Shell Coating   III) Programmable Rupturing

Fig. (2). The printing process and rupturing of the smart capsules as a drug delivery system. I) printing aqueous cores containing therapeutic agents on a solid substrate, II) PLGA solutions composed of gold nanorods are distributed on the cores, III) rupturing of the drug-loaded capsule followed by laser irradiation with a laser wavelength corresponding to the absorption peak of the nanorods (Gupta *et al.*, 2015).

4D bio-printing may be used in pH-responsive materials (Larush *et al.*, 2017), especially for printing implantable drug delivery systems to aid recovery and prevent cancer recurrence. As we said before in chapter 8, various sites of the body have their own pH, such as the gastrointestinal tract, vagina, blood vessels, tumor environment, *etc.* (Gupta *et al.*, 2002). pH-responsive systems can permit the selective release of therapeutic agents in the target site due to the change of the solubility of the vehicle or cleaving of pH-responsive bonds upon the microenvironment pH variation that occurs because of the production of metabolites as lactic acid by the microorganism proliferation (Cicuéndez *et al.*,

2018). For example, a dual-drug-loaded pH-responsive scaffold was fabricated by Sang *et al.* The ciprofloxacin-loaded shell in this study included a mixture of gelatin and sodium bicarbonate (added to provide pH-sensitivity), and the Dox-loaded core was composed of poly(lactide-co-e-caprolactone). This acid-responsive implantable system had a rapid and pH-responsive ciprofloxacin release, and sustained doxorubicin release (Sang *et al.*, 2018). As a result, pH-responsive implantable systems can be fabricated by 4D printing in post tumor resection surgery for localized drug delivery purposes.

In another study, a research group developed a system composed of immobilized glucose oxidase in a pH-responsive polymeric hydrogel, entrapping a saturated insulin solution. An increase in the blood glucose level causes the glucose to penetrate into the membrane. The enclosing glucose oxidase catalyzes the conversion of glucose to gluconic acid, which lowers the pH, resulting in swelling of pH-responsive hydrogels and the release of insulin (Sood *et al.*, 2016, Goldbart *et al.*, 2002). The use of natural pH-responsive polymers has gained great attention recently due to their biodegradable nature, biocompatibility and easy modification by simple chemistry. Dextran, hyaluronic acid, alginic acid, chitosan, and gelatin are the most widely studied natural pH-responsive polymers (Kocak *et al.*, 2017). It should be highlighted that despite the noticeable promise in pH-responsive polymers, it is still extremely necessary to explore pH-responsive drug delivery systems with reduced toxicity (Tang *et al.*, 2019).

Recent studies have focused on the smart release of drugs from Magneto-responsive carriers in response to magnetic fields (Sood *et al.*, 2016). For instance, Zhao *et al.* fabricated a smart porous scaffold that can be remotely controlled by applying a magnetic field to deliver therapeutic agents to the target site at a specific time. This novel delivery system presents a huge deformation and large volume transition of over 70% under a moderate magnetic field, thereby releasing the drug/gene at the target site intelligently (Zhao *et al.*, 2011). Magneto-responsive hydrogels are also able to resemble the native architecture of human tissues. Betsch's *et al.* used a magnetic field during the 4D-printing process to fabricate an articular cartilage-like structure as a multilayer tissue structure. They bio-printed a chondrocyte-loaded bilayer composed of a layer with aligned collagen fibers as the superficial layer. Fiber alignment occurred due to the presence of streptavidin-coated magnetic particles in bioinks. Therefore, collagen fibers may be aligned by applying a magnetic field during bioprinting (Betsch *et al.*, 2018). This method holds a great promise for designing multilayer constructs with complex architecture.

9.5. DESIGNING IN 4D PRINTING

As mentioned before, shape-changing is an important key in 4D printing; this transformation occurs due to material selection and the designing process. Material selection was discussed in the previous section. In this section, we will talk about the importance of the designing process in 4D printing. In general, by changing the orientation of smart materials, it would be possible to control the shape and geometry of the constructs (Firth *et al.*, 2018). Besides, applying multi-material and a suitable design can help the 3D printer fabricate 4D structures with changeable geometries when exposed to appropriate stimuli. So a complex structure is generated from a simple structure through an easy and cost-effective method (Rafiee *et al.*, 2020). This phenomenon paves the way for creating localized drug delivery systems with complex structures.

It should be highlighted that 'active origami' is an important concept in 4D printing and has been utilized to form a three-dimensional and complex structure from a 2D sheet through an easy and cost-effective method. This approach is applied to fabricate 4D retinal implants that can change shape after being implanted in the eye as 2D sheets (Yan *et al.*, 2002). This example shows the great potential of active origami in creating 4D constructs.

Active origami is used to produce self-bending and self-folding structures. These constructs have gained much attention in recent years. The difference between these two mentioned structures is shown in Fig. (**3**). Bending is a global deformation associated with a smoother distributed curvature, whereas folding emphasizes localized deformation with sharp angles in a narrow hinge area. Numerous parameters must be considered in the design of active origamis, including the size of the structure, type of materials, the shape of the final product, and the folding/bending mechanism. Self-folding may be divided into with hinges or without hinges. Self-bending structures can consist of a single, smart component or a combination of several intelligent components (Fig. **3b**). It should be noted that the thickness and dimensions of the different layers in self-bending structures have a serious influence on the bending degree of the printed constructs (Pei and Loh, 2018).

Numerous researches have been carried out on active origami structures. For example, Ge *et al.* printed an active origami composed of shape memory fibers in an elastomeric matrix. The smart hinges in the passive matrix enabled the structure to fold into a complex geometry (Ge *et al.*, 2014). In another study, Bodaghi *et al.* used 4D printing to create self-expanding and self-shrinking structures. These smart constructs were designed by printing two types of shape memory fibers with different glass transition temperatures into a flexible matrix (Bodaghi *et al.*, 2016).

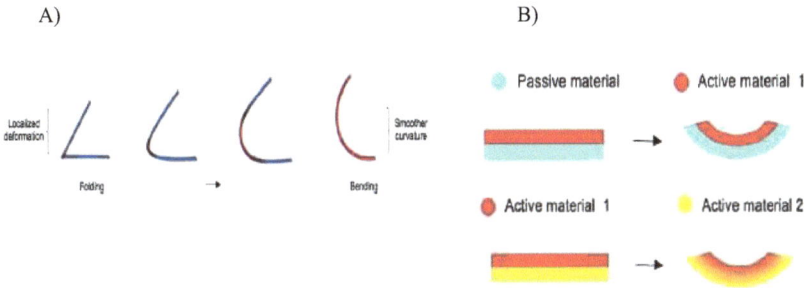

Fig. (3). A) Differences between self-folding and self-bending, **B)** Different self-folding structures: 1) a bilayer of an active and a passive layers, and 2) a heterogeneous composition of two smart layers (open access) (Pei and Loh, 2018).

Many researchers have focused on the 4D printing of more complex structures with the help of designing parameters (Dutta and Cohn, 2017). For example, a group of researchers focused on a structure composed of thermoresponsive gels with photo-responsive fibers. The introduced 4D structure can be reconfigured both remotely and non-invasively. Besides, illumination can be localized to specific sites of the sample, allowing actuation of specified areas, and, therefore, allowing control over local motion (Kuksenok and Balazs, 2016). Fig. (**4**) shows the importance of the design parameters, material selection, and the combination of materials in 4D printing. In fact, in all cases, the main idea is to print samples in a flat shape that is simple to design, and there is no waste of time and material because no support material is needed. Then, by applying a stimulus, the flat constructs are transformed into complex 3D structures with a desired structural shape or stiffness in the final configuration (Ding *et al.*, 2017).

This approach may be used to design smart drug delivery systems with complex geometries. As an instance, Malachowski *et al.* developed a thermoresponsive multi-fingered drug delivery system. This research group used PNIPAm as a thermo-sensitive hinge in a poly(propylene fumarate) matrix. Due to the thermal-responsivity of the gripper, this system reversibly opened and closed around body temperature and may be loaded with therapeutic agents to release them at the target site. The mentioned gripper proposes an active method for sustained release of drugs in the gastrointestinal tract (Malachowski *et al.*, 2014).

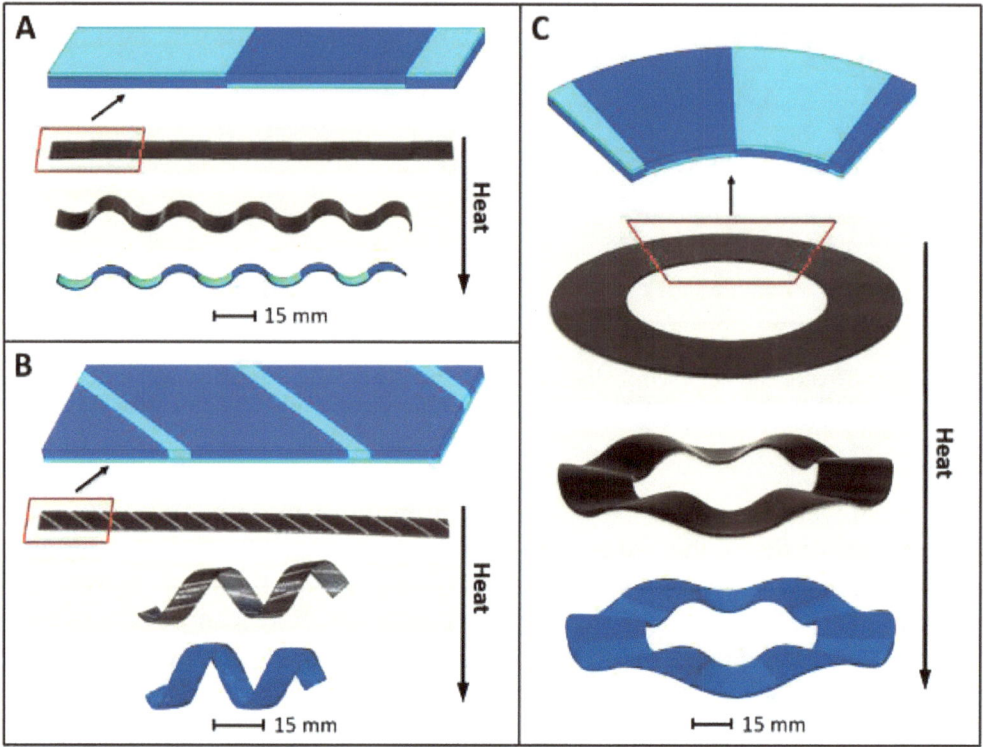

Fig. (4). The importance of design in the final product geometry. (**A**) A printed flat strip that transforms into a wavy structure. (**B**) A printed flat strip that transforms into a helix. (**C**) A ring that transforms into a wavy structure (open access) (Ding *et al.*, 2017).

Despite the huge success of 4D multi-material printing, there are still significant challenges, including limited choice of materials, printing resolution, mechanical properties and dimensional accuracy (Rafiee *et al.*, 2020). Besides, when several smart components are used in a single structure, it will be difficult to predict the final shape and properties of the structure (such as degrees of bending, expansion, shrinkage, *etc.*).

CONCLUSION

3D printing is a powerful technique that may be used to design drug-delivery systems, but it still has its challenges in technology and material selection. Some of these problems may be solved by the development of 4D printing, which is a method for printing dynamic structures.

4D printing is a growing new technique that has attracted attention in recent years, and numerous studies have been done to recognize its benefits, disadvantages and challenges. 4D printing is able to fabricate complex biomedical constructs in a wide range of sizes. It has presented new levels of advanced properties, such as changes in geometry and functionality in correlation with time, which cannot be achieved by other conventional processes like focused ion beam or mechanical machining. 4D printing may have many benefits for the pharmaceutical industry due to its great features. 4D printing can pave the way for the construction of localized drug delivery systems such as complex implantable delivery devices.

Despite all advantages in this field, there are several challenges that need to be solved. The main challenge in 4D printing is material selection. Among all types of materials, which were tested for 4D printing, stimuli-responsive polymers were the most promising. Although there is a wide range of stimuli-responsive materials, the ones which are biodegradable, biocompatible, and safe are considerably limited. Some of these safe polymers are gelatin, alginate, and hyaluronic acid, which demonstrate stimuli-responsive shape transformation. Another important challenge of 4D bio-printing in the pharmaceutical industry is the standardization of processes and materials. Besides, proper mechanical properties of shape-changing structures should be considered. In fact, shape-changing constructs, especially self-folding structures, are usually not tightly closed. The last challenge is the slow and inaccurate actuation and lack of control over intermediary states of deformation. However, it is expected that in the future, more effective methods may be used for the application of stimuli. For example, improving the heat application process in thermo-responsive polymers, or approaches for controlling moisture absorption for hydrogels. Understanding the effects of the scale of structural patterns and the mechanics of transformations will permit more flexibility and applicability, which shows the promise of widespread use and future opportunities in the field of 4D printing.

REFERENCES

Agrawal, A., Gupta, A.K. (2019). 3D printing technology in pharmaceuticals and biomedical: A review. *J. Drug Deliv. Ther., 9*, 1-4.

Ahangar, P., Cooke, M.E., Weber, M.H., Rosenzweig, D.H. (2019). Current biomedical applications of 3D printing and additive manufacturing. *Appl. Sci. (Basel), 9*(8), 1713.
[http://dx.doi.org/10.3390/app9081713]

Algahtani, M.S., Mohammed, A.A., Ahmad, J. (2018). Extrusion-based 3D printing for pharmaceuticals: Contemporary research and applications. *Curr. Pharm. Des., 24*(42), 4991-5008.
[http://dx.doi.org/10.2174/1381612825666190110155931] [PMID: 30636584]

Ashammakhi, N., Ahadian, S., Zengjie, F., Suthiwanich, K., Lorestani, F., Orive, G., Ostrovidov, S., Khademhosseini, A. (2018). Advances and future perspectives in 4D bioprinting. *Biotechnol. J., 13*(12), e1800148.
[http://dx.doi.org/10.1002/biot.201800148] [PMID: 30221837]

Askari, E., Naghib, S.M., Zahedi, A., Seyfoori, A., Zare, Y., Rhee, K.Y. (2021). Local delivery of chemotherapeutic agent in tissue engineering based on gelatin/graphene hydrogel. *J. Mater. Res. Technol., 12*, 412-422.

[http://dx.doi.org/10.1016/j.jmrt.2021.02.084]

Askari, E., Rasouli, M., Darghiasi, S.F., Naghib, S.M., Zare, Y., Rhee, K.Y. (2021). Reduced graphene oxide-grafted bovine serum albumin/bredigite nanocomposites with high mechanical properties and excellent osteogenic bioactivity for bone tissue engineering. *Biodes. Manuf., 4*(2), 243-257.
[http://dx.doi.org/10.1007/s42242-020-00113-4]

Bajpai, A., Baigent, A., Raghav, S., BRáDAIGH, C.O., KOUTSOS, V., RADACSI, N. (2020). 4D Printing: Materials, Technologies, and Future Applications in the Biomedical Field. *Sustainability, 12*, 10628.

Beg, S., Almalki, W.H., Malik, A., Farhan, M., Aatif, M., Rahman, Z., Alruwaili, N.K., Alrobaian, M., Tarique, M., Rahman, M. (2020). 3D printing for drug delivery and biomedical applications. *Drug Discov. Today, 25*(9), 1668-1681.
[http://dx.doi.org/10.1016/j.drudis.2020.07.007] [PMID: 32687871]

Behl, M., Lendlein, A. (2000). Shape-memory polymers. *Kirk☐Othmer Encyclopedia of Chemical Technology*

Betsch, M., Cristian, C., Lin, Y.Y., Blaeser, A., Schöneberg, J., Vogt, M., Buhl, E.M., Fischer, H., Duarte Campos, D.F. (2018). Incorporating 4D into bioprinting: real-time magnetically directed collagen fiber alignment for generating complex multilayered tissues. *Adv. Healthc. Mater., 7*(21), e1800894.
[http://dx.doi.org/10.1002/adhm.201800894] [PMID: 30221829]

Bird, D., Eker, E., Ravindra, N.M. (2019). 3D Printing of Pharmaceuticals and Transdermal Drug Delivery–An Overview. *TMS 2019 148ᵗʰ Annual Meeting & Exhibition Supplemental Proceedings,,* Springer.1563-1573.

Bodaghi, M., Damanpack, A.R., Liao, W.H. (2016). Self-expanding/shrinking structures by 4D printing. *Smart Mater. Struct., 25*(10), 105034.
[http://dx.doi.org/10.1088/0964-1726/25/10/105034]

Camović, M., Biščević, A., Brčić, I., Borčak, K., Bušatlić, S., Ćenanović, N., Dedović, A., Mulalić, A., Osmanlić, M., Sirbubalo, M. (2019). Coated 3d printed PLA microneedles as transdermal drug delivery systems. *International Conference on Medical and Biological Engineering, 735-742.*

Charbe, N.B., McCarron, P.A., Lane, M.E., Tambuwala, M.M. (2017). Application of three-dimensional printing for colon targeted drug delivery systems. *Int. J. Pharm. Investig., 7*(2), 47-59.
[http://dx.doi.org/10.4103/jphi.JPHI_32_17] [PMID: 28929046]

Cheng, G.Z., Folch, E., Wilson, A., Brik, R., Garcia, N., Estepar, R.S.J., Onieva, J.O., Gangadharan, S., Majid, A. (2017). 3D printing and personalized airway stents. *Pulm. Ther., 3*(1), 59-66.
[http://dx.doi.org/10.1007/s41030-016-0026-y]

Chung, J.E., Yokoyama, M., Yamato, M., Aoyagi, T., Sakurai, Y., Okano, T. (1999). Thermo-responsive drug delivery from polymeric micelles constructed using block copolymers of poly(N-isopropylacrylamide) and poly(butylmethacrylate). *J. Control. Release, 62*(1-2), 115-127.
[http://dx.doi.org/10.1016/S0168-3659(99)00029-2] [PMID: 10518643]

Cicuéndez, M., Doadrio, J.C., Hernández, A., Portolés, M.T., Izquierdo-Barba, I., Vallet-Regí, M. (2018). Multifunctional pH sensitive 3D scaffolds for treatment and prevention of bone infection. *Acta Biomater., 65*, 450-461.
[http://dx.doi.org/10.1016/j.actbio.2017.11.009] [PMID: 29127064]

Derakhshanfar, S., Mbeleck, R., Xu, K., Zhang, X., Zhong, W., Xing, M. (2018). 3D bioprinting for biomedical devices and tissue engineering: A review of recent trends and advances. *Bioact. Mater., 3*(2), 144-156.
[http://dx.doi.org/10.1016/j.bioactmat.2017.11.008] [PMID: 29744452]

Ding, Z., Yuan, C., Peng, X., Wang, T., Qi, H.J., Dunn, M.L. (2017). Direct 4D printing *via* active composite materials. *Sci. Adv., 3*(4), e1602890.
[http://dx.doi.org/10.1126/sciadv.1602890] [PMID: 28439560]

Dutta, S., Cohn, D. (2017). Temperature and pH responsive 3D printed scaffolds. *J. Mater. Chem. B Mater.*

Biol. Med., 5(48), 9514-9521.
[http://dx.doi.org/10.1039/C7TB02368E] [PMID: 32264566]

Economidou, S.N., Lamprou, D.A., Douroumis, D. (2018). 3D printing applications for transdermal drug delivery. *Int. J. Pharm., 544*(2), 415-424.
[http://dx.doi.org/10.1016/j.ijpharm.2018.01.031] [PMID: 29355656]

Elkasabgy, N.A., Mahmoud, A.A., Maged, A. (2020). 3D printing: An appealing route for customized drug delivery systems. *Int. J. Pharm., 588*, 119732.
[http://dx.doi.org/10.1016/j.ijpharm.2020.119732] [PMID: 32768528]

Eltom, A., Zhong, G., Muhammad, A. (2019). Scaffold techniques and designs in tissue engineering functions and purposes: a review. *Adv. Mater. Sci. Eng., 2019*, 1-13.
[http://dx.doi.org/10.1155/2019/3429527]

Firth, J., Gaisford, S., Basit, A.W. (2018). *A new dimension: 4D printing opportunities in pharmaceutics. 3D Printing of Pharmaceuticals..* Springer.

Fu, J., Yu, X., Jin, Y. (2018). 3D printing of vaginal rings with personalized shapes for controlled release of progesterone. *Int. J. Pharm., 539*(1-2), 75-82.
[http://dx.doi.org/10.1016/j.ijpharm.2018.01.036] [PMID: 29366944]

Ge, Q., Dunn, C.K., Qi, H.J., Dunn, M.L. (2014). Active origami by 4D printing. *Smart Mater. Struct., 23*(9), 094007.
[http://dx.doi.org/10.1088/0964-1726/23/9/094007]

Ghilan, A., Chiriac, A.P., Nita, L.E., Rusu, A.G., Neamtu, I., Chiriac, V.M. (2020). Trends in 3D printing processes for biomedical field: opportunities and challenges. *J. Polym. Environ., 28*(5), 1345-1367.
[http://dx.doi.org/10.1007/s10924-020-01722-x] [PMID: 32435165]

Goldbart, R., Traitel, T., Lapidot, S.A., Kost, J. (2002). Enzymatically controlled responsive drug delivery systems. *Polym. Adv. Technol., 13*(10-12), 1006-1018.
[http://dx.doi.org/10.1002/pat.275]

Gooneh-Farahani, S., Naghib, S.M., Naimi-Jamal, M.R. (2019). A critical comparison study on the pH-sensitive nanocomposites based on graphene-grafted chitosan for cancer theragnosis. *Multidisciplinary Cancer Investigation, 3*(1), 05-16.
[http://dx.doi.org/10.30699/acadpub.mci.3.1.5]

Gooneh-Farahani, S., Naghib, S.M., Naimi-Jamal, M.R. (2020). A Novel and Inexpensive Method Based on Modified Ionic Gelation for pH-responsive Controlled Drug Release of Homogeneously Distributed Chitosan Nanoparticles with a High Encapsulation Efficiency. *Fibers Polym., 21*(9), 1917-1926.
[http://dx.doi.org/10.1007/s12221-020-1095-y]

Gooneh-Farahani, S., Naimi-Jamal, M.R., Naghib, S.M. (2019). Stimuli-responsive graphene-incorporated multifunctional chitosan for drug delivery applications: a review. *Expert Opin. Drug Deliv., 16*(1), 79-99.
[http://dx.doi.org/10.1080/17425247.2019.1556257] [PMID: 30514124]

Goyanes, A., Chang, H., Sedough, D., Hatton, G.B., Wang, J., Buanz, A., Gaisford, S., Basit, A.W. (2015). Fabrication of controlled-release budesonide tablets *via* desktop (FDM) 3D printing. *Int. J. Pharm., 496*(2), 414-420.
[http://dx.doi.org/10.1016/j.ijpharm.2015.10.039] [PMID: 26481468]

Goyanes, A., Det-Amornrat, U., Wang, J., Basit, A.W., Gaisford, S. (2016). 3D scanning and 3D printing as innovative technologies for fabricating personalized topical drug delivery systems. *J. Control. Release, 234*, 41-48.
[http://dx.doi.org/10.1016/j.jconrel.2016.05.034] [PMID: 27189134]

Gul, J.Z., Memoon, S., Muhammad, M.R. (2018). 3D printing for soft robotics–a review. *Sci. Technol. Adv. Mater., 19*(1), 243-262.

Gupta, P., Vermani, K., Garg, S. (2002). Hydrogels: from controlled release to pH-responsive drug delivery.

Drug Discov. Today, 7(10), 569-579.
[http://dx.doi.org/10.1016/S1359-6446(02)02255-9] [PMID: 12047857]

Hasan, S.M., Nash, L.D., Maitland, D.J. (2016). Porous shape memory polymers: Design and applications. *J. Polym. Sci., B, Polym. Phys., 54*(14), 1300-1318.
[http://dx.doi.org/10.1002/polb.23982]

Hearon, K., Wierzbicki, M.A., Nash, L.D., Landsman, T.L., Laramy, C., Lonnecker, A.T., Gibbons, M.C., Ur, S., Cardinal, K.O., Wilson, T.S., Wooley, K.L., Maitland, D.J. (2015). A processable shape memory polymer system for biomedical applications. *Adv. Healthc. Mater., 4*(9), 1386-1398.
[http://dx.doi.org/10.1002/adhm.201500156] [PMID: 25925212]

Horst, D.J. (2018). 3D printing of pharmaceutical drug delivery systems. *Archives of Organic and Inorganic Chemical Sciences, 1*(2), 65-69.
[http://dx.doi.org/10.32474/AOICS.2018.01.000109]

Huang, W., Zheng, Q., Sun, W., Xu, H., Yang, X. (2007). Levofloxacin implants with predefined microstructure fabricated by three-dimensional printing technique. *Int. J. Pharm., 339*(1-2), 33-38.
[http://dx.doi.org/10.1016/j.ijpharm.2007.02.021] [PMID: 17412538]

Jacob, S., Nair, A.B., Patel, V., Shah, J. (2020). 3D Printing Technologies: Recent Development and Emerging Applications in Various Drug Delivery Systems. *AAPS PharmSciTech, 21*(6), 220.
[http://dx.doi.org/10.1208/s12249-020-01771-4] [PMID: 32748243]

Jamal, M., Kadam, S.S., Xiao, R., Jivan, F., Onn, T.M., Fernandes, R., Nguyen, T.D., Gracias, D.H. (2013). Bio-origami hydrogel scaffolds composed of photocrosslinked PEG bilayers. *Adv. Healthc. Mater., 2*(8), 1142-1150.
[http://dx.doi.org/10.1002/adhm.201200458] [PMID: 23386382]

Kačarević, Ž.P., Rider, P.M., Alkildani, S., Retnasingh, S., Smeets, R., Jung, O., Ivanišević, Z., Barbeck, M. (2018). An introduction to 3D bioprinting: possibilities, challenges and future aspects. *Materials (Basel), 11*(11), 2199.
[http://dx.doi.org/10.3390/ma11112199] [PMID: 30404222]

Kan, Q., LI, J., Kang, G., Zhang, Z. (2018). Experiments and models of thermo-induced shape memory polymers. *Shape-Memory Materials.*

Kim, T.H., Lee, J.H., Ahn, C.B., Hong, J.H., Son, K.H., Lee, J.W. (2019). Development of a 3D-printed drug-eluting stent for treating obstructive salivary gland disease. *ACS Biomater. Sci. Eng., 5*(7), 3572-3581.
[http://dx.doi.org/10.1021/acsbiomaterials.9b00636] [PMID: 33405739]

Kirillova, A., Maxson, R., Stoychev, G., Gomillion, C.T., Ionov, L. (2017). 4D biofabrication using shape-morphing hydrogels. *Adv. Mater., 29*(46), 1703443.
[http://dx.doi.org/10.1002/adma.201703443] [PMID: 29024044]

Knowlton, S., Yenilmez, B., Anand, S., Tasoglu, S. (2017). Photocrosslinking-based bioprinting: Examining crosslinking schemes. *Bioprinting, 5*, 10-18.
[http://dx.doi.org/10.1016/j.bprint.2017.03.001]

Kocak, G., Tuncer, C., Bütün, V. (2017). pH-Responsive polymers. *Polym. Chem., 8*(1), 144-176.
[http://dx.doi.org/10.1039/C6PY01872F]

Kotta, S., Nair, A., Alsabeelah, N. (2018). 3D printing technology in drug delivery: recent progress and application. *Curr. Pharm. Des., 24*(42), 5039-5048.
[http://dx.doi.org/10.2174/1381612825666181206123828] [PMID: 30520368]

Kuksenok, O., Balazs, A.C. (2016). Stimuli-responsive behavior of composites integrating thermo-responsive gels with photo-responsive fibers. *Mater. Horiz., 3*(1), 53-62.
[http://dx.doi.org/10.1039/C5MH00212E]

Kundu, A., Arnett, P., Bagde, A., Azim, N., Kouagou, E., Singh, M., Rajaraman, S. (2020). DLP 3D Printed "Intelligent" Microneedle Array (*i* μNA) for Stimuli Responsive Release of Drugs and Its *in Vitro* and *ex Vivo* Characterization. *J. Microelectromech. Syst., 29*(5), 685-691.

[http://dx.doi.org/10.1109/JMEMS.2020.3003628]

Kwag, H.R., Serbo, J.V., Korangath, P., Sukumar, S., Romer, L.H., Gracias, D.H. (2016). A self-folding hydrogel *in vitro* model for ductal carcinoma. *Tissue Eng. Part C Methods, 22*(4), 398-407.
[http://dx.doi.org/10.1089/ten.tec.2015.0442] [PMID: 26831041]

Kyobula, M., Adedeji, A., Alexander, M.R., Saleh, E., Wildman, R., Ashcroft, I., Gellert, P.R., Roberts, C.J. (2017). 3D inkjet printing of tablets exploiting bespoke complex geometries for controlled and tuneable drug release. *J. Control. Release, 261*, 207-215.
[http://dx.doi.org/10.1016/j.jconrel.2017.06.025] [PMID: 28668378]

Larush, L., Kaner, I., Fluksman, A., Tamsut, A., Pawar, A. A., Lesnovski, P., Benny, O., Magdassi, S. (2017). 3D printing of responsive hydrogels for drug-delivery systems. *Journal of 3D printing in medicine, 1*, 219-229.

Layani, M., Wang, X., Magdassi, S. (2018). Novel materials for 3D printing by photopolymerization. *Adv. Mater., 30*(41), e1706344.
[http://dx.doi.org/10.1002/adma.201706344] [PMID: 29756242]

Li, J., Chen, M., Fan, X., Zhou, H. (2016). Recent advances in bioprinting techniques: approaches, applications and future prospects. *J. Transl. Med., 14*(1), 271.
[http://dx.doi.org/10.1186/s12967-016-1028-0] [PMID: 27645770]

Li, L., Scheiger, J.M., Levkin, P.A. (2019). Design and applications of photoresponsive hydrogels. *Adv. Mater., 31*(26), e1807333.
[http://dx.doi.org/10.1002/adma.201807333] [PMID: 30848524]

Liu, C., Qin, H., Mather, P.T. (2007). Review of progress in shape-memory polymers. *J. Mater. Chem., 17*(16), 1543-1558.
[http://dx.doi.org/10.1039/b615954k]

Liu, J., Yan, C. (2018). 3D printing of scaffolds for tissue engineering. *by Cvetković D. Intech Open, UK, 7*, 137-154.

Lui, Y.S., Sow, W.T., Tan, L.P., Wu, Y., Lai, Y., Li, H. (2019). 4D printing and stimuli-responsive materials in biomedical aspects. *Acta Biomater., 92*, 19-36.
[http://dx.doi.org/10.1016/j.actbio.2019.05.005] [PMID: 31071476]

Lukin, I., Musquiz, S., Erezuma, I., Al-Tel, T.H., Golafshan, N., Dolatshahi-Pirouz, A., Orive, G. (2019). Can 4D bioprinting revolutionize drug development? *Expert Opin. Drug Discov., 14*(10), 953-956.
[http://dx.doi.org/10.1080/17460441.2019.1636781] [PMID: 31282226]

Luzuriaga, M.A., Berry, D.R., Reagan, J.C., Smaldone, R.A., Gassensmith, J.J. (2018). Biodegradable 3D printed polymer microneedles for transdermal drug delivery. *Lab Chip, 18*(8), 1223-1230.
[http://dx.doi.org/10.1039/C8LC00098K] [PMID: 29536070]

Malachowski, K., Breger, J., Kwag, H.R., Wang, M.O., Fisher, J.P., Selaru, F.M., Gracias, D.H. (2014). Stimuli-responsive theragrippers for chemomechanical controlled release. *Angew. Chem. Int. Ed. Engl., 53*(31), 8045-8049.
[http://dx.doi.org/10.1002/anie.201311047] [PMID: 24634136]

Miao, S., Cui, H., Nowicki, M., Lee, S.J., Almeida, J., Zhou, X., Zhu, W., Yao, X., Masood, F., Plesniak, M.W., Mohiuddin, M., Zhang, L.G. (2018). Photolithographic-stereolithographic-tandem fabrication of 4D smart scaffolds for improved stem cell cardiomyogenic differentiation. *Biofabrication, 10*(3), 035007.
[http://dx.doi.org/10.1088/1758-5090/aabe0b] [PMID: 29651999]

Miao, S., Cui, H., Nowicki, M., Xia, L., Zhou, X., Lee, S.J., Zhu, W., Sarkar, K., Zhang, Z., Zhang, L.G. (2018). Stereolithographic 4D bioprinting of multiresponsive architectures for neural engineering. *Adv. Biosyst., 2*(9), 1800101.
[http://dx.doi.org/10.1002/adbi.201800101] [PMID: 30906853]

Mohammed, A., Elshaer, A., Sareh, P., Elsayed, M., Hassanin, H. (2020). Additive manufacturing technologies for drug delivery applications. *Int. J. Pharm., 580*, 119245.

[http://dx.doi.org/10.1016/j.ijpharm.2020.119245] [PMID: 32201252]

Morouço, P., Lattanzi, W., Alves, N. (2017). Four-dimensional bioprinting as a new era for tissue engineering and regenerative medicine. *Front. Bioeng. Biotechnol., 5*, 61.
[http://dx.doi.org/10.3389/fbioe.2017.00061] [PMID: 29090210]

Moussi, K., Bukhamsin, A., Hidalgo, T., Kosel, J. (2020). Biocompatible 3D printed microneedles for transdermal, intradermal, and percutaneous applications. *Adv. Eng. Mater., 22*(2), 1901358.
[http://dx.doi.org/10.1002/adem.201901358]

Moussi, K., Bukhamsin, A., Kosel, J. (2019). ImplanTable 3D Printed Drug Delivery System. *20th International Conference on Solid-State Sensors, Actuators and Microsystems & Eurosensors XXXIII (TRANSDUCERS & EUROSENSORS XXXIII).*, IEEE.2243-2246.

Okwuosa, T.C., Pereira, B.C., Arafat, B., Cieszynska, M., Isreb, A., Alhnan, M.A. (2017). Fabricating a shell-core delayed release tablet using dual FDM 3D printing for patient-centred therapy. *Pharm. Res., 34*(2), 427-437.
[http://dx.doi.org/10.1007/s11095-016-2073-3] [PMID: 27943014]

Okwuosa, T.C., Stefaniak, D., Arafat, B., Isreb, A., Wan, K.W., Alhnan, M.A. (2016). A lower temperature FDM 3D printing for the manufacture of patient-specific immediate release tablets. *Pharm. Res., 33*(11), 2704-2712.
[http://dx.doi.org/10.1007/s11095-016-1995-0] [PMID: 27506424]

Palo, M., Holländer, J., Suominen, J., Yliruusi, J., Sandler, N. (2017). 3D printed drug delivery devices: perspectives and technical challenges. *Expert Review Of Medical Devices, 14*, 685-696.

Pandey, M., Choudhury, H., Fern, J.L.C., Kee, A.T.K., Kou, J., Jing, J.L.J., Her, H.C., Yong, H.S., Ming, H.C., Bhattamisra, S.K., Gorain, B. (2020). 3D printing for oral drug delivery: a new tool to customize drug delivery. *Drug Deliv. Transl. Res., 10*(4), 986-1001.
[http://dx.doi.org/10.1007/s13346-020-00737-0] [PMID: 32207070]

Pei, E., Loh, G.H. (2018). Technological considerations for 4D printing: an overview. *Progress in Additive Manufacturing, 3*(1-2), 95-107.
[http://dx.doi.org/10.1007/s40964-018-0047-1]

Pei, E., Loh, G.H., Harrison, D., Almeida, H.A., Monzón Verona, M.D., Paz, R. (2017). A study of 4D printing and functionally graded additive manufacturing. *Assem. Autom., 37*(2), 147-153.
[http://dx.doi.org/10.1108/AA-01-2017-012]

Persaud, S., Eid, S., Swiderski, N., Serris, I., Cho, H. (2020). Preparations of rectal suppositories containing artesunate. *Pharmaceutics, 12*(3), 222.
[http://dx.doi.org/10.3390/pharmaceutics12030222] [PMID: 32131543]

Placone, J.K., Engler, A.J. (2018). Recent advances in extrusion-based 3D printing for biomedical applications. *Adv. Healthc. Mater., 7*(8), e1701161.
[http://dx.doi.org/10.1002/adhm.201701161] [PMID: 29283220]

Prasad, L.K., Smyth, H. (2016). 3D Printing technologies for drug delivery: a review. *Drug Dev. Ind. Pharm., 42*(7), 1019-1031.
[http://dx.doi.org/10.3109/03639045.2015.1120743] [PMID: 26625986]

Quan, H., Zhang, T., Xu, H., Luo, S., Nie, J., Zhu, X. (2020). Photo-curing 3D printing technique and its challenges. *Bioact. Mater., 5*(1), 110-115.
[http://dx.doi.org/10.1016/j.bioactmat.2019.12.003] [PMID: 32021945]

Rafiee, M., Farahani, R.D., Therriault, D. (2020). Multi-Material 3D and 4D Printing: A Survey. *Adv. Sci. (Weinh.), 7*(12), 1902307.
[http://dx.doi.org/10.1002/advs.201902307] [PMID: 32596102]

Rahmanian, M., seyfoori, A., Dehghan, M.M., Eini, L., Naghib, S.M., Gholami, H., Farzad Mohajeri, S., Mamaghani, K.R., Majidzadeh-A, K. (2019). Multifunctional gelatin–tricalcium phosphate porous nanocomposite scaffolds for tissue engineering and local drug delivery: *In vitro* and *in vivo* studies. *J. Taiwan*

Inst. Chem. Eng., 101, 214-220.
[http://dx.doi.org/10.1016/j.jtice.2019.04.028]

Sang, Q., Li, H., Williams, G., Wu, H., Zhu, L.M. (2018). Core-shell poly(lactide-co-ε-caprolactone)-gelatin fiber scaffolds as pH-sensitive drug delivery systems. *J. Biomater. Appl., 32*(8), 1105-1118.
[http://dx.doi.org/10.1177/0885328217749962] [PMID: 29295656]

Saritha, D., Boyina, D. (2021). A concise review on 4D printing technology. *Mater. Today Proc., 46*, 692-695.
[http://dx.doi.org/10.1016/j.matpr.2020.12.016]

Schmidleithner, C., Kalaskar, D.M. (2018). *Stereolithography.* IntechOpen.

Seoane-viaño, I., Gómez-LADO, N., Lázare-IGLESIAS, H., García-OTERO, X., Antúnez-López, J.R., Ruibal, Á., Varela-correa, J.J., Aguiar, P., Basit, A.W., Otero-espinar, F.J. (2020). 3D Printed Tacrolimus Rectal Formulations Ameliorate Colitis in an Experimental Animal Model of Inflammatory Bowel Disease. *Biomedicines, 8*, 563.

Skowyra, J., Pietrzak, K., Alhnan, M.A. (2015). Fabrication of extended-release patient-tailored prednisolone tablets *via* fused deposition modelling (FDM) 3D printing. *Eur. J. Pharm. Sci., 68*, 11-17.
[http://dx.doi.org/10.1016/j.ejps.2014.11.009] [PMID: 25460545]

Sood, N., Bhardwaj, A., Mehta, S., Mehta, A. (2016). Stimuli-responsive hydrogels in drug delivery and tissue engineering. *Drug Deliv., 23*(3), 758-780.
[http://dx.doi.org/10.3109/10717544.2014.940091] [PMID: 25045782]

Sun, H., Hu, C., Zhou, C., Wu, L., Sun, J., Zhou, X., Xing, F., Long, C., Kong, Q., Liang, J., Fan, Y., Zhang, X. (2020). 3D printing of calcium phosphate scaffolds with controlled release of antibacterial functions for jaw bone repair. *Mater. Des., 189*, 108540.
[http://dx.doi.org/10.1016/j.matdes.2020.108540]

Tan, D.K., Maniruzzaman, M., Nokhodchi, A. (2019). Development and optimisation of novel polymeric compositions for sustained release theophylline caplets (PrintCap) *via* FDM 3D printing. *Polymers (Basel), 12*(1), 27.
[http://dx.doi.org/10.3390/polym12010027] [PMID: 31877755]

Tang, H., Zhao, W., Yu, J., Li, Y., Zhao, C. (2018). Recent development of pH-responsive polymers for cancer nanomedicine. *Molecules, 24*(1), 4.
[http://dx.doi.org/10.3390/molecules24010004] [PMID: 30577475]

Tetsuka, H., Shin, S.R. (2020). Materials and technical innovations in 3D printing in biomedical applications. *J. Mater. Chem. B Mater. Biol. Med., 8*(15), 2930-2950.
[http://dx.doi.org/10.1039/D0TB00034E] [PMID: 32239017]

Tomatsu, I., Peng, K., Kros, A. (2011). Photoresponsive hydrogels for biomedical applications. *Adv. Drug Deliv. Rev., 63*(14-15), 1257-1266.
[http://dx.doi.org/10.1016/j.addr.2011.06.009] [PMID: 21745509]

Trenfield, S.J., Awad, A., Madla, C.M., Hatton, G.B., Firth, J., Goyanes, A., Gaisford, S., Basit, A.W. (2019). Shaping the future: recent advances of 3D printing in drug delivery and healthcare. *Expert Opin. Drug Deliv., 16*(10), 1081-1094.
[http://dx.doi.org/10.1080/17425247.2019.1660318] [PMID: 31478752]

Tsuji, T., Tamai, H., Igaki, K., Kyo, E., Kosuga, K., Hata, T., Nakamura, T., Fujita, S., Takeda, S., Motohara, S., Uehata, H. (2003). Biodegradable stents as a platform to drug loading. *Int. J. Cardiovasc. Intervent., 5*(1), 13-16.
[http://dx.doi.org/10.1080/14628840304609] [PMID: 12623560]

Uddin, M.J., Scoutaris, N., Klepetsanis, P., Chowdhry, B., Prausnitz, M.R., Douroumis, D. (2015). Inkjet printing of transdermal microneedles for the delivery of anticancer agents. *Int. J. Pharm., 494*(2), 593-602.
[http://dx.doi.org/10.1016/j.ijpharm.2015.01.038] [PMID: 25617676]

Uziel, A., Shpigel, T., Goldin, N., Lewitus, D. Y. (2019). Three-dimensional printing for drug delivery devices: a state-of-the-art survey. *Journal of 3D Printing in Medicine, 3*, 95-109.

Ventola, C.L. (2014). Medical applications for 3D printing: current and projected uses. *P&T, 39*(10), 704-711.
[PMID: 25336867]

Vikram Singh, A., Hasan Dad Ansari, M., Wang, S., Laux, P., Luch, A., Kumar, A., Patil, R., Nussberger, S. (2019). The adoption of three-dimensional additive manufacturing from biomedical material design to 3d organ printing. *Appl. Sci. (Basel), 9*(4), 811.
[http://dx.doi.org/10.3390/app9040811]

Wallis, M., Al-Dulimi, Z., Tan, D.K., Maniruzzaman, M., Nokhodchi, A. (2020). 3D printing for enhanced drug delivery: current state-of-the-art and challenges. *Drug Dev. Ind. Pharm., 46*(9), 1385-1401.
[http://dx.doi.org/10.1080/03639045.2020.1801714] [PMID: 32715832]

Wang, J., Goyanes, A., Gaisford, S., Basit, A.W. (2016). Stereolithographic (SLA) 3D printing of oral modified-release dosage forms. *Int. J. Pharm., 503*(1-2), 207-212.
[http://dx.doi.org/10.1016/j.ijpharm.2016.03.016] [PMID: 26976500]

Wang, K., Strandman, S., Zhu, X.X. (2017). A mini review: Shape memory polymers for biomedical applications. *Front. Chem. Sci. Eng., 11*(2), 143-153.
[http://dx.doi.org/10.1007/s11705-017-1632-4]

Wang, Q., Sun, J., Yao, Q., Ji, C., Liu, J., Zhu, Q. (2018). 3D printing with cellulose materials. *Cellulose, 25*(8), 4275-4301.
[http://dx.doi.org/10.1007/s10570-018-1888-y]

Wang, Y., Sun, L., Mei, Z., Zhang, F., He, M., Fletcher, C., Wang, F., Yang, J., Bi, D., Jiang, Y., Liu, P. (2020). 3D printed biodegradable implants as an individualized drug delivery system for local chemotherapy of osteosarcoma. *Mater. Des., 186*, 108336.
[http://dx.doi.org/10.1016/j.matdes.2019.108336]

Wischke, C., Lendlein, A. (2010). Shape-memory polymers as drug carriers--a multifunctional system. *Pharm. Res., 27*(4), 527-529.
[http://dx.doi.org/10.1007/s11095-010-0062-5] [PMID: 20127394]

Xie, Z., Gao, M., Lobo, A.O., Webster, T.J. (2020). 3D Bioprinting in Tissue Engineering for Medical Applications: The Classic and the Hybrid. *Polymers (Basel), 12*(8), 1717.
[http://dx.doi.org/10.3390/polym12081717] [PMID: 32751797]

Xu, X., Goyanes, A., Trenfield, S.J., Diaz-Gomez, L., Alvarez-Lorenzo, C., Gaisford, S., Basit, A.W. (2021). Stereolithography (SLA) 3D printing of a bladder device for intravesical drug delivery. *Mater. Sci. Eng. C, 120*, 111773.
[http://dx.doi.org/10.1016/j.msec.2020.111773] [PMID: 33545904]

Yan, W., Wang, C.H., Zhang, X.P., Mai, Y.W. (2002). Effect of transformation volume contraction on the toughness of superelastic shape memory alloys. *Smart Mater. Struct., 11*(6), 947-955.
[http://dx.doi.org/10.1088/0964-1726/11/6/316]

Yi, H.G., Choi, Y.J., Kang, K.S., Hong, J.M., Pati, R.G., Park, M.N., Shim, I.K., Lee, C.M., Kim, S.C., Cho, D.W. (2016). A 3D-printed local drug delivery patch for pancreatic cancer growth suppression. *J. Control. Release, 238*, 231-241.
[http://dx.doi.org/10.1016/j.jconrel.2016.06.015] [PMID: 27288878]

Yoshida, K., Nezu, K., Khosla, A., Makino, M., Kawakami, M., Furukawa, H. (2020). Behaviors of 3D-printed objects made of thermo-responsive hydrogels: motion in flow and molecule release ability. *Microsyst. Technol.*, 1-6.

Zarek, M., Mansour, N., Shapira, S., Cohn, D. (2017). 4D printing of shape memory-based personalized endoluminal medical devices. *Macromol. Rapid Commun., 38*(2), 1600628.
[http://dx.doi.org/10.1002/marc.201600628] [PMID: 27918636]

Zeinali Kalkhoran, A.H., Naghib, S.M., Vahidi, O., Rahmanian, M. (2018). Synthesis and characterization of

graphene-grafted gelatin nanocomposite hydrogels as emerging drug delivery systems. *Biomed. Phys. Eng. Express, 4*(5), 055017.
[http://dx.doi.org/10.1088/2057-1976/aad745]

Zeinali Kalkhoran, A.H., Vahidi, O., Naghib, S.M. (2018). A new mathematical approach to predict the actual drug release from hydrogels. *Eur. J. Pharm. Sci., 111*, 303-310.
[http://dx.doi.org/10.1016/j.ejps.2017.09.038] [PMID: 28962856]

Zhang, B., Gao, L., Ma, L., Luo, Y., Yang, H., Cui, Z. (2019). 3D Bioprinting: A novel avenue for manufacturing tissues and organs. *Engineering (Beijing), 5*(4), 777-794.
[http://dx.doi.org/10.1016/j.eng.2019.03.009]

Zhang, D., George, O.J., Petersen, K.M., Jimenez-Vergara, A.C., Hahn, M.S., Grunlan, M.A. (2014). A bioactive "self-fitting" shape memory polymer scaffold with potential to treat cranio-maxillo facial bone defects. *Acta Biomater., 10*(11), 4597-4605.
[http://dx.doi.org/10.1016/j.actbio.2014.07.020] [PMID: 25063999]

Zhao, X., Kim, J., Cezar, C.A., Huebsch, N., Lee, K., Bouhadir, K., Mooney, D.J. (2011). Active scaffolds for on-demand drug and cell delivery. *Proc. Natl. Acad. Sci. USA, 108*(1), 67-72.
[http://dx.doi.org/10.1073/pnas.1007862108] [PMID: 21149682]

Zhou, G., Liu, W., Zhang, Y., Gu, W., Li, M., Lu, C., Zhou, R., Che, Y., Lu, H., Zhu, Y., Teng, G., Cheng, Y. (2020). Application of three-dimensional printing in interventional medicine. *Journal of Interventional Medicine, 3*(1), 1-16.
[http://dx.doi.org/10.1016/j.jimed.2020.01.001] [PMID: 34805900]

CHAPTER 10

Conclusion and Future Outlooks

Drug delivery (DD), which plays a crucial role in disease treatment, is a method or process to deliver pharmaceutical compounds in order to achieve therapeutic effects in patients (Tiwari *et al.*, 2012). Drugs can be administered through a wide range of conventional systems (DDSs), which exist either in bulk, micro, or nanoforms, such as lotions, mixtures, solutions, ointments, powders, creams, suppositories, suspensions, injectables, pills, immediate-release capsules, tablets, *etc.* (Nayak *et al.*, 2018, Gundloori *et al.*, 2019).

In general, DDSs can be classified based on the route of administration (*i.e.*, the path by which the therapeutic drug is taken into the body) or the intended site of action (*i.e.* where in the body the therapeutic cargo ends up). In this context, these can be both systemic or local. It should be highlighted that administration and site of action are not the same, for instance, there are DDSs applied into the systemic circulation with a local effect that can deliver therapeutic agents to a target site in the body. Besides, the systemic effect can also be achieved by local administration (Ji and Kohane, 2019).

However, the systemic effect is routinely achieved after intravenous injection and oral administration (Serwer *et al.*, 2010). Oral drug administration suffers from numerous disadvantages, including poor stability in the gastric environment, low solubility, low bioavailability, drug expulsion *via* intestinal drug transporter, and the continuous secretion of mucus, which is known to prevent drug absorption and penetration (Mehta and Pawar, 2018, Herlem *et al.*, 2019, Mohammadzadeh and Javadzadeh, 2018, Ensign *et al.*, 2012). Besides, the amount of therapeutic agents that reach the site of disease should be sufficient to obtain desired therapeutic effect (Aj *et al.*, 2012). On the other hand, intravenous injection has some limitations such as discomfort, stress to patients, high cost, and high risk of hospital-acquired infections. Besides, in most cases, for achieving therapeutic effects in patients, frequent injections are needed due to the short duration of drug action (Batra *et al.*, 2019, Aj *et al.*, 2012).

It should be highlighted that systemic delivery affects both healthy and diseased cells in all areas of the body; as an example, conventional chemotherapy cargoes are not tumor-specific and commonly, their nature leads to significant toxic effects on healthy tissues (Campbell and Smeets, 2019, Palumbo *et al.*, 2013). So, one of the considerable challenges in systemic drug delivery systems is to get the desired drug concentration at the specific organ, while reducing side effects, and preventing drug inefficiency. Researchers have studied numerous approaches, such as developing 'localized drug delivery systems' to overcome these drawbacks (De Jong and Borm, 2008).

Localized drug delivery is a specific form of targeted drug delivery, in which a high concentration of therapeutic agents is locally delivered to the disease site. In fact, local delivery systems allow for reduced movement and subsequent absorption into the bloodstream, therefore these systems minimize side effects toward other tissues and provide controlled drug release (Askari *et al.*, 2020, Rolfes *et al.*, 2012).

Among the current depot delivery systems for localized therapy, several systems attracted great attention:

1) Implantable delivery systems, including passive and dynamic implants (such as scaffolds, stents, vaginal delivery systems, pumps, MEMS and NEMS-based systems, patches and transdermal films, *etc.*) (Stewart *et al.*, 2018, Yi *et al.*, 2016, Fu *et al.*, 2018, Kim *et al.*, 2019, Herrlich *et al.*, 2012, Solanki *et al.*, 2010, Grayson *et al.*, 2004).

2) Injectable delivery systems (*in-situ* forming implants) (Bae *et al.*, 2006).

3) Sprayable systems (Askari *et al.*, 2020).

In this regard, polymers are interesting materials for developing localized drug delivery systems, specifically for developing implantable devices. Natural polymers such as dextran, chitosan, alginates, collagen, albumin, gelatin, and synthetic polymers, such as poly(ε-caprolactone), Poly lactic acid (PLA), poly glycolic acid (PGA) polyethylene glycol, poly(lactic-co-glycolic acid), have been used for polymeric local drug delivery systems (Kim *et al.*, 2014). Synthetic polymers show significant potential as localized delivery systems due to customization and high level of control in their chemical and mechanical properties, and minimal risk of immunogenicity and disease transmission, a particular concern in the use of natural polymers (De Souza *et al.*, 2010).

The key parameter in developing polymer-based implantable drug delivery systems is their degradation mechanisms that consist of nondegradable, chemical degradation – hydrolysis, oxidation, and enzymatic and physical degradation. The degradation ratio in polymer-based systems depends on 3 main parameters, including chemical structure, pH, and water uptake (Solorio *et al.*, 2014).

Nondegradable implantable delivery systems have a fixed geometry and will not degrade or erode during long-term exposure to the patient body environment. These systems can be categorized into one of two structure classes: reservoir systems (composed of a compact drug core entrapped within a permeable polymer membrane) or matrix systems (where the cargoes are homogeneously dispersed throughout the polymer network). However, the removal of nondegradable delivery systems could be difficult and incomplete due to the formation of fibrous tissue around the implant and implant fracture, respectively. In comparison with non-biodegradable delivery systems, biodegradable systems are more patient-friendly without the need for surgical removal and with more control over the drug release profile. These degradable implants have challenges and one of the biggest challenges in these systems is related to the toxicity caused by the degradation of by-products (Solorio *et al.*, 2014).

In the past decade, nanomaterials and smart materials have been used for developing localized delivery systems (Kamaly *et al.*, 2016). In this regard, a wide range of nanomaterials including polymer-based nanoparticles (such as, polymeric micelles and Vesicles, liposomes, polymeric nanogels, and dendrimers), metallic nanoparticles (such as gold nanoparticles, and magnetic nanoparticle), graphene, quantum dots, fullerene, carbon nanotubes, *etc.*, can be used as carriers for developing localized drug delivery systems (Kong *et al.*, 2017).

On the other hand, smart materials or stimuli-responsive materials can be used for creating smart delivery systems that can be administered through a wide range of systems (DDSs), such as injectable *in-situ* forming implants (*e.g.*, a system introduced into the body as injectable fluid in which the liquid-gel transition occurs at body environment in response to a stimulus), smart nanodevices, smart scaffolds, and *etc.* In these smart systems, the payloads are released at the treatment site, and at the appropriate time. This triggered release occurs due to the changes in the system structure or chemistry in response to endogenous and/ or exogenous stimulus leading to the local effect and release of the drugs at the disease site. The endogenous triggers such as pH, redox, enzyme concentration, and bio-molecules are related to the disease pathological characteristics. Whilst in exogeneous-triggered delivery, drug/gene release is controlled by external stimuli such as temperature, light, magnetic and electric field, or ultrasound. Some of the nanoparticles are liposomes, micelles, hydrogels, nanogels, nanoemulsions, mesoporous silica, nanocomposites, *etc.* can be used as stimuli-responsive drug delivery systems (Torchilin, 2018).

The unique features of nanomaterials make them a good candidate for localized delivery. These features include their small size which permits penetration of cell membranes and escape the endosome/lysosome system, a large surface that allows the carry of many classes of therapeutic agents such as drugs, probes, and proteins, modulate drug release, leading to the triggered release of drugs at the site of disease, and deliver several therapeutic agents simultaneously (De Jong and Borm, 2008). In general, nanomaterials can be used as localized delivery systems with two approaches: 1) nanomaterial-based targeted drug delivery systems, or 2) nanomaterial-based smart drug delivery systems.

The first approach is categorized into two main classes, including 'active' and 'passive' targeting. The term 'passive targeting' has been defined as nanoparticle accumulation in diseased sites with affected and leaky vasculature (infarcted sites, tumors, and inflammations) because of the enhanced permeability and retention (EPR) effect. This phenomenon can lead to the deposition of therapeutic agents within target cells (Attia *et al.*, 2019). On the other hand, the term, 'active targeting' commonly refers to the nanoparticle that has been decorated with targeting moieties (such as peptides, antibodies, aptamers, small molecules, saccharides, and proteins) to augment their homing toward receptors overexpressed onto the desired target cells (Vallet-Regí *et al.*, 2018).

In the second approach, the stimuli-responsive nanomaterials can be engineered to release their payloads in response to cellular or extracellular stimuli. It is worth to note that in both approaches, the surface chemistry, shape, and size of nanoparticles, play a vital role in designing localized delivery systems for specific functions.

In addition to the aforementioned systems, multistimuli-responsive drug delivery systems (Mura *et al.*, 2013) or combining targeting ligands with stimuli-responsive systems (Torchilin, 2018, Wang *et al.*, 2015) can provide better control over the delivery of therapeutic agents while minimizing side effects.

So, localized drug delivery with any of these mechanisms can lead to enhanced drug release at the target site in its therapeutic concentration, reducing local toxicity and side effects, controlling the drug release profile, reducing the need for repeated administrations, and increasing patient compliance. Besides these systems can be used for the treatment of a wide range of diseases including many types of cancers, diabetes, cartilage damage, cardiovascular diseases, bacterial/viral infection, autoimmune diseases, and *etc.* (Lombardo *et al.*, 2019).

Localized delivery systems can be manufactured using a number of techniques, including Emulsification-solvent evaporation, electrospraying, microfluidics, emulsion techniques, injection molding, solvent casting, hot melt extrusion, and, more recently, 3D printing and 4D printing. Recently, numerous studies have been done to recognize 4D printing benefits as a helpful method for designing localized drug-delivery systems. This technique has presented new levels of advanced properties, such as changes in geometry and functionality in correlation with time, which cannot be achieved by other conventional processes. So, the construction of localized delivery systems such as complex implantable delivery devices could be possible with 4D printing. However, all of these manufacturing techniques have their own advantages and challenges, and various factors need to be considered when choosing one of them for the production of a localized delivery system such as cost, standardization of process, challenges, efficiency, differences in properties of the products, and *etc.*

In summary, there are numerous studies that illustrate the benefits of localized drug delivery systems, but many disadvantages remain for their clinical application in many indications.

One main challenge is that most major research in the field of localized delivery systems is achieved as 2D *in vitro* models, and there is a poor relationship between such results and *in vivo* animal studies. Besides, the animal models may not mimic the human environment for which the devices are being developed. Therefore these incompatibilities can lead to the failure of numerous local delivery systems in *in vivo* and clinical studies (Abdo *et al.*, 2020). The second challenge which causes serious problems, is related to the lack of degradability or insufficient biocompatibility of most materials, specifically stimuli-responsive materials, that are used in local delivery systems (Alsehli, 2020).

The third drawback is the high cost of the manufacturing process and tests to provide acceptable proof of the effectiveness of the localized delivery systems (Lind, 2017, Hamid and Manzoor, 2020). Besides, innovative development is often performed by small pharmaceutical companies that cannot support themselves on current revenues (Emerich and Thanos, 2007).

Another challenge is related to nanoparticle-based systems that are trickier to achieve FDA approval from, and less information exists on their toxicity concern in the patient body. So, a wide range of safety/toxicity tests need to be done for assessing their safety. Besides, large-sized particles (>150nm) will end up in the lungs, liver, kidney, and spleen (Campbell and Smeets, 2019).

The complexity and often the over-complexity of payload release from localized delivery systems still remains a matter of concern, and until now, these systems have been unable to completely fulfill the promise of localized drug delivery. As a result, clinical safety evaluations are needed to improve the future of localized drug delivery systems and numerous investigations are required for designing perfect and non-invasive devices. Once these challenges are addressed, localized drug delivery has a great potential to significantly improve therapeutic efficacy and toxicity profiles in the treatment of a wide range of diseases.

REFERENCES

Abdo, G. G., Zagho, M. M., Khalil, A. (2020). Recent advances in stimuli-responsive drug release and targeting concepts using mesoporous silica nanoparticles. *Emergent Materials,* 1-19.

Aj, M.Z., Patil, S.K., Baviskar, D.T., Jain, D.K. (2012). Implantable drug delivery system: a review. *Int. J. Pharm. Tech. Res., 4,* 280-292.

Alsehli, M. (2020). Polymeric nanocarriers as stimuli-responsive systems for targeted tumor (cancer) therapy: Recent advances in drug delivery. *Saudi Pharm. J., 28*(3), 255-265.
[http://dx.doi.org/10.1016/j.jsps.2020.01.004] [PMID: 32194326]

Askari, E., Seyfoori, A., Amereh, M., Gharaie, S.S., Ghazali, H.S., Ghazali, Z.S., Khunjush, B., Akbari, M. (2020). Stimuli-responsive hydrogels for local post-surgical drug delivery. *Gels, 6*(2), 14.
[http://dx.doi.org/10.3390/gels6020014] [PMID: 32397180]

Attia, M.F., Anton, N., Wallyn, J., Omran, Z., Vandamme, T.F. (2019). An overview of active and passive targeting strategies to improve the nanocarriers efficiency to tumour sites. *J. Pharm. Pharmacol., 71*(8), 1185-1198.
[http://dx.doi.org/10.1111/jphp.13098] [PMID: 31049986]

Bae, J.W., Go, D.H., Park, K.D., Lee, S.J. (2006). Thermosensitive chitosan as an injectable carrier for local drug delivery. *Macromol. Res., 14*(4), 461-465.
[http://dx.doi.org/10.1007/BF03219111]

Batra, H., Pawar, S., Bahl, D. (2019). Curcumin in combination with anti-cancer drugs: A nanomedicine review. *Pharmacol. Res., 139,* 91-105.
[http://dx.doi.org/10.1016/j.phrs.2018.11.005] [PMID: 30408575]

Campbell, S., Smeets, N. (2019). *Drug delivery: localized and systemic therapeutic strategies with polymer systems. Functional polymers. Polymers and polymeric composites: a reference series..* Cham: Springer.

de Jong, W.H., Borm, P.J. (2008). Drug delivery and nanoparticles: Applications and hazards. *Int. J. Nanomedicine, 3*(2), 133-149.
[http://dx.doi.org/10.2147/IJN.S596] [PMID: 18686775]

De Souza, R., Zahedi, P., Allen, C.J., Piquette-Miller, M. (2010). Polymeric drug delivery systems for localized cancer chemotherapy. *Drug Deliv., 17*(6), 365-375.
[http://dx.doi.org/10.3109/10717541003762854] [PMID: 20429844]

Emerich, D.F., Thanos, C.G. (2007). Targeted nanoparticle-based drug delivery and diagnosis. *J. Drug Target., 15*(3), 163-183.
[http://dx.doi.org/10.1080/10611860701231810] [PMID: 17454354]

Ensign, L.M., Cone, R., Hanes, J. (2012). Oral drug delivery with polymeric nanoparticles: The gastrointestinal mucus barriers. *Adv. Drug Deliv. Rev., 64*(6), 557-570.
[http://dx.doi.org/10.1016/j.addr.2011.12.009] [PMID: 22212900]

Fu, J., Yu, X., Jin, Y. (2018). 3D printing of vaginal rings with personalized shapes for controlled release of progesterone. *Int. J. Pharm., 539*(1-2), 75-82.
[http://dx.doi.org/10.1016/j.ijpharm.2018.01.036] [PMID: 29366944]

Gundloori, R.V., Singam, A., Killi, N. (2019). *Nanobased intravenous and transdermal drug delivery systems. Applications of Targeted Nano Drugs and Delivery Systems..* Elsevier.

Hamid, R., Manzoor, I. (2020). Nanomedicines: nano based drug delivery systems challenges and opportunities. *Alternative Medicine..* IntechOpen.

Herlem, G., Picaud, F., Girardet, C., Micheau, O. (2019). Carbon nanotubes: synthesis, characterization, and applications in drug-delivery systems. *Nanocarriers for drug delivery.,* 469-529.

Herrlich, S., Spieth, S., Messner, S., Zengerle, R. (2012). Osmotic micropumps for drug delivery. *Adv. Drug Deliv. Rev., 64*(14), 1617-1627.
[http://dx.doi.org/10.1016/j.addr.2012.02.003] [PMID: 22370615]

Ji, T., Kohane, D.S. (2019). Nanoscale systems for local drug delivery. *Nano Today, 28*, 100765.
[http://dx.doi.org/10.1016/j.nantod.2019.100765] [PMID: 32831899]

Kamaly, N., Yameen, B., Wu, J., Farokhzad, O.C. (2016). Degradable controlled-release polymers and polymeric nanoparticles: mechanisms of controlling drug release. *Chem. Rev., 116*(4), 2602-2663.
[http://dx.doi.org/10.1021/acs.chemrev.5b00346] [PMID: 26854975]

Kim, J.K., Kim, H.J., Chung, J.Y., Lee, J.H., Young, S.B., Kim, Y.H. (2014). Natural and synthetic biomaterials for controlled drug delivery. *Arch. Pharm. Res., 37*(1), 60-68.
[http://dx.doi.org/10.1007/s12272-013-0280-6] [PMID: 24197492]

Kim, T.H., Lee, J.H., Ahn, C.B., Hong, J.H., Son, K.H., Lee, J.W. (2019). Development of a 3D-printed drug-eluting stent for treating obstructive salivary gland disease. *ACS Biomater. Sci. Eng., 5*(7), 3572-3581.
[http://dx.doi.org/10.1021/acsbiomaterials.9b00636] [PMID: 33405739]

Kong, F.Y., Zhang, J.W., Li, R.F., Wang, Z.X., Wang, W.J., Wang, W. (2017). Unique roles of gold nanoparticles in drug delivery, targeting and imaging applications. *Molecules, 22*(9), 1445.
[http://dx.doi.org/10.3390/molecules22091445] [PMID: 28858253]

Lind, K.D. (2017). Understanding the market for implantable medical devices. *Insight.*

Lombardo, D., Kiselev, M.A., Caccamo, M.T. (2019). Smart nanoparticles for drug delivery application: development of versatile nanocarrier platforms in biotechnology and nanomedicine. *J. Nanomater., 2019*, 1-26.
[http://dx.doi.org/10.1155/2019/3702518]

Mehta, P.P., Pawar, V.S. (2018). *Electrospun nanofiber scaffolds: technology and applications. Applications of nanocomposite materials in drug delivery..* Elsevier.
[http://dx.doi.org/10.1016/B978-0-12-813741-3.00023-6]

Mohammadzadeh, R., Javadzadeh, Y. (2018). An overview on oral drug delivery *via* nano-based formulations. *Pharmaceutical and Biomedical Research, 4*, 1-7.
[http://dx.doi.org/10.18502/pbr.v4i1.139]

Mura, S., Nicolas, J., Couvreur, P. (2013). Stimuli-responsive nanocarriers for drug delivery. *Nat. Mater., 12*(11), 991-1003.
[http://dx.doi.org/10.1038/nmat3776] [PMID: 24150417]

Nayak, A.K., Ahmad, S.A., Beg, S., Ara, T.J., Hasnain, M.S. (2018). *Drug delivery: present, past, and future of medicine. Applications of Nanocomposite Materials in Drug Delivery..* Elsevier.

Palumbo, M.O., Kavan, P., Miller, W.H., Jr, Panasci, L., Assouline, S., Johnson, N., Cohen, V., Patenaude, F., Pollak, M., Jagoe, R.T., Batist, G. (2013). Systemic cancer therapy: achievements and challenges that lie ahead. *Front. Pharmacol., 4*, 57.
[http://dx.doi.org/10.3389/fphar.2013.00057] [PMID: 23675348]

Richards Grayson, A., Scheidt Shawgo, R., Li, Y., Cima, M.J. (2004). Electronic MEMS for triggered delivery. *Adv. Drug Deliv. Rev., 56*(2), 173-184.
[http://dx.doi.org/10.1016/j.addr.2003.07.012] [PMID: 14741114]

Rolfes, C., Howard, S., Goff, R., Iaizzo, P. A. (2012). Localized drug delivery for cardiothoracic surgery. *Current concepts in general thoracic surgery.,* InTech Open Access Chapter.279-304.

Serwer, L., Hashizume, R., Ozawa, T., James, C.D. (2010). Systemic and local drug delivery for treating diseases of the central nervous system in rodent models. *J. Vis. Exp.,* (42), 1992.
[http://dx.doi.org/10.3791/1992] [PMID: 20736920]

Solanki, H.K., Thakkar, J.H., Jani, G.K. (2010). Recent advances in implantable drug delivery. *Int. J. Pharm.*

Sci. Rev. Res., 4, 168-177.

Solorio, L., Carlson, A., Zhou, H., Exner, A.A. (2014). Implantable drug delivery systems. In: Bader, R.A., Putnam, D.A., (Eds.), *Engineering Polymer Systems for Improved Drug Delivery.*

Stewart, S., Domínguez-Robles, J., Donnelly, R., Larrañeta, E. (2018). Implantable polymeric drug delivery devices: Classification, manufacture, materials, and clinical applications. *Polymers (Basel), 10*(12), 1379. [http://dx.doi.org/10.3390/polym10121379] [PMID: 30961303]

Tiwari, G., Tiwari, R., Bannerjee, S.K., Bhati, L., Pandey, S., Pandey, P., Sriwastawa, B. (2012). Drug delivery systems: An updated review. *Int. J. Pharm. Investig., 2*(1), 2-11. [http://dx.doi.org/10.4103/2230-973X.96920] [PMID: 23071954]

Torchilin, V. P. (2018). Fundamentals of stimuli-responsive drug and gene delivery systems. [http://dx.doi.org/10.1039/9781788013536-00001]

Vallet-Regí, M., Colilla, M., Izquierdo-Barba, I., Manzano, M. (2017). Mesoporous silica nanoparticles for drug delivery: Current insights. *Molecules, 23*(1), 47. [http://dx.doi.org/10.3390/molecules23010047] [PMID: 29295564]

Wang, Y., Zhao, Q., Han, N., Bai, L., Li, J., Liu, J., Che, E., Hu, L., Zhang, Q., Jiang, T., Wang, S. (2015). Mesoporous silica nanoparticles in drug delivery and biomedical applications. *Nanomedicine, 11*(2), 313-327. [http://dx.doi.org/10.1016/j.nano.2014.09.014] [PMID: 25461284]

Yi, H.G., Choi, Y.J., Kang, K.S., Hong, J.M., Pati, R.G., Park, M.N., Shim, I.K., Lee, C.M., Kim, S.C., Cho, D.W. (2016). A 3D-printed local drug delivery patch for pancreatic cancer growth suppression. *J. Control. Release, 238*, 231-241. [http://dx.doi.org/10.1016/j.jconrel.2016.06.015] [PMID: 27288878]

SUBJECT INDEX

A

Ablation 30, 35
  photothermal 30
Abnormal dynamics 101
Acid(s) 6, 25, 26, 33, 34, 38, 39, 49, 50, 52,
    53, 54, 57, 59, 60, 61, 62, 63, 73, 84, 86,
    87, 96, 97, 102, 126, 130, 136, 139, 154,
    158, 164, 170, 189, 190, 192, 195, 198,
    216, 224, 225, 229, 239
  alginic 225
  amino 38, 59, 63, 130, 195
  carboxyl 73
  carboxylic 190
  chlorogenic (CA) 97
  deoxyribonucleic 198
  dicarboxylic 59
  fatty 154
  folic (FA) 25, 97, 102, 136, 189, 190, 195
  gambogic 97
  gluconic 170, 225
  glycolic 52, 53, 54
  hyaluronic 49, 61, 62, 63, 126, 225, 229
  hypochlorous 158
  lactic 50, 52, 54, 130, 224
  lactic-co-glycolic 192, 239
  maleic 84
  nucleic 6, 26, 33, 34, 39, 54, 60, 61, 139
  oleic 86
  polyglycolic (PGA) 52, 53, 54, 87, 164, 239
  polylactic-co-glycolic 96
  ribonucleic 198
  salicylic 216
  suberic 57
Acidic 160, 162
  conditions, normal non-menstrual 162
  metabolic waste products 160
Acrylateoligolactide 130
Acrylonitrile 80
Active targeting 26, 102
  methods 102
  therapy 26

Activity 7, 32, 62, 167, 219, 224
  anti-cancer 7
  anti-tumor 62
  bactericidal 32
  hemolytic 32
Actuators, pneumatic 213
Adsorption 26, 27, 33, 35, 71, 188
  exfoliation 71
  near-NIR 26
Agents 3, 5, 6, 8, 13, 15, 26, 33, 54, 64, 65,
    132, 133, 139, 162, 154, 182, 196, 155,
    215, 218, 219
  antibacterial 162, 218, 219
  antibiotic 183, 196, 219
  anti-HIV 162
  anti-inflammatory 3, 54, 162
  antimicrobial 5, 65, 196
  anti-microbial 219
  antitumor 26, 65
  nanotherapeutic delivery 8
  organic 182
  photochromic 132, 133
  toxic 15
  toxic photocuring 215
  ultrasound contrast 139
Albumin 100, 108, 195, 239
  bovine serum 108
  human serum 100
Alternating magnetic field (AMF) 191, 192
Aminated guar gum (AGG) 193
Amorphous 106, 195
  calcium phosphate (ACP) 195
  solid dispersions (ASD) 106
Amphiphilic 61, 106, 140, 156
  block copolymers 140
  chitosan 61
Andrographolide 195
Angiogenesis 101, 102, 158
Angiography 59
Antibodies 3, 26, 62, 103, 108, 182, 188, 189,
    198, 241
  electrosprayed 108

H

I

www.ingramcontent.com/pod-product-compliance
Lightning Source LLC
Chambersburg PA
CBHW050821220326
41598CB00006B/282